Cosmic Nutrition

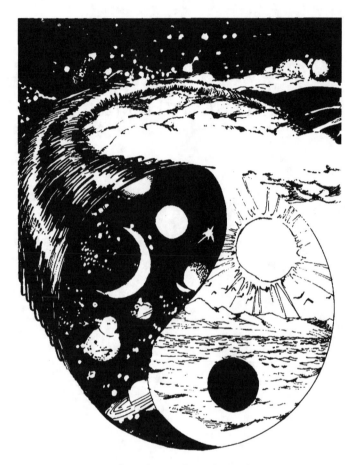

Infinite heavenly realm and
yin and yang of the physical world

Cosmic Nutrition

The Taoist Approach to Health and Longevity

Mantak Chia
and
William U. Wei

Destiny Books
Rochester, Vermont • Toronto, Canada

Destiny Books
One Park Street
Rochester, Vermont 05767
www.DestinyBooks.com

Text stock is SFI certified

Destiny Books is a division of Inner Traditions International

Library of Congress Cataloging-in-Publication Data
Chia, Mantak, 1944–
  Cosmic nutrition : the Taoist approach to health and longevity / Mantak Chia
and William U. Wei.
      p. cm.
  Originally published: Thailand : Universal Tao Publications, 2011.
  Includes bibliographical references and index.
  ISBN 978-1-59477-470-6 (pbk.) — ISBN 978-1-59477-688-5 (e-book)
  1. Nutrition—Religious aspects—Taoism. 2. Health—Religious aspects—
Taoism. I. Wei, William U. II. Title.
  RA784.C4749 2012
  613.2—dc23

2011045078

Printed and bound in the United States by Lake Book Manufacturing, Inc.
The text stock is SFI certified. The Sustainable Forestry Initiative® program promotes sustainable forest management.

10 9 8 7 6 5 4 3 2 1

Text design and layout by Priscilla Baker
This book was typeset in Janson, with Futura and Present used as display typefaces

Photographs by Sopitnapa Promnon
Illustrations by Udon Jandee

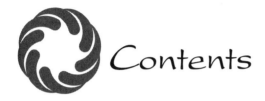# Contents

Acknowledgments

The Universal Tao Publications staff involved in the preparation and production of *Cosmic Nutrition* extend our gratitude to the many generations of Taoist masters who have passed on their special lineage, in the form of an unbroken oral transmission, over thousands of years. We thank Taoist Master Yi Eng for his openness in transmitting the formulas of Taoist Inner Alchemy. We also wish to thank the thousands of unknown men and women of the Chinese healing arts who developed many of the methods and ideas presented in this book.

We offer our eternal gratitude to our parents and teachers for their many gifts to us. Remembering them brings joy and satisfaction to our continued efforts in presenting the Universal Healing Tao System. For their gifts, we offer our eternal gratitude and love. As always, their contribution has been crucial in presenting the concepts and techniques of the Universal Healing Tao.

Thanks to Juan Li for the use of his beautiful and visionary paintings, illustrating Taoist esoteric practices. We offer our gratitude to Bob Zuraw—without whom the book would not have come to be—for sharing his kindness, healing techniques, inspiration, and Taoist understandings.

For their efforts to clarify the text and produce this handsome new edition of the book, we thank the editorial and production staff at Inner Traditions/Destiny Books. We also thank Nancy Yeilding for her line edit of the new edition.

We wish to thank the following people for their assistance in producing the original edition of this book: Bob Lewanski for his editorial work and writing and our fellow instructors Colin Drown and Shashi Solluna for their insightful contributions.

A special thanks goes to our Thai production team: Hirunyathorn Punsan, computer graphics; Saysunee Yongyod, photography; Udon Jandee, illustrations; and Saniem Chaisarn, production design.

Putting Cosmic Nutrition into Practice

The practices described in this book have been used successfully for thousands of years by Taoists trained by personal instruction. Readers should not undertake the practice without receiving personal transmission and training from a certified instructor of the Universal Healing Tao, since certain of these practices, if done improperly, may cause injury or result in health problems. This book is intended to supplement individual training by the Universal Healing Tao and to serve as a reference guide for these practices. Anyone who undertakes these practices on the basis of this book alone does so entirely at his or her own risk.

The meditations, practices, and techniques described herein are *not* intended to be used as an alternative or substitute for professional medical treatment and care. If any readers are suffering from illnesses based on mental or emotional disorders, an appropriate professional health care practitioner or therapist should be consulted. Such problems should be corrected before you start training.

This book does not attempt to give any medical diagnosis, treatment, prescription, or remedial recommendation in relation to any human disease, ailment, suffering, or physical condition whatsoever.

Neither the Universal Healing Tao nor its staff and instructors can be responsible for the consequences of any practice or misuse of the information contained in this book. If the reader undertakes any exercise without strictly following the instructions, notes, and warnings, the responsibility must lie solely with the reader.

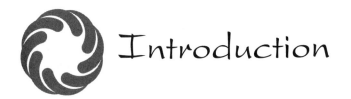 Introduction

The ancient sages and philosophers long ago discovered the secret of regeneration. But still we search for outward cures, when all the time the solution to the riddle of health lies within: we find it by living in harmony with the natural laws of the universe.

From the health teachings passed down to our time has come the momentous discovery that the premature aging process, which so quickly mars the human body, is not divinely caused; it is a chronic disease, caused by bad living habits. Aging arises from the breaking of natural health laws, resulting in chronic conditions. From this understanding it follows that the aging process must be subject to the universal law of cause and effect. To stop the symptoms of aging, which are sickness and decrepitude, remove the causes. At the present writing, most if not all the causes of aging and disease seem to have been clearly worked out. Most importantly, every one of these known causes is found to be preventable.

A fact long known to science is that the living tissue cells of our bodies are constantly wearing out and being replaced by new ones. The ancient sages, however, maintained that all human tissue is entirely renewed within seven years. If this is so, it means that every human body is actually a new body every seven years and, moreover, that if our bodies could be protected from the conditions that we know gradually bring about aging, they could live on indefinitely (barring accidents), in changeless youth and strength. On the other hand, by natural analogy, it would appear that no human or other body can be expected to live forever, even if all the secrets of life were known to science. All things have a certain time during which they exist on the earth. If a person's time to stay is over, he or she will have to die. But many die before their time is over, not by a visitation of Providence, but because they are ignorant of the laws controlling their nature.

We must all learn from nature, our supreme teacher, and never subject ourselves to any fanatical, rigidly enforced one-sidedness. Air, sun, water, food, exercise, fasting, sleep, and relaxation are all necessary and natural rejuvenating factors, each of equal value, each complemented by and completing the others. It is our everyday task and duty to make use of them, at the right time and place, so that our vitality can be strengthened, our health promoted, our well-being increased, and our ability to work preserved until the end of our days. If we carry out nature's plan properly, we shall not meet with an early, unnatural end thrust upon us by illness; we shall rather fade away in old age, without pain or torment of death, and find eternal peace.

Health is the most precious jewel and greatest possession. Your future health depends upon your daily personal habits of eating, living, and thinking in the present. Reflect upon this ancient wisdom: if you will pay the small price now in learning and disciplining your body, mind, and spirit, you will soon come to experience the joy of living in its truest sense. Life could be indefinitely prolonged if the problem of intestinal autointoxication could be solved; the two-hundred-year-old person could be a result of the science of the immediate future.

Medical science as a body, however, is still skeptical about procedures designed to prolong youth or rejuvenate aging. This need not be taken as discouraging. The history of medicine and science teems with records of organized opposition to new and revolutionary developments. The accepted medical and scientific attitude toward such things has always had and will always have three stages. First, it ignores them. Second, it becomes sarcastic and irritated about them. Third, it accepts them and forgets that it has not always done so. But this organized resistance to new things works also for the good, in that it warns and protects, so far as it can, the innocent citizen against fraudulent (licensed) doctors and other quick cure con men. These dishonest quacks should not be mistaken for the honest health practitioner or decent doctor.

Let us be warned by the mistakes of our scientific past and try to be open-minded—but not credulous—toward this ancient yet up-to-date knowledge of prolonging youth, preventing disease, and creating a state of super health. Remember that the present advancement of science admonishes us against defining limits to possible human longevity; it increasingly supports the words of an ancient sage written two thousand years ago: "Man does not die; he kills himself." The ancients speak of regeneration (renewing youth) by living in accordance with universal law, the Tao. The wise person of today will also maintain youthful health and prevent disease as taught by ancient cultures.

In the following pages you will learn not only the ancient and modern secrets of prolonging youth, preventing disease, and building health but also the philosophy behind wholesome living. This comprehensive health program should serve a very useful purpose both in securing better nutrition for those in need of it and as a practical philosophy for those seeking a better way of living. This book can be heartily recommended for old and young, rich and poor. Our station in life does not change our biological, emotional, mental, and spiritual needs.

We all have the desire to be healthy. But most people feel below par with no energy, vitality, or zest for living. Perhaps you too have to drag your weary, exhausted body out of bed every morning and are always tired throughout the day. Or maybe you need ten cups of coffee to keep you going from morning until night, or you are plagued with constant headaches, colds, aches, pains, and sick nauseated feelings. Unfortunately, many people believe that they cannot live a life without disease; they think a healthy, vibrant life is impossible, and they give up in despair.

It is generally believed that sound health arises out of thin air and that practically nothing can be done about it. With this apathetic public attitude toward personal health and physical fitness, is it any wonder that so few individuals radiate good health? There must be a cause for all of this suffering and disease.

Observe closely what people are consuming in the name of food. You will find them consuming tons of white sugar, white flour and its products, salt, oils, fried foods, canned foods, TV dinners, cakes, pop, candy, alcohol, meat, cigarettes, spices, drugs, and chemically treated food in boxes and packages. Nothing more needs to be said. Americans may lead the world in science and technology, but American health is declining. Our average life span is only seventy some years, less than in more than thirty other countries of the world and far below that of healthful living people. Disease is on the increase. Mental and nervous disturbances, heart disease, TB, MS, diabetes, kidney and liver disease, cancer, blood disorders, poor eyesight, and so on are evidenced more than ever before. Sickness and suffering affect almost the entire population. Annually, billions are poured into disease research, new wonder drugs, and hospitals. But Americans are not becoming healthier.

Which are the truly civilized peoples of the world? Are they the industrialized countries, or the Okinawans, Hunzas of Pakistan, Russian peasants of the Black Sea area, Watusi tribes of Africa, and Bulgarian mountain dwellers? These cultures have one thing in common: a long average life span, with many members who live to at least one hundred years, in good health and able to work and enjoy life until the day they die. A truly civilized nation is created by excellent physical, mental, emotional, and spiritual health.

The ancient sages, philosophers, and wise men and women of antiquity lived to an advanced age, as they taught and practiced the universal secrets and principles of the Tao. The ancient Taoist masters of China related that they received their knowledge even before recorded history, from highly spiritual beings called Sons of Reflected Light, who brought the healing arts known as the Eight Strands of the Brocade. The eight strands are:

1. Diagnosis
2. Yin/yang diet and exercise
3. Herbal therapy
4. Hydrotherapy
5. Acupuncture
6. Acupressure
7. Massage
8. Meditation or the way of contemplation

The focus of this book is on nutritional therapy, which can be used alone or combined with other treatments. Ancient Taoist theory is the foundation for two popular nutritional systems: (1) macrobiotics, which is concerned with the balance and harmony between yin and yang, and (2) five-element nutrition, which provides a more detailed look into the health of each organ system. Macrobiotics has been highly developed in Japanese culture, whereas five-element nutrition is more widespread in China. Each can be used alone or the systems can be integrated. You will find our own thorough interpretation of the fundamentals of balancing yin and yang and of five-element nutrition in the pages of this book.

Awaiting you is a rare experience. You will find this book like a passport to a wonderful new style and attitude of life. It is strange that science has largely neglected studying those of advanced age. It would seem that if more were known about the habits of those who reach one hundred, physicians could better advise those of us aspiring to such an age. Common sense dictates that long life must be more than chance and happenstance. There must be a combination of factors that increase a person's chances of living to an advanced age, and the sooner this formula becomes common knowledge, the longer many of us can hope to survive.

Here in this enlightening, inspiring, and informative book you will discover the formulas and secret teachings that have been taught throughout the ages. For the first time, in one volume, you will be given specific step-by-step instructions of exactly what you can do, with complete confidence, to help yourself and your loved ones to a superior way of living and to build a long, useful, satisfying life of health, success, and happiness far into advanced age.

This creative book bridges the gap between Eastern philosophy and Western science, thus treating ancient health teachings in a new light and presenting new ideas from a unique but authentic point of view. The rare combination of simplicity and mastery of subject that the authors share is the result of years of experience, research, observation, and practice in the fields of natural health, new age psychology, spiritual culture, and physical culture. The final section contains invaluable information on attaining inward calm for mental and spiritual happiness and success in life. This philosophy is a practical and positive method to attain peace of mind, emotional stability, and a vibrant state of health. What you want in life will seek you out, but when it comes, it is up to you to seize it.

Persistent research into the vast mysteries of health, from all parts of the world, enables us to assure you that you can master all of your respective afflictions with the most gratifying results through correct nutrition and through proper application of the physical, mental, and spiritual teachings set forth in this book. Here you will be introduced to proven principles, the personal application of which can literally transform your life for the better. With these safe teachings you can progress as far as you wish to go in regaining or maintaining superb health, beauty, strength, and fitness.

This book shares with you confidential disclosures about how to build the kind of magnificent health you are entitled to possess. And these secrets of *Cosmic Nutrition* are all so simple and easy to follow. However, health is a condition you have to personally earn for yourself. No one can do it for you. In fairness to yourself, decide to apply these life principles faithfully, patiently, persistently, and joyously. Stick to these advanced teachings with conviction. Believe and know that all will be well for you over a long and richly rewarding life. Nothing else can pay you so well. All the teachings in this tremendous volume are fully endorsed by time-tested understandings. It is a genuine pleasure for us to unhesitatingly recommend that you adopt these rejuvenation teachings and make them a vital part of your life.

Every day that you apply these health teachings, you will build and improve your well-being. So why not start today, right now, and decide that you too can benefit by all of these wonderful restorative methods. Discover for yourself what a dramatic transformation they will bring into your life! Then let others marvel at the results you have achieved. May the Tao be with you as you activate three of the greatest words in the English language, "Do It Now!"

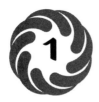

Philosophy of Health

CHARACTERISTICS OF GOOD HEALTH, YOUR NATURAL BIRTHRIGHT

The individual who is in excellent health has a smile on his face, while the sick person wears a frown. Good health carries with it poise, power, self-confidence, courage, and success. Poor health leads to irritability, weakness, lack of confidence, fear, and failure.

Good health develops personal attractiveness, for nothing adds so much to the appearance of a man or woman as a wholesome condition of mind and body. People who are well can concentrate upon their work and can keep at it day after day with no sense of fatigue, depression, or discouragement. Those in ill health work spasmodically and are unable to bring to their work the energy and enthusiasm that begets success and fortune. Good health encompasses physical, mental, emotional, and spiritual health.

Physical Health

Physical health requires a natural diet of pure wholesome foods (organically grown if possible), which include a daily balance of proteins, fats, carbohydrates, vitamins, and minerals; sufficient exercise, such as jogging, swimming, yoga, weightlifting, Chi Kung, walking, massage, Tai Chi, breathing techniques, and cycling; fresh outside air and sunshine daily; fasting when necessary; adequate sleep (at least eight hours);

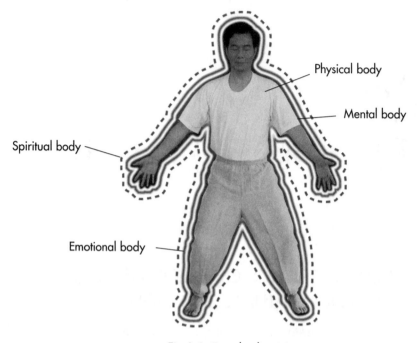

Fig.1.1. Four bodies in one

resting when tired; and drinking pure water (distilled, rain water, or spring water).

The development of good physical health requires several years, depending upon the person's initial physical condition. The wheels of nature grind slowly but, nevertheless, surely. Time and healthful eating and living habits are the primary requirements for attaining good physical health. The human body, like all phenomena in nature, possesses the inherent power of self-regeneration when the conditions of healthful existence are adopted.

Emotional Health

Emotional turmoil is the result of ill health and confusion in the mental realm, brought about by overwork, lack of rest and sleep, jealousy, greed, hate, worry, fear, and a life of constant debauchery. People in a state of emotional confusion have little or no control in any department of their lives. They react in a negative way and become emotionally upset when the world around them is not catering to their every whim or desire.

Emotional calmness under trying circumstances marks the person of dynamic health and personal magnetism. Good emotional health leads to lofty spiritual attainment.

Mental Health

Good physical health is the foundation for the development of sound mental health. The ancients teach us to remain calm and to refrain from hindering or interfering with another's life. Chinese Taoist Professor Chee Soo states:

> Do fish in the water complain that it is cold or dirty? Of course not. Do they complain because the sea becomes rough, or envy or try to exploit each other? No. They live in harmony constantly, never envying or hating anything. Life for them is simply living . . . The way to the spirit is through constant good thoughts and good deeds, now and every minute of each day, and through this way of life everything becomes an "open door" and the Tao becomes apparent to you in everything you do, and in every thought that passes through your head.

A calm mental attitude is necessary to carry us through the trials of everyday life. Living in harmony with the universal rhythm of life (moderation in every undertaking) produces a healthy mental state.

Spiritual Health

Here we have the culmination and synthesis of the first three characteristics of true health: physical, mental, and emotional. Spirituality can be developed only when all conditions, circumstances, and difficulties in the game of life have been mastered. When all selfishness, greed, thoughts of hate, fear, anger, worry, and anxiety are vanquished, it can then be said that you are on the road to spirituality. A spiritual person expresses total love to all people everywhere, whether they are good or bad, black or white, rich or poor, and so on. They are unattached to worldly or material possessions and are happy with or without these possessions. For them, happiness comes from realizing that nothing in this world brings happiness except *peace of mind.*

It is our human destiny to live in harmony with the order of the universe and attain good health, otherwise we attract mental and physical suffering and pain. Health cannot be purchased. It cannot be conferred by another. Health, happiness, and a successfully abundant life cannot be voted in by a government legislature. Neither king, queen, nor congress can guarantee the delivery of health, vitality, and happiness to you. You must earn it through your own efforts, hour by hour and day by day. Only then will you have learned the joy of living as taught by the ancients.

We urge all those who are interested in living a better life to always keep an open mind and to constantly study, making improvements where necessary. This is the only way possible to arrive at any kind of scientific truth. We can learn something new every day if we have the desire to do so. Let us search together now and hopefully we will meet at the golden gates of truth. Disease is an unnatural state to one living a natural existence. To those who live unnaturally and surround themselves with artificial circumstances, disease is natural, for the laws of cause and effect decree that normalcy shall generate normalcy and abnormality produce its kind. Hence all disease is seated in some shortcoming that opens the individual to such afflictions.

Four Bodies in One

If you look at a fan when it is still, you can see its blades. When you start up the fan at the first speed, the blades will move and you will see the blades. If you turn up the speed, the blades will move faster and you will just barely be able to see them. Then if you turn it up to its highest speed, you will not see the blades anymore. But the blades are still there. This is similar to our first four bodies: they are really just one body with four different frequencies (physical, mental, emotional, and spiritual). If you work on one body (frequency), you work on all of them at the same time.

The Taoist approaches healing by first focusing on the physical body because it exists in time and space and we can access it with our five senses. By working with the physical body through cosmic nutrition we can heal and balance the mental, emotional, and spiritual bodies at the same time. We can also access our other bodies (etheric, astral, and so on) through further advanced Taoist practices with our sixth and seventh

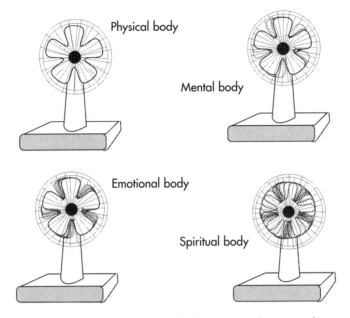

Physical body

Mental body

Emotional body

Spiritual body

Fig.1.2. The four frequencies of a fan are similar to our four
bodies (physical, emotional, mental, and spiritual) in one.

senses (clairvoyance and telepathy), but again we work on all the bodies at
the same time when we work on the physical body, because all the bodies
are one body.

TOXEMIA AND DISEASE

Oliver Wendell Holmes, M.D., that scholarly gentleman, who was far
ahead of the medical world, so aptly voiced his verdict upon his own
medical profession when he once stated: "I firmly believe that, if the
whole *materia medica* could be sunk to the bottom of the sea, it would be
all the better for mankind and all the worse for the fishes."

Disease in and of itself is a remedial process, a response to a "crisis of
toxemia," as defined by Dr. J. H. Tilden, a medical doctor, in his skillfully
penned 1926 book *Toxemia Explained*. He notes that both cell-building
anabolism and cell-destroying catabolism are involved in the process of
tissue-building metabolism. The broken-down tissue is toxic. In health,
when nerve energy is normal, toxins are eliminated from the blood as
fast as they are generated. When nerve energy is dissipated as a result of

any cause, such as physical or mental excitement or bad habits, the body becomes enervated and elimination is checked, which causes toxemia, a retention of toxins in the blood.

A thousand and one enervating habits of living are the primary causes of toxemia. Without proper and adequate nerve energy, our food is not digested and assimilated properly, cellular elimination and renewal is checked, and metabolic wastes are retained in the system, causing toxemia. Every so-called disease is a crisis of toxemia, which means that toxic matter has accumulated in the blood above the point of toleration. Disease is a crisis of elimination in a system overloaded with toxic waste and auto-generated poisons. It comes as the end point of years of enervating habits, consumption of poor foods, overeating, alcohol consumption, smoking, lack of exercise, stress, little sleep, and so on.

The organism's attempts to eliminate or discharge that which is harmful to it are the symptoms of disease, which are generally accom-

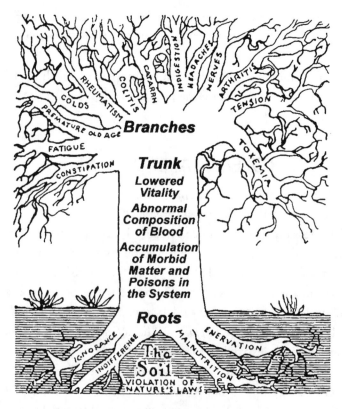

Fig. 1.3. Tree of toxemia

panied by our early warning system called pain. If pain is heeded and the proper natural therapy applied, including correct eating and health habits, disease and the symptoms of disease can be overcome. Nature is endeavoring to rid the body of toxin. A fast, rest in bed, and the giving-up of enervating habits, mental and physical, will allow nature to eliminate the accumulated toxin; then, if rational living habits are adopted, health will come back to stay. Any treatment that obstructs this effort of elimination baffles nature in her efforts at self-curing.

DRUGS DO NOT CURE

The following statement is a universal law of healing: Medicines do not heal or cure the body. The true cure lies in the removal of the causes of disease and adopting rational and healthful living habits. When this path is followed, the body will then have the energy and power to regenerate, recuperate, and heal itself. We then become free from the causes and symptoms of disease. We can discover new wonder cures every day, but we can never escape from the natural law of cause and effect: whatever we sow, so shall we reap. Disease is created by diseased habits; health is created by natural health habits and principles.

Acute diseases are short-termed. Their symptoms are often violent, but only temporary. Acute symptoms indicate that the body possesses sufficient vital nerve force and energy to eliminate internal toxic conditions, such as colds, flu, mumps, measles, acne, and so on. On the other hand, chronic diseased conditions, such as cancer, are of a more long-standing nature, in which pathological degeneration of the cells, tissues, and organs has taken place.

Suppressing acute symptoms of disease with drugs, if continued for many years, will result in chronic ailments. Acute disease symptoms should be allowed to run their course, without being suppressed by drugs. Drugs create chronic pathology by suppressing the natural channels of elimination: kidneys, bowels, lungs, and skin.

The indiscriminate use of medication when the body is already diseased (toxic) is an unwise gesture. If the organism has the inherent power of self-healing, self-cleansing, and self-regeneration, what then is the purpose of introducing drug medication in an attempt to cure? There is no return to health with such a practice. Human beings are the willing guinea pigs for drug experimenters. The cures may come and the cures may go, but the curing goes on forever. The billions of dollars involved in the research and the sale of drugs also goes on forever.

This outmoded suppression treatment does not stop the cause of sickness, cannot prevent further illness, and certainly plays no part in the building and maintenance of healthy cells and tissues. It is not the Creator's intention that we should live by the aid of crutches (drugs and other artificial remedies) or turn this planet into one vast hospital for the sick.

Proper elimination is prevented by drugs, feeding, fear, and continuing to work. These conditions cause a cold to be driven into chronic catarrh; flu may be forced to take on an infected state; pneumonia may end fatally if secretions are checked by drugs; typhoid will be forced into

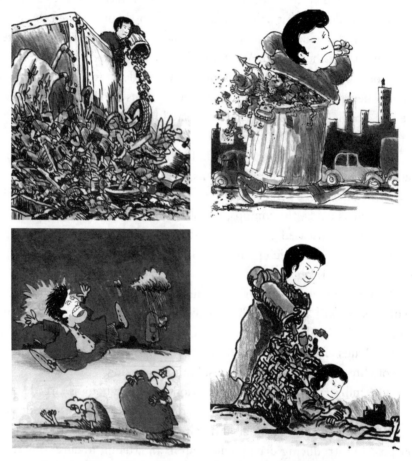

Fig. 1.4. Toxic physical, emotional, mental, and spiritual bodies

a septic state and greatly prolonged, if the patient is not killed. Drugging pain of any kind checks elimination and prevents the human organism from cleaning house.

Cancer, tuberculosis, Bright's disease, and all chronic diseases were once innocent colds that were "ameliorated" by drugs, only to return and be ameliorated again and again. Each time they were accompanied by greater constitutional enervation and toleration for toxin-poisoning. This required a greater requisition of mucous membrane through which to eliminate the toxin. To find the cause of cancer, start with colds and catarrh, and watch the pathology as it travels from irritation, catarrh, inflammation, induration, and ulceration to cancer.

Disease is perverted health. The proper way to study disease is to study health and every influence favorable or unfavorable to its continuance. Any influence that lowers nerve energy becomes disease-producing. Disease cannot be its own cause; neither can it be its own cure, and certainly not its own prevention. Heroic treatment of disease with drugs is disease-building. Of the action of drugs we know little, yet we put them into bodies about which we know less, to cure disease of which we know nothing at all.

Drug Toxicity

Treating the sick with drugs only adds more to the existing toxemia within the body. Chemical drugs merely palliate the symptoms of disease; they impair the body's self-healing process and drive the disease toxins deeper into the organs and tissues. Drugs destroy red blood cells, cause anemia, and create a false illusion of being cured. The drugged patient returns again and again for stronger doses of medication and more experimental treatment.

Drugs produce "side effects," which are very often far worse than the original toxic disease. The side effects of drugs indicate that the body is using its vital energy in an attempt to eliminate the drug poison through the internal organs or other body parts. Medicines only relieve the "temporary" symptoms of disease, pain, and distress; they do not overcome disease or improve a person's state of health and well-being. Drugs do not possess the quality or power to act in a living organism; the living organism acts or reacts to any drug or poison in an attempt to expel it before it causes any possible internal damage. The key word here is *living*. The human body cell is a living intelligence, and as a unit of life it knows when it is being ill-treated or poisoned by dead and inert substances inimical to its existence. Thus, we observe the side effects of drugs when the living, acting body goes into action against them.

Dr. H. M. Shelton, a leading health researcher, writes that the so-called physiological effects of drugs are symptoms of disease. No pharmacologist, no pathologist, no physician will deny this. He says that when a drug is vomited, it is an action of the living organism and not of the lifeless drug. It is absurd to write of the physiological actions of poisons: first, because they cannot act; and, second, because their presence always occasions pathological action. Dr. Anthony J. Sattilaro, who cured himself of cancer through diet, writes: "If we can at least show that people can live better in their lifetimes, rather than suffering all the iatrogenic effects of the standard modalities that we have in Western medicine, I think we will have made a great contribution."

Western medicine too often tends to look at disease in small parts, forgetting that the whole body functions together as an entire unit. Instead of merely treating a particular symptom of disease, we must learn to look for the cause of disease and eradicate it. The real error arose when pharmacology began to be joined with morphology (form and structure of living things) to treat disease. That resulted in an organ being treated with a drug or an organ being transplanted. Such measures only temporarily palliate the symptoms of disease. The body functions as a whole and will regenerate itself if properly cared for; it was never meant to be taken apart or artificially poisoned. The organs work in a system within the body to overcome disease and regain a state of equilibrium. Fostering this is the thrust of holistic medicine.

The treatment of disease is so simple that it staggers those who believe in curing with drugs. It consists in this: find in what way nerve energy is wasted, and stop it. Then returning to normal is a matter of time, in which nature attends to all repairs herself. And nature resents medical officiousness. Health is built through everyday healthy eating and living habits. In addition, health can be restored by applying nature's holistic therapies such as fasting, herbs, acupuncture, massage, sunshine, oxygen, hydrotherapy, exercise therapy, and so on.

GERM THEORY: MYTH OR REALITY?

The germ theory of disease will be laughed at during the next century as the crowning folly of the present. This foolishness all began in the mid-seventeenth century, when Leeuwenhoek and O. F. Muller studied and reported on several forms of bacteria. Early investigations were badly handicapped by poor microscopes and the lack of understanding and accuracy. Then, around 1830, microbes were separated and grouped into species and genera by German naturalist Ehrenberg.

Louis Pasteur became famous as a result of the controversial research he conducted on the germ theory of disease. He is known mostly for the Pasteur treatment of hydrophobia and pasteurization. Pasteur claimed the body was like a barrel of beer. He said that, like beer, our bodies were at the mercy of, or subject to, invasion from germs and bacteria. He pronounced the germ theory of disease, asserting that each type of germ (microorganism) is responsible for creating its own specific type of disease or sickness, and that diseases are due to an outside invasion of specific germ organisms. This theory was merely an announcement or conjecture by Pasteur, but it was, unfortunately, heralded as the final answer and great advancement in science, though the theory had absolutely no foundation in fact. If this theory were true, and proved scientifically, we would all be dead immediately as a result of germ invasion.

More than a century later Dr. Robert O. Young made an important discovery while working with the dark field phase-contrast microscope, a high-powered microscope that can magnify objects up to 28,000 times, enabling a clear view of bacterial and fungal forms in the blood in exact detail. He noticed that a dying cell reverted back to a living cell when the internal environment of the cell changed from an acid state to an alkaline state. He was so overwhelmed that he researched all the data on the germ theory dating back more than 150 years. He discovered that the bloodstream and the inside of the body (cells) have a landscape or terrain that, in a diseased state, becomes too acidic. This imbalance sets the stage for chaos and disease when the body is not getting the raw materials (nutrients) it needs for maintenance and repair to change the terrain back to normal. He concluded that symptoms are the actions of germs thriving in an unbalanced terrain.

Dr. Young also discovered that Antoine Bechamp (1816–1908), a

French professor of medical chemistry and pharmacy, had described the process of fermentation for what it is: a process of digestion by microscopic beings. He was also the first to assert that the blood is not a liquid but a flowing tissue. In 1866 he brought to the world the profound revelation that the elementary granules that constitute the cells are living ferments. He renamed them *microzymas*, meaning "small ferments," independently living elements within all living things that build, recycle, and destroy organisms. In a state of health, the microzymas act harmoniously and fermentation occurs normally. But in the condition of disease, microzymas become disturbed and change their form and function. Then they become poised to recycle the physical body into the earth upon death (dust to dust).

Bechamp found microzymas to be physiologically imperishable and autonomously alive, with the ability to adapt to any circumstance while maintaining their purpose to enhance and organize life, whether for the host or for themselves. Bechamp stated that the microzyma was thoroughly impressionable and the only living entity capable of receiving an impression. The understandings of Bechamp and Young, about microzymas and the balancing of the pH factor, concur with the Taoist understandings of the cosmic dust particles (star dust) that give life to all beings and the importance of the balance of yin (-) and yang (+) in the body for health and well-being.

Pasteur himself, despite his previously heralded announcement, became convinced that the germ was secondary and the disease came first. At a later date he proved the fallacy of the germ theory to his entire satisfaction. He said: "The presence in the body of a pathogenic agent is not necessarily synonymous with infectious disease." In the mid-1880s he opened his eyes to the fundamental fact that germs and bacteria change their forms according to their environment. Since this departed from his first discovery, it was suppressed. The investigations of Cohn, Pasteur, Koch, Nageli, Kurth, and others were totally overlooked. They proved that bacteria are affected by the medium in which they are cultivated, and not only are the forms modified but also the physiological activity varies in degree and time. The stage was set, the propaganda had already begun, the lie perpetuated, and the error, unfortunately, has continued up to the present day.

The Truth about Germs

There is no question that certain bacteria are associated with specific diseases, but the big question science must face is: are these germs the accompaniment of the disease or are they the cause of the diseased condition?

The idea that bacteria of a certain specific kind were the accompaniment of a disease was ruled out because it was found that in any particular disease the same type of bacteria was always found. In order to satisfy a doubting public and furnish an answer to the question, "What makes me sick?" the medical profession answered "Germs, of course." However, in view of the scientific research that has been cast aside by medicine, it is just as reasonable to assume that the maggots and flies found in a manure pile caused the manure pile as it is to assume that the various kinds of germs and bacteria, bacilli, or micro-organisms, by whatever name you may call them, found in a thoroughly filthy body poisoned with (bad) food, drugs, and bad habits caused the condition of ill health.

Long ago it was demonstrated that the living tissues of a healthy body exert actions that are antagonistic to parasitic invaders. More recent bacteriological research shows that the mere admission of a germ or bacteria into an animal does not necessarily cause disease. For example, Dr. Rawlins claimed that 2 percent of the population are diphtheria carriers, with diphtheria germs in their noses and throats, and yet have no diphtheria. How then can the germ theory as the cause of disease be correct?

We constantly breathe in some 14,000 germs and bacteria per hour. We cannot keep them out of our bodies; they are everywhere. Why, then, do we not all have some form of disease? Why are some people immune to many diseases and others susceptible? It was proven many years ago by Dr. Bosenow of the Mayo Clinic that bacteria change their form according to the medium in which they live. For example, he was able to "reduce the pneumococcus (germ) to a streptococcus, and a streptococcus back to a staphylococcus," simply by changing the medium and environment in which they lived. This is very important for you to understand, for it will liberate you from the fear that germs can cause a disease. When you understand that both health and disease are created by your own living and eating habits, you will no longer fear the ever-present germ.

It is a scientifically known fact that: 1) germs take on a form in accordance with their environment; 2) so long as the internal environment and health of the body remains sound and vigorous, it will be completely immune; 3) germs and bacteria are the lowest form of scavengers and they thrive and multiply in waste matter and filth within the system; 4) disease germs and bacteria are not capable of affecting healthy living cells and tissues, for they do not have the strength or power to change or alter a higher living life form than themselves (that is, germs only feed on the lifeless waste of an unhealthy and broken down condition of the body); 5) bacteria are not the cause of disease, but may be considered as accessory factors or tertiary causes, analogous to the common garbage fly or vulture, who feed only when the refuse is placed in the garbage receptacle or an animal dies in the wild.

Germs: A Necessary Benefit for All Life

Microbes are spread throughout nature; in fact, they are ubiquitous. They are in the food we eat, the water we drink, and the air we breathe. We are reared in an environment laden with them. We cannot escape them. We can destroy them only to a limited extent. We must accept them as one of the joys of life.

Germs are saprophytes, that is, they live off dead inorganic matter. They are omnipresent scavengers in nature's great laboratory, transforming dead organic matter into forms appropriate to the nourishment of growing vegetation. Without them, neither plant nor animal could long exist, and the earth would rapidly become encumbered with dead bodies. In a septic tank, they reduce sewage until it finally passes out as pure water in which fish may live. From both the aesthetic and economic viewpoint, they are benefactors.

We live in a balanced and interdependent world, which is too complex for us to ever fully understand. However, our dependence upon the symbiotic support of germ life is at least partly known. In the body they perform the same function that is ascribed to them everywhere else in nature—they break up and consume dead and dying cells and discharges from the tissues. Viewed from this angle, they are purifying and beneficial agents.

Germs are really our best friends. All living matter and human health are totally and completely dependent upon bacterial presence. They are fundamental to the existence of all higher organic life. Earth's atmosphere is 80 percent nitrogen but no plant or animal can use nitrogen directly, with the sole exception of nitrogen-fixing bacteria. Soil bacteria convert nitrogen, with other elements, into nitrates and nitrites, thus providing material for plants to use to develop protein. We obtain our nitrogen from the plants, and the plant gets it from the soil with the help of these bacteria.

Scientific experiments have shown that small animals placed in completely germ-free containers fail to develop normally: under such conditions the intestinal tract becomes abnormal, the liver deformed, the lungs fail to develop properly, and many deformities and ill-health follow. Bacteria are essential for normal development and health. For example, an infant at birth is totally sterile, but in twenty-four hours there are millions of bacteria in the gastrointestinal tract, which are necessary for the utilization of mother's milk.

Complete and adequate digestion of food is dependent upon a natural abundant supply of intestinal flora, providing what is referred to as bacterial enzyme activity. They are necessary for the breakdown, assimilation, and absorption of all food material. When health is normal the digestive secretions are sufficient protection against germs and parasites. It is true, for example, that germs may cause putrefaction after a meal of lobsters when enervation prevents digestion. However, when digestion is normal, the bacilli are utilized as food along with the lobster. All of the digestive juices are germicidal, and normal digestion digests germs as readily as it does apples or bread.

Germs Do Not Cause Disease

If germs are powerless against a healthy body, the logical preventative is the cultivation of health. If the body manufactures its own antiseptics and antitoxins, it should be supplied with the proper elements of sun, air, water, (natural) food, exercise, rest, and so on, out of which it can build these protective potencies, instead of being subjected to the present madhouse efforts to produce artificial immunity.

Even Pasteur said: "In a state of health the body is closed against the action of disease germs." It is a mistake to single out one of the correlated factors that constitute cause and hold it responsible for pathology. Germs alone can no more produce pathology than a seed alone can produce a tree. Just as a seed must have fertile soil, moisture, air, water, warmth, and sunshine, if it is to grow into a tree, so the germ, if it is to add its complicating influence to an evolving pathology, must find certain essential conditions existing in the bodies of those it enters, before it can do the slightest harm. Normal nerve energy and pure blood (in a word, good health) are proof against germs of all kinds.

Impaired health provides suitable soil for germs to thrive and grow. The soil is more important than the germ. Infection and degeneration can set in only when the soil is badly fertilized by inappropriate nutrition. Germs are coagitators, but always secondary; a possible reinforcing or contingent cause, but never a primary cause.

A universal cause comes first, then the fermenting agent, in the form of a germ, gains access to the weakened tissues and attempts to assist the removal of undesirable material by liquefying it. The morbid material generated by this activity is more a by-product of the disintegrating tissue than a virulent poison resulting from bacterial maliciousness. Germ activity, in this view, is an outside accessory that facilitates the removal of auto-generated filth. Germs may complicate matters when there is a perversion of chemistry. But the germs of the so-called specific diseases never take on specificity until the vitality of the different tissues is lowered and nutrition perverted because the chemistry of the blood fails to supply the essential elements. Then germs, previously innocent, take on virulence in keeping with the general enervation and systemic toxemia of the individual.

Four Postulates

Many years ago, the famous bacteriologist Dr. Koch concluded that the mere presence of a germ or bacteria in a cell, tissue, or organ is not adequate proof that it causes the disease. He stated four requirements that must be met before any causal relationship between germs and disease could be admitted:

1. Specific bacteria or germs must be found in every case of the disease.
2. Bacterium must never be discovered apart from the disease.
3. It should be possible to isolate the bacteria, culture them in a medium, and observe that they are capable of independent existence.

4. The introduction of a small amount of a pure germ culture should produce signs and symptoms of a specific disease in a healthy organism or body.

For the germ theory to be valid, all four conditions must be met, whereas all four postulates have been disproved.

First Postulate: It is a scientifically known fact that specific bacteria are not found in every case of a specific disease. Koch's first condition is not fulfilled in tuberculosis, diphtheria, typhoid fever, pneumonia, or any other disease. The well-known physician Sir William Osier reported that the diphtheria bacillus is absent in 28 to 40 percent of cases. And, according to *Green's Medical Diagnosis*, "Tubercule bacilli may be present early, more often late, or in rare instances be absent throughout."

Second Postulate: It is a medically known fact that bacteria and germs are found in bodies, human and animal, that exhibit no signs or symptoms of any disease, proving beyond any doubt that the lowly innocent germ is not causing a disease. Healthy, disease-free people of all ages, upon examination, will be found to harbor bacteria associated with many different diseases. They do not have, have not had, and do not subsequently develop the diseases these germs are supposed to cause.

Third Postulate: Germs and bacteria are not capable of independent existence, as they totally depend on the human or animal organism for their survival. If germs depend on the "host organism" for survival, they cannot be considered as direct causes of disease. Therefore, Koch's third postulate, just as the first two, fails to meet the test that would support the germ theory of disease.

Fourth Postulate: Introducing germ cultures in a healthy body or organism does not produce signs and symptoms of the disease. The Biochemical Society of Toronto conducted a number of very interesting experiments in which pure cultures of typhoid, diphtheria, pneumonia, tuberculosis, and meningitis germs were consumed by the millions in food and drink by a group of volunteers. Tuberculosis germs were fed in water, milk, bread, cheese, butter, and potatoes; meningitis germs were swabbed into the nostrils, tongues, and tonsils; diphtheria germs were taken in large doses. The results of these tests showed absolutely no signs of disease or any ill effects whatsoever. The fourth postulate that germs cause disease is a complete failure.

Germs versus Disease

If you have a particular disease, what should you do about it? What we want you to understand is that you do not need to do anything about it. Instead, you need to do something about the causes. That's most important. The disease represents the effort of resistance on the part of your body against the causes. It is the causes of disease that bring about changes within the body; it is the causes of disease that bring about degeneration; it is the causes of disease that kill you, not the disease. The disease is the body's attempt to combat, overcome, and destroy the causes. Disease is the process of resistance, of remedial, defensive, or adaptive action. Germs contribute positively to the remedial process by breaking down certain decomposed organic products and by the partial digestion of the body's degenerated tissue. The bacteria themselves elaborate enzymes that digest damaged and unhealthy tissue.

As a patient's health status changes, bacteria found in the organism also change. Normal flora change into pathogenic as a result of a change of health. For example, a person can be in a hospital with normal or average bacteria flora in the body, but within a matter of hours after a cardiac arrest, the bacterial flora change and pathogenic bacteria will be present. This indicates clearly that the person first develops the disease and then the bacteria change and proliferate. At that point they may perhaps contribute, as secondary factors, by elaborating their own toxins, which the body has to deal with. In this way they are associated with certain diseases, but not as causes.

Obviously, we can do nothing about germs in the way of destroying them. If it were possible to destroy them, we would also destroy the rest of organic existence. We should try to understand the interrelationships between microorganisms and humans and not be forever in fear of them or pursuing methods and mechanisms of destroying them. It is, indeed, difficult to understand why a whole profession has gone insane on the subject of bugs, to the utter neglect of those states of metabolism and nutrition which, when vitiated, constitute the universal cause of all disease.

The medical profession believes that the blood can be immunized. Normal blood does not need it, and the process lowers its resistance. The victim of low-resistance toxemia is further deteriorated by such treatment. An unreasoning way to rid the victim of germs and parasites is to destroy them with germicides and parasiticides. After killing them off, what is to be done about their habitat, the patient? Even if medical men are still trying to kill venereal germs with drugs, the fact still remains that they damage their patients more than they do the germs. If I had my life to live over again, I would devote it to proving that germs seek their natural habitat, diseased tissue, rather than being the cause of diseased tissue, just as mosquitoes seek stagnant water but do not cause a pool to become stagnant.

Germ Theory Conclusions

The great fact remains that germs, bacteria, and microbes are our best friends instead of our worst enemies. They are necessary in both health and diseased conditions. In health, they are friendly fermenting agents (enzymes) that ensure the proper digestion and assimilation of foods; in diseased conditions, they become active and assist in the removal of undesirable material (dead cells, cellular wastes, and filth) by liquefying it. Germ activity, in this view, is an outside accessory that facilitates the removal of auto-generated filth, which, if not released, will cause the dissolution of the body. With the filth go the germs.

It is now known generally that the juices of a healthy body provide for far greater powers of immunity than any antibiotic that can be made. Instead of hunting for a magic pill, powder, or medicine to kill off "germs," it would be more intelligent to study the requirements and conditions that bring about a state of health. If you live in a super state of health, you need not worry about resisting noxious bacteria, for you will once and for all rid your (temple) body of the filthy soil that is required for the life and propagation of germ scavengers. Then you and germs will be living together on friendly basis.

TAKE CHARGE OF YOUR HEALTH

The entire philosophy of health is expressed in these words: "Keep clean internally and externally, and learn to control and stay within the magnetic margins of your vitality and health." The health-building suggestions provided in the rest of this book, if followed faithfully, will reward you with superior health, vitality, energy, and a zest for living far into advanced age. You will have no fear of germs, for through understanding you will gain knowledge, wisdom, and the power to master the drama of life, including the lowly microbe. You should not attempt to cure the body without the soul, for the cure of many diseases is unknown to the physicians who are ignorant of the whole, and the part can never be well unless the whole is well.

True understanding dispels fear. When we understand health and disease, in its whole form, we can no longer place the blame for our ill health on the lowly germ or bacteria. We then look within for the answers to build our health force. No sane person wants to be ill; we all desire to be healthy and vibrant. It is tragic to witness loved ones in pain and suffering. Unfortunately, too few people understand or adhere to the natural laws that govern health and life. The ancients referred to sowing and reaping as karma or cause and effect. One may sow (cause) good karma by adhering diligently to the habits that create health. Conversely, one may also sow (cause) illness by ignoring the habits of natural health.

These are only a few of the basic causes of health and disease. Open your mind, for you can always learn more about life; keep the channels of your mind ever open for new causes. The mind is like a parachute, which functions only when open.

NERVE FORCE PRINCIPLE

Are you nervous, irritable, and fidgety? Do you easily lose your temper? Do you entertain thoughts of fear and suspicion? How often do you take headache-relieving drugs and medicines? Do you suffer from nervous butterflies, and do you constantly pity yourself? Are you sleeping soundly? Did you know that your low moods are the result of a depleted, destroyed, and malnourished nervous system? Damaged and half-starved nerves impair digestion and cause headaches, mental anguish, heart

CAUSES OF HEALTH	CAUSES OF DISEASE

Correct eating:
  Balancing yin and yang foods
  Acid and alkaline balance
  Chewing food well
  Eating only when hungry and thirsty
  Eating foods in season; for climate
	Incorrect eating:
	  Eating extreme yin and yang foods
	  Acid and alkaline imbalance
	  Malnutrition
	  Overeating and drinking
	  Eating foods out of season; not for climate

Personal cleanliness	Poor personal hygiene
Fasting or eliminative diet	Toxemia (from enervating habits)
Intestinal cleanse	Constipation
Sufficient exercise	Excess or insufficient exercise
Proper posture	Incorrect posture
Stretching	Insufficient stretching
Plenty of fresh air	Indoors too much
Adequate sunshine	Lack of sunshine or overexposure
Pure water	Impure water
Deep breathing; exhaling sufficiently	Insufficient exhaling
Moderation; temperance in habits	Use of prescription or recreational drugs or alcohol
Correct reading and close work	Incorrect reading and excessive close work
Comfortable clothing	Restrictive clothing
Sufficient rest and sleep	Insufficient rest and sleep
Relaxation	Overwork; working at night
Meditation and prayer	Nervousness
Self-control	Lack of self-control
Knowing what you want; positive thinking	Fear and doubt; self-pity
Confidence	Discouragement
Compassion	Self-righteousness
Honesty	Confusion
Cheerfulness	Gloominess
Thankfulness	Fault-finding
Forgiveness and love	Vengeance and hate
Freedom	Tension and worry

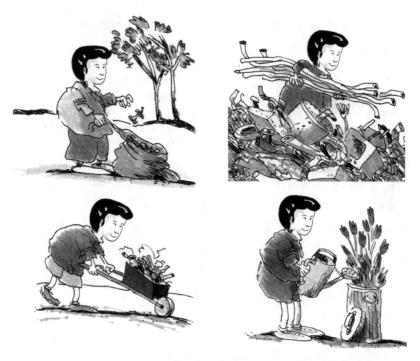

Fig. 1.5. Learn to work with the causes of health.

disease, impotence, mental illness, nerve disorders, and a host of other physical ills. Poor nerve health and constant nerve leakage can destroy friendships and put an end to your love life and marriage. No matter how wealthy, influential, or successful you are, if your nerves are jangled, starved, and weak, you cannot be happy in life.

Our super-fast style of living, constantly rushing and on the go from morning until night, tends to drain and weaken nerve force faster than it can be recharged and energized. Nerve force can be drained away quickly by the following habits:

1. Immoderation: Overworking, overeating, and overdoing anything.
2. Poor posture: Slouched sitting posture and bent standing posture.
3. Malnutrition: Irritants to the nerves include coffee, alcohol, drugs, marijuana, tobacco, salt, white flour foods, white sugar, and sugared foods.

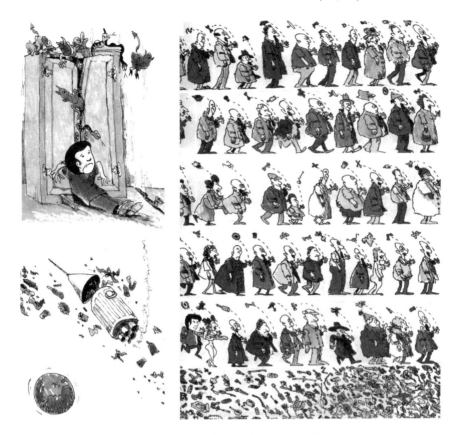

Fig. 1.6. Learn to work with the causes of disease.

4. Lack of proper exercise: No daily exercise program and not getting enough pure outdoor oxygen after meals and throughout the day results in sluggish nerve flow and poor nerve nourishment due to lack of adequate circulation of the blood to all body parts.

5. Insufficient rest and sleep: Lack of sufficient rest and sleep can result in rapid nerve loss and nervous disorders. No known remedy can rejuvenate a sleep- and rest-starved body. Proper sleep and rest is one of the quickest ways to restore lost nerve power.

6. Lack of mental poise: This is the result of immoderation, poor nutrition, lack of exercise, rest, and sleep. People lacking emotional poise have the least nerve power and lead miserable and unhappy lives.

Every act of living uses up or drains away a certain amount of nerve force daily. The more nerve force we can accumulate within the system, the healthier, stronger, and younger we will remain. People who are constantly ill possess very low nerve force, and they deplete it faster than it can be replenished. To attain the highest level of health, we must conserve our energy and learn how to accumulate, recharge, and rebuild our internal batteries to acquire powerful nerve force vitality.

Conserve Nerve Force Energy

Nerve energy and personal magnetism are conserved and accumulated within the body by the practice of controlling body movements and motions. Constant fidgeting, excessive and nervous hand and leg motions while sitting, temper tantrums, constant talking and chattering, and irritability must be controlled. All of these useless motions cause a serious leakage of nerve energy away from the body. If this nerve energy were not squandered away in wasted motions and other immoderate habits, we could easily acquire a high degree of health.

While walking, relax and make all your movements smooth and easy; refrain from jerky motions and use only the muscles required for the task. It is best to sit down with both feet on the floor and in correct posture, relaxing without unnecessary motions. During the day, when time permits, lie down and relax in a dead still position for a few moments; it may be the refreshing lift you need. If we constantly strive to be self-controlled, our vital nerve force energy and health can improve by leaps and bounds. Here is an excellent nerve exercise that can help you gain self control and personal magnetism.

Dead Still Paper Exercise

This exercise helps to control and stop nerve energy leakage and will enable you to gain control of your body and mind. It forces the body and mind to concentrate and be still, while conserving and accumulating a supply of nerve force. While performing this exercise, do not cease breathing or eye blinking; just relax and be calm!

1. Take a standing position. Grasp a sheet of blank paper by the lower right hand corner between the thumb and first two fingers; hold it in front of your chest with the elbow away from the body.

2. Next, locate a tiny spot or small point somewhere on a wall and hold the paper so that the upper opposite edge of the paper is in exact line with your eye and the spot on the wall. Control it in this position for 15 seconds without any kind of shaking. At first, the paper may shake uncontrollably, but keep practicing in spare moments, and you will finally succeed in not moving in the slightest degree during the 15 seconds.

It may take a few weeks to master this technique, but eventually nervousness will vanish and relaxation and control will follow. You will gain personal magnetism that will be noticed.

Nerve Force Health Rating System

The age of a person does not determine a health rating; his or her daily health habits do. You can be old at the age of twenty or young and healthy at the age of a hundred. Time or calendar years is not a prime factor in developing degenerative disease or super health. In fact, you can develop a super health rating at any age if you persistently follow the teachings in this book.

Level One: Degenerative Disease

The individuals in this category have lost their health and vitality, and have very low nerve force energy. They suffer from every known degenerative disease, such as cancer, rheumatoid arthritis, Parkinson's disease, heart disorders, tuberculosis, multiple sclerosis, muscular dystrophy, diabetes, colitis, blood disorders, nephritis, and extreme fatigue. Many young children born today of unhealthy, alcoholic, drug-addicted, and junk-food-eating parents are coming into this world with level-one health or degenerative diseases. Many are lucky to have average health, and very few children or adults are fortunate to be blessed with good health. It is possible to build health from level one to level three or four, but only by following the level-five formula very strictly.

Level Two: Poor Health

People at this level generally have poor health, and are constantly fatigued and lack energy. They suffer with chronic conditions such as kidney, liver, and organic problems that have not yet reached the degenerative state, such as asthma, eczema, psoriasis, sciatica, back problems, nerve disorders, hypoglycemia, mental problems, sexual impotence, frigidity, chronic fatigue, and chronic visual and hearing problems. The majority of this group are past the age of fifty. However, an increasing number of younger people have been developing these same chronic disease symptoms and therefore fall into the level-two category of poor health. A poor constitution and poor health are either inherited from the parents or conditioned by poor eating and living habits early in life. They can, however, be improved.

Level Three: Average Health

This is the category of average health into which most Americans fall. Their nerve force energy runs from high to low on any given day. Average health includes poor eyesight and hearing, colds, flu, hay fever, and sinus problems. Colds, flu, and so on are vital signs of internal elimination, which indicates that the body still has sufficient nerve force power to eliminate toxins and prevent degenerative conditions, such as arthritis, heart trouble, cancer, and so on. Suppressing acute conditions such as colds will eventually lead to chronic disease. Today many children are born in the third-level health category, while many years ago they were born with fifth-level super health because of better food and healthier environmental conditions.

Level Four: Good Health

People at this level possess a great deal of energy and good health. They retire evenings only slightly fatigued and arise the following morning full of energy and nerve force, ready for a full day of activity and excitement. They possess normal sight, hearing, digestion, elimination, and good organic health. Few people over the age of twenty attain a level-four rating. Health begins to decline from age twenty to thirty. Those over the age of twenty or thirty who possess the level-four rating are either living and eating properly or were born of extremely healthy parents into a fifth-level health category.

Level Five: Super Health

Super health is the ultimate reward of those possessing a fifth-level rating. The individuals in this elite classification enjoy an abundance of vitality, nerve force, and human energy mentally, physically, emotionally, and spiritually, and do not know what it is to be fatigued or worn out. Such people are endowed with the following qualities: hair shines, eyes sparkle, skin glows, teeth are glossy white, muscles are firm, the posture is perfect, and they radiate a wealth of energy, confidence, and happiness.

Level-five people retire evenings with a reserve of energy, and arise at the crack of dawn with a zest for living, ready to conquer the world. Their health is far above the norm; they suffer neither digestive problems nor organic disease, enjoy excellent sight, hearing, sexual magnetism, and a clear voice. They are self-motivators and great leaders in their respective fields, setting high standards for the world to follow. To possess the level-five nerve force health rating is a grand accomplishment in itself, and it is a very worthwhile goal for all, for it is the closest reality to developing super bionic men and women, endowed with superior spiritual, mental, emotional, and physical health. That is the goal of creation.

Six Formulas to Increase Your Nerve Force

Take care of your health; you do not have the right to neglect it and thus become a burden to yourself, and perhaps to others. If you follow these six formulas, the nerve force principle will help build a healthy, strong, and powerful nervous system: nerves of steel responding to your every command.

1. Moderation in all the good things of life
2. Super nutrition
3. Correct posture
4. Adequate daily exercise
5. Sufficient rest and sleep
6. Mental and emotional poise

Following these six formulas can lead you to happiness and success far beyond your highest expectations. As you gain in super-health and nerve force, you will become poised, emotionally balanced, and in complete control of your life. You will have developed complete mastery in the drama and circumstances of your earthly existence.

Moderation

Moderation basically consists of this one key point: expend no more energy than what has been accumulated each day. By not going to extremes we will automatically maintain our reserve energy supply and enjoy excellent health. Overstepping our energy bounds can easily lead to nerve leaks and consequent failing health. It is similar to saving money; if the bank account is overdrawn, there will be no funds in reserve to live on. Likewise with energy: the more energy we conserve, the more we will accumulate in the body to be utilized for reserve and emergency purposes.

Powerful nerve force can never be built by going to extremes or immoderation in eating, working, studying, exercising, sleeping, reading, sexual indulgence, and so on. Super health will be an impossibility for a person who continually depletes, drains, and destroys his or her nerve force. People with level-one health possess very little nerve force, and if they are injured or wounded, they heal very slowly or not at all. On the other hand, people at level four or five possess an abundance of recuperative power and heal very quickly.

On the pathway to super health, you must learn how to regulate and conserve your own energy supply. You may accomplish this by adhering closely to the law of rhythm, which teaches balance. For example, when you've had enough to eat, your body rhythm alerts you by taking away hunger until more food is required; if you do not sleep or rest when tired or exhausted, you have ignored your body rhythm, and you may collapse from nerve exhaustion. Moderation is the key that unlocks the door to greater nerve force.

Super Nutrition

To build powerful nerve force we need an abundance of essential nutrients in the form of vitamins, minerals, proteins, carbohydrates, trace minerals, enzymes, and fats. However, the nerves must not only be fed, they must also be cleansed. A detoxification diet of three to five days or a short fast of a few days will help tremendously in cleansing the cells and tissues of the body for a more perfect and smooth nerve flow. Be sure to follow the cleansing period with eating highly nourishing foods. The following food minerals will rebuild, feed, and protect the nerves. They are absolutely necessary in your quest for super health.

Calcium	Iron	Phosphorus
Chlorine	Magnesium	Sodium
Iodine	Manganese	

Correct Posture

Correct posture is a vitally important factor in restoring our nerve force vigor. A slumped back and shoulder position while sitting or standing is a sure way of cutting off nerve supply from the spinal cord to the entire body. The head, chest, and shoulders should be held up.

A bent over, stooped position broadcasts to the world that life feels too difficult for you to cope with; it is the appearance of a coward and makes you actually feel like one. You will never see or hear stooped over individuals singing "happy days are here again," because it is contrary to their nature. A flabby, clumsy, stooped body and a protruding abdomen detract greatly from the beauty and efficiency of the body. Poor posture can lead to headaches, backaches, tiredness, and fatigue. Incorrect posture hinders good breathing, affects the digestion, and is a prime cause of constipation. It develops spinal curves, weakens the internal organs, and forces out the pelvic joints, which is a major cause of prolapsed organs.

A proper and correct posture will instill in you an attitude of courage and confidence that will be noticed by all those around you. Proper posture ensures excellent circulation throughout the body, which means greater nerve force, more energy, and a higher health rating. An abundance of proper exercise tends toward the building up of an erect, well-proportioned body.

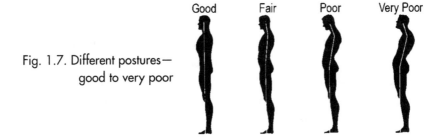

Fig. 1.7. Different postures— good to very poor

Good   Fair   Poor   Very Poor

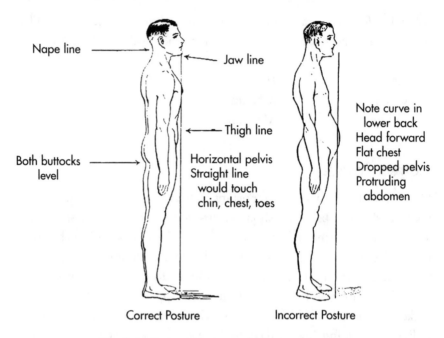

Fig. 1.8. Correct posture and incorrect posture

The road to perfect posture lies in the daily practice of sitting and standing as upright as we possibly can. Always sit with hips and back firmly against the back of a chair. While writing in a sitting position, bend from the hips, but do not round the back while doing so; this maintains the lumbar and sacral vertebrae in perfect alignment. Here follows an excellent exercise to assist in developing a straight standing posture.

Lower Back Wall Exercise

The idea of this exercise is to maintain an upright posture without the lower back curving inward and away from the wall. Strive to relax in this exercise and remain free from strain and tension.

1. Stand against a straight wall with the heels about two inches away from the base of the wall, with the buttocks, shoulders, and lower back all touching the wall. The lower back should be flat and in line with the hips, not curving inward in a swayback position. You should not be able to place a hand between the lower back and the wall. Flat-

ten the lower hips against the wall; this will remove the lower back curve.

2. Practice this exercise for a few minutes 2 or 3 times a day and strive to maintain this correct posture daily. A perfect posture will allow the internal organs to remain in their proper place. Good posture enables the organs to function normally and the muscles to become firm and strong; you will be able to completely relax and become less fatigued while working.

Delsarte Hook

This is another posture exercise that will help you to gain a perfect upright carriage.

1. Imagine a fully expanded and suspended balloon. Think of the lungs as a large balloon and the chest as a collapsible aerodrome, with the ribs as the rafters. The rafters must be lifted up completely away from the balloon. This is done by standing erect, then placing an imaginary hook where your breast bone is and a pulley in the ceiling above you; then imagine yourself pulling the rope through the pulley, to lift up that portion of the anatomy (rib cage), which will leave the arms free to swing loosely, shoulders relaxed back and down. The entire body will fall in proper alignment. In this correct posture you will be able to breathe easily and naturally.

2. Always remember to keep the shoulders back and down and the chest out. Stand with the knees locked (abdomen and back flat). This is the correct standing posture. If you suffer from back problems, consult a chiropractor for instruction on the proper care and exercise of your spine and back.

Adequate Daily Exercise

Proper daily exercise is as necessary to life as is food and nutrition. Exercise tones up the internal and external organs and muscles; it helps to circulate the nutrients to the nerves, muscles, and vital organs. Exercises that leave us breathless are a great tonic to the body, inspiring us with courage, strength, and confidence; they impart a fresh feeling of energy and nerve power to every cell in our body. There is nothing like daily exercise to lift our spirits and set us on the path to super health. An adequate amount of daily exercise, together with proper rest and sleep, is vitally important in building powerful nerve force and energy.

The best type of exercises are those that reach all the joints, spinal area, and muscles of the body. The cells and tissues automatically go through a system of contraction and relaxing. When they contract they squeeze out their waste matter; when they relax they absorb their nutrients. Here are a couple of suggestions.

Standing Spinal Twist and Stretch

This exercise can be performed any time during the day when you need a quick energy boost.

1. Stand with both feet on the floor, raise arms over head, lock fingers together, turn palms out, keep knees stiff, and stretch forward as far as possible.

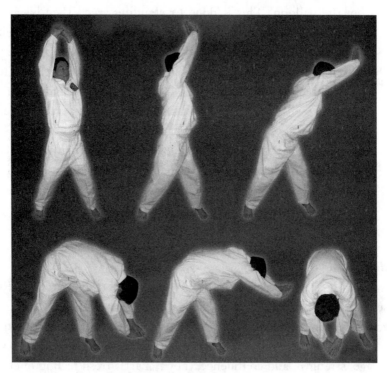

Fig. 1.9. Wide circle phase of standing spinal twist and stretch

2. After bending forward, return back to the erect position with the hands above the head.

3. Now bend backward slowly and feel the muscles relaxing.

4. Repeat the two movements 5 or 6 times.

5. Next, for waist reduction and stomach, liver, and kidney stimulation, stretch and swing the body in a complete circle 3 to 5 times in each direction, with hands interlocked. Inhale in upright position, and exhale slowly and completely while making a wide circle as shown.

Stretching the Neck

The neck where the cervical vertebrae are located is an area of much congestion and interference with blood flow and nerve energy to the eyes, ears, and nasal cavities. This exercise will help to remove some of that congestion.

1. Stretch neck by leaning head backward and forward as far as possible. Repeat 6 times.

2. Next, stretch the neck from side to side by attempting to lay your head on each shoulder. Repeat 6 times.

3. Then turn head from one side to the other, looking over each shoulder. Repeat 6 times.

4. Next rotate the head in a circular motion, clockwise and counter clockwise, each 6 times.

5. Stretch the muscles, then relax them.

This type of joint exercise should be performed with other body parts as well; for example, you can twist, stretch, flex, and rotate your shoulders, wrists, ankles, hips, knees, fingers, and arms. You can stimulate nerve and blood circulation to your face by squeezing, stretching, and making face contortions; this will keep the face looking young and firm. The hands, feet, and toes may be squeezed, rotated, and stretched for better circulation. Stretching before arising in the morning is an excellent method of awakening vital nerve force for the day ahead. All of these various circulation exercises are beneficial to all the organs, cells, blood, and nerves of the body, building powerful nerve health.

Sufficient Rest and Sleep

Sleep and rest are vitally necessary to restore powerful nerve force in the body. It is during sleep that the body repairs itself; resting during the day recuperates the nerve energy lost during daily activity. For sound sleep, your room should be well ventilated for the complete circulation of air. Fresh night air vitalizes the body during sleep and prevents carbon monoxide poisoning from your own exhalation. However, the room temperature should be neither hot nor cold.

Most people require from six to nine hours of sound sleep for the maintenance of health and repair of cells, tissues, and nerves. Lack of sufficient rest and sleep is a prime cause of a drawn-out haggard look, wrinkles, loss of vitality, poor memory, grouchiness, and loss of beauty. Some people try to get by on only a few hours of sleep a night; others in their mad rush for wealth, fame, and power neglect proper rest and sleep. Nervous exhaustion is usually their reward.

When fatigued and sleepy, stop all activity—that is, reading, watching television, and so on. Retire to bed. For proper spinal nerve flow, the bed should be firm and not soft. Old, worn-out, soft mattresses create spinal curvatures and impinge the nerves. Relax your muscles, starting from the toes and loosening all body parts up to your head, feeling each body part relaxing in turn as you free it from tension. Think of your body as an extremely heavy weight sinking deeper and deeper into the mattress while relinquishing from your mind all thoughts of worry, anxiety, and tension. Now fill your mind with beautiful and serene thoughts of love, happiness, and peace. Spend a few minutes mentally forgiving everyone, and send thoughts of love, happiness, and peace to the far corners of the world. By mentally blessing and forgiving the world, you send out healing energy, which returns its blessings in health, success, and sound sleep. Also, mentally picture yourself attaining your heart's desires and success. These few sleeping secrets will help to give you a peaceful night's rest. The next morning you will feel fit and ready to face the world with courage, confidence, and love.

It is generally believed that there is little harm in lying down or sleeping after meals, but this idea is entirely false. When you lie down or sleep after eating, the gastric juices do not flow readily. The main objective of sleep is to repair and replenish the nerves and tissues, but if we consume food directly before retiring at night, the body spends its energy on digestion instead of repair. The result will be a lack of vitality, health, and strength. Because of poor elimination, it can result in anemia. It is best to eat no later than three or four hours before going to sleep. If hungry at bedtime, a piece of fruit before retiring will do no harm, as it will be very quickly digested.

No-Exercise Super Beauty Treatment

This super exercise is so simple that you expend absolutely no energy in performing it; all you do is lie down in bed and sleep! Sounds too easy, doesn't it? Try this no-exercise health and beauty treatment and see and feel the results for yourself.

1. Here is what you do before retiring to bed: raise the foot end of your bed about two inches off the floor with a wooden block.
2. Leave the bed in this raised position from now on. After a few days you will become accustomed to this position and begin to see and feel the results in better muscle tone, brighter complexion, smoother internal functions, and firmer facial skin.

What does this simple exercise accomplish? It reverses the downward pull of gravity on facial muscles, skin, and internal organs. When the lower part of the body is raised a few incher higher than the upper body while lying down, the bloodstream gently courses down to the head, stimulating the ductless glands to pour out their rejuvenating and beautifying juices to all parts of the face and body. This sleeping position gives the vital organs an opportunity to fall back into their proper position, allowing them to function at peak efficiency to keep you young and vigorous.

Mental and Emotional Poise

The wisdom of the ancient sages passed down through the centuries has taught humans that mental poise or peace of mind is one of the greatest assets a person may possess. The sages tell us not to worry about the future, not to overly concern ourselves about employment, marriage, possessions, or losses. They advise us to live the best we can in the present; this will ensure our future success and happiness while giving us mental and emotional poise in life.

Freedom from worry is a vitally important factor in cleansing the mind and attaining mental poise. Do you worry about a certain problem and then discover that the problem was hardly a problem at all? Worrying about the future or over trivial matters prevents us from accomplishing our best in the present; it stops us from doing the things we could and should do but fail to do, because of our incessant worry about the things we cannot do.

Many people constantly dwell on some future desire, thinking that when they achieve their desires and goals, happiness will be guaranteed. This is generally not the case. Dwelling on future desires will not bring happiness but only anxiety and mental torment. For example, many people believe that they would be happy and contented as a president or executive of an organization. How many of these executives do you know are happy with their tremendous responsibilities?

Happiness is a result of the right attitude of mind. If we have a negative attitude toward our present life and activities we will be unhappy; if we have a positive attitude toward life we will remain enthusiastic and enjoy our successes and achievements. When we let go of the idea that we must have something to be happy, we automatically let go of envy, jealousy, revenge, hate, pride, and in their place will appear true happiness and mental poise. We then become master of our emotions. Perfect mental poise will open the inner door to our higher mind. This greater power will guide us to peace, health, harmony, happiness, success, a good marriage, and true friends. The Supreme Architect knows your every need. To have faith is the highest high you may ever achieve. A mind brimming with faith and love is a tonic to the nerves and entire system. Perfect mental poise will regenerate your body, which is a major step toward super health.

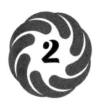

Yin and Yang in Health and Longevity

The secrets of health, life, and longevity have been known and passed down from generation to generation by the ancient sages and wise men throughout history. The universal laws of yin and yang were formulated by the Taoist masters of the mysterious East who observed all physical phenomena on Earth as being dual in nature; that is, for every force, object, or occurrence, there exists its polar opposite. The Taoist creation story is that Oneness, or Wu Chi, the source of all, manifests into this life of duality that we observe. Five thousand years ago the *Huang Ti Nei Ching Su Wen (Yellow Emperor's Classic of Chinese Medicine)*, an ancient Chinese manuscript on the subjects of health, healing, and medicine, described the beginning of all in this way:

> The Oneness (Wu Chi) splits and becomes two. These two are the poles and energies of yin and yang. They emerge continuously from this point within the expanse of infinity as a result of the endless movement within the primal sea. By their combination and interplay, the yin and the yang give rise to all the forms that inhabit the world of the relative universe. Thus, all antagonistic-complementary dualisms of the phenomenal world are but the two faces of the front and the back of one ultimate reality.

Life unfolds as a spiral from the infinite One to the relative world, then to the phenomenal world, material world, elements, minerals, then organic life, including vegetable, animals, and human beings.

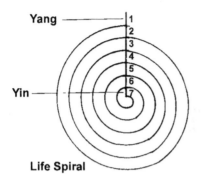

1. Infinity (Wu Chi), the Tao
2. Yin and yang—relative world begins
3. Energy, emotion, and thought—phenomenal world begins
4. Fire, preatomic—material world formed
5. World of elements and minerals is formed
6. Vegetable organic world begins
7. Human beings and animal kingdom begin

Fig. 2.1. Yin and yang in life's spiral

Nature is a perfect manifestation of Wu Chi, so we can learn a lot about life by observing, understanding, and living according to nature's laws. The microcosm reflects the macrocosm. By understanding nature's flows we can understand our own internal alchemy and also the dynamics of the universe. One of the first aspects of nature we can observe is duality: the existence of apparent opposites. For example, we see night and day; we can feel the difference between winter and summer; we experience both light and dark; we can feel warmth and coldness. These apparent opposites are not separate from one another but are the same energy at different stages of a cycle. Thus we can observe the seasonal cycle taking us from the coldest part of winter through to the warmest part of summer and back again.

Figure 2.2 is a clairvoyant's picture of the heart of the universe, with the ultimate physical atom seen as a manifestation of pure light force spinning perpetually through itself, interacting in the opposites of yin and yang.

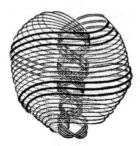

Fig. 2.2. Yin and yang cosmic energy vortex

NATURE OF YIN AND YANG

From the interaction of the Subtle Origin in the Mysterious Mother and the balanced energy of yin and yang, all phenomena of life came forth. Yang energy is subtle and spiritual and is referred to as Heaven. It is positive, and action is its nature. Yin is coarse and physical and is referred to as Earth. It is negative, and receptiveness is its nature. Both energies are equal and support each other in perfect harmony.

YIN	YANG
Night	Day
Winter	Summer
Dark moon	Full moon
Dark	Light
Introvert	Extrovert
Intuition	Analysis
Rest	Activity
Feminine	Masculine
Body	Spirit
Material	Immaterial
Contracted	Expanded

While we can compare opposite pairs as yin and yang, it is important to remember that these opposites are not separate: they are one entity at different stages of its cycle, or Oneness reflected as two. We would not know darkness (yin) without light (yang); heat (yang) without cold (yin); male (yang) without female (yin); hardness (yang) without softness (yin); and life (yang) without death (yin).

Yin describes the feminine principle of life and energy in its most contracted form. Winter, nighttime, and the dark moon are all examples of energy at its most contracted. In winter we feel like staying inside more (we contract socially). At night we sleep (we contract our activity levels). At dark moon we become introspective (we contract psychologically). When energy contracts it becomes solid. Thus all things manifest and solid, such as the body, the blood, and the earth, are described as yin.

Yang describes the masculine principle of life and energy in its most expanded form. Summer, daytime, and full moon are all examples of

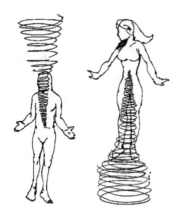

Fig. 2.3. Contracting centripetal forces from the upper atmosphere toward the center of the earth produce the yang male organism. Expanding centrifugal forces from the center of the earth upward produce the yin female organism.

energy at its most expanded. In summer we feel lively and sociable. During the daytime we are at our most active. At full moon we feel more inclined to go out and connect with others. When energy expands it becomes more intangible (just as when water is heated it becomes a gas). Thus all things that are less solid are described as yang, such as the spirit, the chi, and Heaven.

Yin and Yang Create Physical Change

Change in the physical realm is inevitable; it manifests itself in a dual nature of yin and yang, which are opposite yet complementary. Neither one is absolute, and the interplay between them is a constant give and take, like the ebb and flow of the ocean tides, acting and reacting, day flowing into night, summer (yang) slowly giving way to winter (yin).

The Canon of Medicine provides us with many examples of this interchange between yin and yang and of the duality preserved within a single thing. The most concrete example of this duality is man. As a male, man belongs to yang; as a female, man belongs to yin. Yet both, male and female, are products of two primary elements, hence both qualities are contained in both sexes.

The principle of yin and yang is the basis of the entire universe. It is the principle of everything in creation. It brings about the transformation to parenthood; it is the root and source of life and death. Heaven was created by an accumulation of yang; Earth was created by an accumulation of yin. The ways of yin and yang are to the left and to the right. Water and fire are the symbols of yin and yang. Yin and yang are the source of power and the beginning of everything in creation (alpha and omega). Yang ascends to Heaven; yin descends to Earth. Hence the universe (Heaven and Earth) represents motion and rest, controlled by the wisdom of nature. Nature grants the power to beget and to grow, to harvest and to store, to finish and to begin anew.

Seven Principles of the Order of the Universe

1. All things are the differentiated apparatus of one infinity.
2. Everything changes.
3. All antagonisms are complementary.
4. There is nothing identical.
5. What has a front has a back.
6. The bigger the front, the bigger the back.
7. What has a beginning has an end.

Nei Ching continues:

Everything in creation is covered by Heaven and supported by the Earth. When nothing has as yet come forth the Earth is called the place where yin dwells. It is also known as the yin within the yin. Yang supplies that which is upright, while yin acts as a ruler of yang. The affinity of yin and yang to each other was held to have a decisive influence upon man's health. Perfect harmony between the two primogenitors meant health; disharmony or undue preponderance of one element brought disease and death. But man is not helplessly exposed to the whims of yin and yang. Man received the doctrine of the Tao as a means of maintaining perfect balance and to secure for himself health and long life.

Here, and throughout this book, *Tao* does not represent the masculine or father image. It refers instead to the supreme creative force of the universe. As mentioned earlier, it is also the one that creates the yin and yang, negative and positive, centrifugal and centripetal, alkaline and acid, electron and proton, and the polar opposites that manifest on the physical plane.

The I Ching states: "The yang and the yin of the universe are called Tao. This knowledge of the Tao and of the workings of yin and yang was considered even strong enough to counteract the effect of age." Thus, we find it said in the *Nei Ching:* "Those who have the true wisdom remain strong, while those who have no wisdom grow old and feeble." The official view of the Chinese government regarding yin and yang states that "it contains an original, spontaneously dialectical, and simple materialistic doctrine; it is free of superstition; it approximates scientific formulation; and it represents a progressive way of thinking."

Taoist Principles of Life within Yin and Yang

1. All phenomena exist within infinite space.
2. All phenomena are interrelated.
3. All phenomena are relative.
4. Everything has energy or vibration.
5. Everything is in a constant state of change.

The conception of yin and yang is not a fabricated theory of recent origin; it began with the conception of the universe and our physical world. It is an inescapable principle of life, a duality stemming from infinity itself and manifesting in the physical world of polar opposites. The nature of health and diet is intimately connected and interrelated to the universal laws and operations of yin and yang. To understand electricity, we must learn how to use positive and negative fields. Similarly, we need to know how we can personally use the laws of yin and yang in our daily lives to improve our diet, health, and mental makeup.

Yin Flows into Yang; Yang Flows into Yin

As a way of reminding us that the apparent opposites of yin and yang are not separate entities but in continuous flow, the ancient Taoists created a symbol called the Tai Chi, which shows the spiraling and dynamic nature of this flow. One dot of black appears on the white half and a white dot in

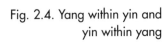

Fig. 2.4. Yang within yin and yin within yang

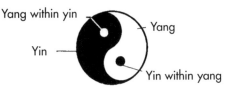

Yang within yin

Yang

Yin

Yin within yang

the black half. This symbolizes that no phenomena is purely yin or purely yang. Extreme yin contains the seed of yang, and vice versa. Although many people have difficulty understanding this part of the theory, looking to nature can help us to grasp it. In the middle of winter, it is hard to see the seed of summer! Yet after mid-winter (winter solstice, December 21) the days begin to get longer each day. This is the seed of summer.

Because each opposite contains the seed of the other, when we push to an extreme, we find we suddenly shift to the opposite. Thus if we push something to extreme yang, it will become yin, and vice versa. In this constantly changing world, nothing remains the same forever. Yin and yang flow into each other like night and day or inhaling and exhaling. For example, when we are cold, we contract and become still; we can describe this as yin. In the summer we feel more flexible and active; this is described as yang. But in extreme cold we begin to shiver, moving very fast: extreme yin has become yang. In the hottest part of a hot summer we may simply lie motionless under a tree: extreme yang has turned to yin.

Another example of the extremes is when we become a workaholic and work excessively hard (yang), we may suddenly have a breakdown and develop fatigue (yin). Likewise, people who are forced into a yin state of not being able to be active, such as being confined into a small space, become very restless (yang).

It takes wisdom and intelligence to understand and apply the universal laws of yin and yang. The more they are applied, the more you will be guided in life by the Tao. The ultimate key to this unifying principle is very simple. Moderation or adhering to the middle path in life and avoiding extremes in activity will automatically create a yin and yang balance. This will lead to harmony in body, happiness in mind and soul, and success in life.

There can be a tendency to try to perceive yin and yang as being separate when we try to understand Oriental theory through the dualistic modern mind: this leads automatically to judgment. We may try to choose between yin and yang, almost subconsciously, to decide which one is good and which one is bad. Our cultural bias tends to be toward labeling all yin aspects as bad and yang as good. The whole purpose of the Tao path is to transcend dualistic thought and to recognize that all of life is indeed One. Therefore, we need to be careful not to make judgments but rather to see how apparent opposites are simply different stages of the cycle or reflections of the whole.

By observing nature, we can begin to eliminate such judgments. When we have developed a deep relationship with nature, we cannot choose between winter and summer or between sunset and sunrise. Rather we begin to embrace all and see it as one cycle that has different stages. Nature can teach us how to live in a harmonious way. Nature has no resistances to what is; the tree does not try to hold on to its leaves when autumn comes; the rock does not fight the ocean waves that break against it but gently wears away. Thus we can learn to accept what is and yet to walk our path: the path is the Way; it is the Tao.

Twelve Theorems of the Unifying Principle

1. One infinity differentiates itself into yin and yang, which are the poles that come into operation when the infinite arrives at the geometric point of bifurcation.
2. Yin and yang result continuously from the infinite.
3. Yin is centrifugal. Yang is centripetal.
4. Yin attracts yang. Yang attracts yin.
5. Yin repels yang. Yang repels yin.
6. The force of attraction and repulsion is proportional to the difference of the yin and yang components. Yin and yang combined in varying proportion produce energy and all phenomena.
7. All phenomena are ephemeral, constantly changing their constitution of yin and yang components.
8. Nothing is solely yin or solely yang. Everything involves polarity.
9. There is nothing neuter. Either yin or yang is in excess in every occurrence.
10. Large yin attracts small yang. Large yang attracts small yin.
11. At the extremes, yin produces yang and yang produces yin.
12. All physical forms and objects are yang at the center and yin at the surface.

YIN AND YANG CHARACTERISTICS

YIN	YANG
Alkaline	Acid
Centrifugal	Centripetal
Negative	Positive
Potassium	Sodium
Cold	Hot
Moon	Sun
Water	Fire
Dark	Light
Night	Day
Moist	Dry
Fall and winter	Spring and summer
Female	Male
Rest	Activity
Vegetable	Animal
Expansion	Contraction
Outward tendency	Inward tendency
Narrow	Wide
Space	Time
Purple	Red
Soft	Hard
Mental	Physical
Periphery	Center
Earth's surface	Earth's center
Raw food	Cooked food
West and north	East and south
Sour, sweet, spicy	Salty, bitter
Tall	Short
Slow	Fast
Passive	Active
Weak	Strong
Chronic disease	Acute disease
Even numbers	Odd numbers
Parasympathetic nervous system	Sympathetic nervous system
Catabolism	Anabolism
Fruitarian	Carnivore
Electron	Proton
Abdomen	Back

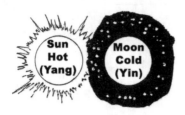

Fig. 2.5. Yin and yang principle (cold and hot)

The ancient mystery schools teach what we have not been taught in our modern schools. The general list of yin and yang classifications and attributes on the previous page will help you to understand what the ancients taught and will clarify your thinking on this most vast subject. Remember: the yin and yang principle is the law of opposites in the physical realm. For example, in the celestial realm (Heaven) the moon is considered yin (cold) and the sun is yang (hot). On Earth cold winter weather is yin and hot summer weather is yang. Study this chapter and subsequent ones to thoroughly acquaint yourself with the infinite variety and characteristics of yin and yang that abound in our midst.

YIN AND YANG IN FOOD AND ENVIRONMENT

By studying and understanding the yin and yang foods and weather conditions we can know what to eat, how to eat, when to eat, and how much to eat at any given time of the day or year. The key is to balance the yin and yang and the acid and alkaline in the diet.

Hot (yang) climates produce expanded (yin) fruits, vegetables, flowers, and plants, with the aid of much rain, which is yin and expansive. This climate produces food that is large, watery, sweet, with an abundance of the potassium element. These are cooling (yin) foods, which should be eaten in hot (yang) weather. If you are in a southern area or in the tropics, the natural tendency is to consume more of the yin foods grown in that climate. These foods are also considered alkaline or base-forming elements.

Cold (yin) climates produce more contracted (yang) foods such as smaller grains and vegetables and fruits with less liquid within them. Cold climates require more warming foods in the diet, such as cooked grains, soups, bread, and other cooked foods. Foods grown in northern climates contain an abundance of the sodium element (yang), which is necessary to keep the body warm and contracted during the cold winter months.

YIN AND YANG FOOD SCALE
(From yin to yang in this order)

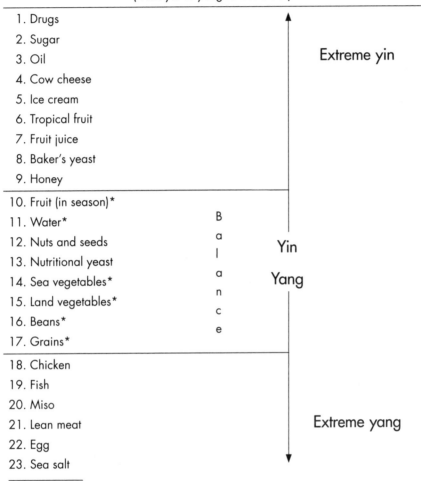

1. Drugs		
2. Sugar		Extreme yin
3. Oil		
4. Cow cheese		
5. Ice cream		
6. Tropical fruit		
7. Fruit juice		
8. Baker's yeast		
9. Honey		
10. Fruit (in season)*		
11. Water*	B	
12. Nuts and seeds	a	Yin
13. Nutritional yeast	l	
14. Sea vegetables*	a	Yang
15. Land vegetables*	n	
16. Beans*	c	
17. Grains*	e	
18. Chicken		
19. Fish		
20. Miso		
21. Lean meat		Extreme yang
22. Egg		
23. Sea salt		

*Staple foods to be used daily in season.

Yang foods, such as grains, eggs, and meat are considered acid-forming.

Chapter 7 offers you detailed guidance for rebalancing. Generally, you should eat more yang foods during the cold (yin) winter and reverse in summer; that is, you should eat about 60 to 85 percent yang foods and 10 to 30 percent yin foods in winter and 60 to 85 percent yin foods and 10 to 30 percent yang foods in summer. Sun, heat, and activity are yang. The moon, cold, and rest are yin. The sun and heat bring on summer outdoor activity. Cold weather is yin, passive, tending toward indoor activity.

In balancing the diet, we also need to learn to listen to that small inner voice within, our body intelligence, which instinctively instructs us as to the proper choice of foods in various environments. If we can tune in to our true bodily needs, yin and yang balance can easily be achieved, resulting in superior health.

Extreme yin substances such as drugs, marijuana, medicine, sugar, and alcohol tend to dissipate and expand the cells and tissues of the body and brain, causing light-headedness or a spaced-out feeling and lack of judgment. Since yin is centrifugal and expanding outward, it requires a great deal of yang binding and contracting force to equalize the extreme expansion caused by excessive yin foods and yin mind-expanding substances. Salt, time, heat, and pressure create yang conditions in nature and in food preparation. Salt preserves food and in the body it contracts (yang) the cells and keeps them from expanding. Yang foods counteract yin (expansion).

YIN AND YANG OF HEALTH

In Taoist healing we are always looking at the balance between yin and yang as a measure of health. It is said that when yin and yang finally separate, death occurs. The yin body returns to Earth and the yang spirit ascends to Heaven. Thus the work of a Taoist healer is to maintain a balance between yin and yang in order to preserve life. Healing is about becoming whole. In order to feel balanced and healthy, we have to have a flow between our yin aspects and our yang aspects.

Yin: ability to stay calm; rejuvenation; detoxification; sleep
Yang: ability to take action; exercise; movement; zest for life

If these are out of balance, then health problems may follow: physical, mental, or emotional. We can see this immediately by observing the extreme cases. If a person is excessively yin without enough yang—such as sitting at home on the couch all day watching TV, getting no exercise, and not working—soon enough such a person may suffer from overweight, fatigue, and depression. If a person is excessively yang without enough yin—such as working long hours, spending time off working out fanatically in a gym, always rushing about and never resting—such a person may sooner or later suffer from panic attacks, hyperactivity, sleeping problems, and heart problems.

Just as night and day do not have to coexist, but each has its own time and they flow one into one another in a smooth cycle, yin and yang do not have to be in balance at any one moment. But they must flow in a smooth and regular cycle for health to ensue. There is no problem with being busy, as long as you take time to unwind and relax later. Likewise, there is no problem with completely relaxing and being still, as long as you take time to exercise and move later on.

In terms of health, there are some signs of imbalance that indicate we are overly yin (or do not have enough yang) and others that indicate we are overly yang (or do not have enough yin). Some imbalances are a result of our constitutional traits and others are due more to our lifestyle factors. Here are some examples of symptoms that may indicate that we are becoming either overly yin or overly yang:

OVERLY YIN	OVERLY YANG
Excessively cold	Excessively hot
Deficient chi	Excess chi
Fatigued	Hyper
Weak	Rigid
Excess fluids	Dryness in the body
Low blood pressure	High blood pressure
Slow respiratory rate	Fast respiratory rate

Health is about harmony: smooth flow and overall balance. If we experience one of these symptoms (such as feeling cold), it is not necessarily a problem unless it is consistent and unbalanced. The more we connect to nature, the more we can see how we flow harmoniously with nature's cycles. For example, human beings naturally operate well when they are awake and active during the daytime and rest and sleep during the night. We are more comfortable if we stay in more during the winter months and spend more time outdoors during the summer.

Thus, if you are very active during the day, this does not mean you have an overly yang problem. But if it persists and you are unable to sleep well at night, then this indicates an imbalance. If you are cold during the winter, no problem. But if you continue to feel cold even in the summer months, there may be a deeper problem. Likewise, when we force our bodies out of harmony with nature for extended periods, we usually fall ill. A prime example is that of the night-shift worker. Even though a person may be sleeping a full eight hours every day, if he or she always works at night, then the person is acting against the natural flow. It is not uncommon for night-shift workers to begin to experience imbalances.

Yin and yang theory gives us a dynamic model to understand health and illness. Many models of health make the mistake of using a static model: assuming that there is a point of good health to attain. It is very difficult, indeed impossible, to reach a static goal of health. Our bodies are constantly changing and evolving, responding to the world around us. For example, our bodies tend to put on a little extra weight during colder months and become lighter in the summer. Thus if we are trying to stick to a single static weight, we are fighting against nature. The Oriental therapies give us a more fluid model, yet a model with very clear ways of understanding our health and illness.

YIN ORGANS	YANG ORGANS
Hollow	Dense
Absorption	Blood filled
Discharge	Regulate
Store energy	Transport energy
Gallbladder	Liver
Small Intestine	Heart
Stomach	Spleen/Pancreas
Large Intestine	Lung
Bladder	Kidney

YIN AND YANG OF ILLNESS

We can also view different illnesses in terms of yin and yang, though it must be remembered that the suggestions given here are only an approximation and do not apply to every case. In ancient times when Oriental therapy was used, the names of diseases were often not known. A Chinese doctor would simply look at the symptoms and examine the person's energy to decide how to treat them. However, we can see that there are often similar patterns in particular diseases, and thus we can make an estimation of yin and yang imbalances. It is always important to look at the individual's expression of the illness and his or her unique symptoms (such as heat, cold, and weakness).

OVERLY YIN	OVERLY YANG
Headaches (front of head)	Headaches (back of head)
Diabetes II	Syndrome X
Colitis	Duodenal ulcers
Asthma	Gout
Hypothyroid	Hyperthyroid
Meningitis	Appendicitis

In Chinese medicinal theory, it is known that there are different underlying situations that can create each surface appearance. An overly yin situation may be caused by either excess yin or deficient yang. In other words, it may be that the person has built up an excess of yin energies, habits, or foods, or it may be that the person does not have enough yang qualities to balance his or her yin. We can understand this by making simple charts to demonstrate. Balanced yin and yang would look like this:

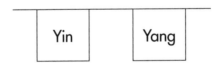

Fig. 2.6. Balanced yin and yang

Yin may become excessive. This may be our constitutional tendency, or it may result from our behavior, such as if we take too many cold watery foods and drinks, which are yin. It could be that we are in a very cold damp environment and thus develop an excessively yin situation. There are a number of ways that we can develop too much yin, which can be illustrated like this:

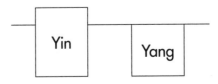

Fig. 2.7. Excess yin

The other scenario that externally appears the same is deficient yang. This may be due to our constitution or may develop out of our behaviors. For example, we may lose yang when we avoid stimulating activities and sports. If we are lazy and sedentary, we may become deficient in yang, or if we do not spend enough time with other people we can develop a deficiency. Deficient yang may be illustrated like this:

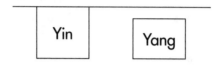

Fig. 2.8. Deficient yang

Thus excess yin and deficient yang externally appear the same, but under the surface there is a slightly different cause. Excess is always the result of too much of something (e.g., too many iced drinks) and deficiency a result of a lack (e.g., not enough exercise).

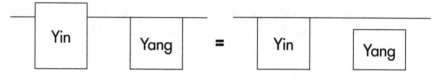

Fig. 2.9. Excess yin equals deficient yang

The same can be found when we examine an overly yang situation. This has two possibilities, one of excess yang and the other of deficient yin. It may be that we have built up an excess of yang energies, habits, or foods, or it may be that we do not have enough yin qualities to balance our yang. For example, if we eat too many rich and spicy foods then we can develop excess yang. It can be illustrated like this:

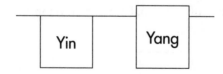

Fig. 2.10. Excess yang

Deficient yin may be constitutional or we may develop it from not nourishing our yin qualities. For example, if we do not take enough rest, do not take enough time alone, and do not surrender into relaxing pastimes, we may develop a lack of yin. This can be illustrated like this:

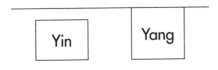

Fig. 2.11. Deficient yin

Thus we can see that from the surface level, excess yang and deficient yin look the same, though they have different underlying patterns.

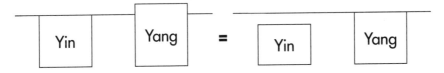

Fig. 2.12. Excess yang equals deficient yin

In Oriental theory, we distinguish between different underlying patterns so that we can understand the situation even deeper and know how to respond to it in an appropriate way.

Thus in the two main types, the yin and the yang, there are four different subgroups. The following table shows the four different groups identified in yin and yang diagnostics:

	OVERLY YANG	OVERLY YIN
YIN IMBALANCES	Deficient yin	Excess yin
YANG IMBALANCES	Excess yang	Deficient yang

The external appearances indicate two groups: overly yang and overly yin. The internal imbalances may take four different forms, depending on whether it is a predominantly yin imbalance or a predominantly yang imbalance. Understanding our health problems from this perspective can help us to gain deeper insight into the nature of our issue. To a certain extent we can treat overly yin and overly yang situations the same. However, this deeper insight can show us how we can treat the situation even more effectively.

DIAGNOSING YIN AND YANG CONDITIONS

As mentioned, there are two factors to consider in diagnosing: inherited constitution and the present health condition. Each individual is born with a certain body type, a yin or yang constitution, but no person or phenomena is exclusively yin or yang. The yin and yang principle is variable, and there are varying degrees of both yin and yang people. On a scale from 1 to 10, 1 is yang, 10 is yin, and 5 is balanced. People are called yin or yang because one or the other of these forces dominate in the body. Body conditions can be diagnosed in a general overall way, but to diagnose accurately and precisely, each body organ and body part must be diagnosed separately.

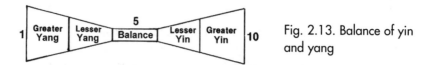

Fig. 2.13. Balance of yin and yang

There are five classifications of yin and yang conditions: greater yang and lesser yang, greater yin and lesser yin, and healthy balanced yin and yang. The balanced person does not exhibit extreme yin or yang symptoms. When people show greater yin (or yang) signs, they are referred to as yin-full (or yang-full); when they show lesser yin (or yang) signs, we refer to them as yin-empty (or yang-empty). This tells us how much vitality or energy a person possesses. A yang-full person is much more active; a yin-full person is less active and energetic.

We can alter our yin or yang condition by the way we eat and live. A simple way to apply Oriental dietary therapy is to eat a little more of

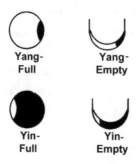

Fig. 2.14. Empty and full yin and yang

the foods that will rebalance us, until we feel harmonized again. Those who are too yin can assist their body with the addition of a few more contractive foods to build strength and stamina. Those who are too yang can assist their body by eating a few more expansive foods. Try to listen to your body as you adapt your diet to hear how it responds to different foods. This is about rebalancing: you do not want to move to another extreme. Therefore, just try gently altering your diet, rather than making sudden and dramatic changes.

The Yang-Full Person

A yang-full person has certain characteristics, which indicate the kind of diet needed to bring about yin/yang balance.

Symptoms of a Yang-Full Person

Overenergetic	Reddish complexion
Round, fleshy face, wide jaw	Overweight, strong pulse
Fat, strong abdomen muscles	Overactive organs
Yang liver and kidneys	Heart disorders
High blood pressure	Circulatory diseases
Strong digestion and appetite	Eats meat, dairy, salt, and eggs
Likes alcoholic drinks	Generally constipated
Needs little sleep	Energetic and strong talk
Enjoys cold weather	Positive and aggressive
Works hard and heals quickly	

The dietary recommendations for yang-full people are:

- Eat less cooked food and more raw fruit and vegetables.
- Use much less salt, tamari, and miso.
- Use thinner broth soups.
- Use watermelons, grapefruit, lemons, celery, parsley, cucumber, sprouts, radishes, and greens.
- Avoid fats, cheese, red meat, alcohol, oils, fried foods, ice cream, pastries.
- Drink more liquid, particularly herb teas.

- Recommended herbs: juniper berries, dandelion leaf, Oregon grape root, asparagus, sage, chaparral, gravel root.
- Exercise and sweat more.

To balance the yang-full person in extreme yang conditions: induce diarrhea, sweating, and vomiting. This diminishes excess energy in the body.

The Yang-Empty Person

A yang-empty person has certain characteristics, which indicate the kind of diet needed to bring about yin/yang balance.

Symptoms of a Yang-Empty Person

Overactive, energetic	Tan to brown skin
Tight skin	Thin, square, or bony face
Contracted eyes	Slim to underweight
Flat abdomen and firm muscles	Athletic prowess
Kidney and liver trouble	Nervous condition
Weaker digestion and appetite	Moderate drinker
Yang constipation	Easily fatigued
Needs more rest and sleep	Energetic talk
Positive and aggressive	Takes longer to heal

The dietary recommendations for yang-empty people are:

- Eat less salt, miso, and so on.
- Eat softer cooked foods; chew food 30 to 40 times.
- Drink a moderate amount of liquid.
- Eat warm foods.
- Eat more cooked vegetables.
- Eat less protein and fat.
- Eat fruits and vegetables in season.
- Avoid fats, meat, cheese, ice cream, alcohol, oils, ungerminated seeds and nuts, citrus fruits.
- Recommended herbs: chamomile, comfrey, yarrow, juniper berry, parsley leaf, dandelion leaf, alfalfa, sage, yam, plantain, chaparral.

To balance the yang-empty person in extreme yang conditions: keep warm; avoid noise and inharmonious surroundings; obtain sufficient sleep and rest. In extreme yang-empty conditions, the person should eat more yin-quality food. For a yang-empty person with constipation, diarrhea and sweating should be induced and vomiting avoided.

The Yin-Full Person

A yin-full person has certain characteristics, which indicate the kind of diet needed to bring about yin/yang balance.

Symptoms of a Yin-Full Person

Does not like exercise	Round fleshy face
Blue or yellow color	Overweight
Loose flesh	Bruises easily
Prolapsed abdomen, falling organs	Underactive thyroid
Underactive organs	Yin liver and kidneys
Weak heart	Low blood pressure
Menstrual difficulties	Eats too much sugar, fat,
Cold hands and feet	cold drinks, pastries
Likes warm weather	Poor memory and thinking

The dietary recommendations for yin-full people are:

- Use less salt, less liquid.
- Eat less protein and fat.
- Eat warm soup broths.
- Eat some fresh raw fruits and vegetables, including some citrus.
- Eat slowly, chew well.
- Avoid pastries, ice cream, milk, cheese, coffee, sugar products, ungerminated nuts.
- Use mushrooms, potato, radish, lettuce.
- Recommended herbs: oatstraw, horsetail, watercress, nettle, marsh mallow root, licorice, garlic, slippery elm.

To balance the yin-full person in extreme yin conditions: sweat to induce harmony; avoid fasting; regularly eat whole cooked grains and vegetables; get daily exercise and do deep breathing.

The Yin-Empty Person

A yin-empty person has certain characteristics, which indicate the kind of diet needed to bring about yin/yang balance.

Symptoms of a Yin-Empty Person

Inactive, low energy	Lack of exercise
Anemic and pale complexion	Underweight, thin
No strength, weak muscles	Weak heart and internal organs
Yin liver and kidneys	Can develop TB
Hypoglycemia	Hyperactive thyroid
Poor digestion and assimilation	Eats too much yin food
Cold hands and feet	Poor memory and thinking
Likes warm weather	

The dietary recommendations for yin-empty people are:

- Eat grains.
- Eat thick vegetable and grain soups (avoid liquid broth soups).
- Eat less raw foods.
- Drink yang beverages.
- Eat slowly and chew well.
- Avoid juices, tropical fruit, ice cream, dairy products.
- Use slightly more salt, miso, or tamari.
- Recommended herbs: oatstraw, horsetail, watercress, nettle, marsh mallow root, licorice, garlic, slippery elm, ginseng, burdock.

To balance the yin-empty person in extreme yin conditions: the body should be kept warm and much energy provided; fasting should be avoided; living environment must be harmonious. Very light internal exercises should be begun and the person should work up slowly to more muscular movements over several months.

The Yin/Yang Balanced Person

A yin and yang healthy balanced person is moderate in all activities, neither too slow nor fast, but even-tempered in thought and action. This person can eat a wide variety of natural foods in moderation, and digestion and internal organs function properly.

Symptoms of a Yin/Yang Balanced Person

Transparent (glowing) complexion	Good muscle tone
Neither underweight nor overweight	Never overeats
Eats seasonally	No craving for extreme yin or yang junk foods
No constipation	Moderate internal and external exercises daily and weekly
Meditates daily	

The balanced yin/yang person is gentle, kind, helpful, giving, loving, and will inspire others. Such a person walks the middle path to truth, enlightenment, good deeds, and wisdom, ever listening to the Tao within to learn the secrets of the universe.

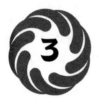

Signs of Health and Disease

Many people really do not know what good health is or what causes it and the lack of it. Many individuals honestly do not take the time and effort necessary to discover who and what they are or make a deep study of the universal laws of health and life. It is almost a tragedy to hear people boastfully claim that they are in perfect health, when visible diagnostic symptoms indicate the complete opposite.

People do not see that their skin is pale and anemic or their complexion is waxy, yellow, or pimply and their eyes are dull and listless. They do not notice their body is weak and fatigued after the least exertion. They do not pay attention to the fact that their hearing is impaired or their eyesight failing, resulting in the need for eyeglasses. They do not understand when they are plagued with insomnia, worry, hate, fear, nervousness, irritableness, pessimism, and anger. These are signs and symptoms of failing health and diagnostic conditions of disease.

According to ancient Chinese and Japanese physicians, physical diagnosis is the observation of a person's external condition, which stems from internal organic disorders. We are living in a universe of cause and effect. Disease is an outcome (effect) of our daily eating and living habits (cause), along with our heredity, which is the effect of our ancestors' living and eating habits. We all inherit constitutional weaknesses and strengths from our parents; our habits and nutrition since birth make us what we are today. This is the just law of nature and no person can escape its consequences. We can, however, live in relative harmony with the Tao or nature and reap the benefits of good health.

The causes of illness are many. There are no simple spontaneous causes or quick remedies. The human body is not attacked by disease; disease is the process of degeneration and the symptoms can easily be diagnosed before chronic conditions develop. Every body organ affects every other organ, which in turn affects the entire system and manifests itself in observable physical symptoms. Our external physical conditions—such as our voice, skin tone, hair, nails, and daily vitality—depend on the condition of our blood, skeletal, organ, and nervous systems, which in turn depend on our total daily eating and living habits.

FOUR PHASES OF ORIENTAL DIAGNOSIS

It is possible to detect malfunctions in the body by knowing how and what to look for: the biological changes the body goes through under various conditions of health, disease, and the aging process. Oriental diagnosis has four phases:

1. *Bo-Shin:* The art of observational diagnosis, using the eyes to detect and observe imbalances in the face, hands, nails, posture, skin tone and color, eyes, and general habits of living and eating.
2. *Bun-Shin:* The art of diagnosing by sounds, such as voice texture, tone, tempo, pitch, and breathing.
3. *Mon-Shin:* Diagnosing by questioning a person about personal habits, diet, family history, employment problems, and psychological tendencies.
4. *Setsu-Shin:* The art of touch diagnosis, such as acupressure, acupuncture points, pulse diagnosis, skin texture, and sense of touch.

The balance of this chapter will primarily cover the art of observational diagnosis, with a brief overview of the art of diagnosing by sounds/voice. With some conscientious study and research, both of these methods are helpful in discovering and overcoming many diagnosable conditions. Diagnosing by questioning and touch require deeper technical research and study, so are more appropriate for the use of doctors, health practitioners, and others involved in clinical patient care.

GENERAL BODY SYMPTOMS

Belching, heartburn, nausea, loss of appetite, and dyspepsia are caused by an overloaded stomach and excessive fats, proteins, oils, and sugars in the diet. Toxemia and fermentation result from overeating, disorderly eating, and various other enervating living habits. Constipation is usually present.

A swollen abdomen, itching about the anus and genitals, and an offensive bad breath indicate pin worms or tape worms in the stomach or intestines, constipation, and general body toxemia. Disorderly eating, overeating, and extremes in diet are general causes of this condition. A pain in the lower back, in many cases, can be attributed to yang (over-worked) kidneys; the kidneys are located just above the right and left hipbones in the lower back region. An excessive intake of animal protein contracts (yang) the kidneys and causes pain in the lower back.

An unlively, slow, and mincing walk, when habitual, indicates premature nerve degeneration or senility. This can happen at any age, depending on the individual's living and eating habits. You can be young, active, and full of vitality at eighty, or burned out and aged at thirty or forty; it all depends on your health habits and attitude. Constant colds, flu, or sinus trouble is a definite indication of an excessive intake of fatty foods, cheeses, oils, fruits, liquids, sugars, and animal protein. Excessive fruit eating can also lower stomach acids, depress kidney and lung activity, and result in chronic mucus. Nuts, cheese, milk, and fruits can cause colds and mucus just as fast as junk food.

FACIAL DIAGNOSIS

Facial Symptoms and Indications

The following symptoms indicate the specific conditions as noted:

Forward bulging forehead indicates inactive internal secretions and poor body circulation.

Hollow and sunken cheeks indicate weak lungs and digestive organs, improper nutrition or malnutrition, physical exhaustion, and poor endurance.

A hollow area in front of the ear opening denotes subnormal secretion of saliva and inefficient food assimilation.

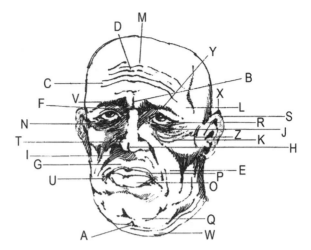

Fig. 3.1. Facial symptoms of disease

Facial Symptoms of Disease

A. Cleft chin: strong constitution and amorous
B. Vertical line between eyebrows: yang liver
C. Horizontal forehead lines: denotes excess intake of liquids, expanded large intestine and kidneys
D. Broken and uneven forehead lines: small intestine disorders, yin condition
E. Cheeks sunken in: malnutrition, poor assimilation
F. Horizontal line on nose bridge: denotes yang liver condition, excessive animal foods
G. Swollen area above upper lip: shows expanded (yin) condition of pancreas, sex glands, spleen, and stomach
H. Cleft on nose lip: heart and circulatory disease
I. Horizontal line above upper lip: female sex gland and organ weakness
J. Bags under eyes: expanded (yin) kidneys
K. Puffy half circles (bags) an inch below eyes: intestinal toxemia and weak lungs
L. Spleen area: weak stomach
M. Bladder area: lines indicate a yin bladder
N. Dark blue under eyes: kidney, bladder, and sexual disorders
O. Swollen/projecting lower lip: intestinal toxemia/constipation
P. Stomach area: swollen, cracked, or inflamed (redness) indicates stomach disorders and expanded (yin) condition
Q. Massiveness: strong, protruding chin denotes persistence and determination, amorous nature
R. White under iris: sanpaku ("three whites") indicates extreme yin condition in body
S. Kidney area: ears red or swollen show kidney disorders
T. Wide nostrils: strong lungs, vitality/Narrow nostrils: weak lungs
U. Duodenum area: cracked or swollen corners indicate diseased duodenum
V. Pancreas area: red, swollen, or veined denotes pancreatic disease
W. Double chin: denotes excessive cholesterol in system and yin condition
X. Pointed ears: excessive meat (yang) intake and disordered eating
Y. Sparse eyebrows: degenerative condition and weak vitality
Z. Hollow on front of ear: poor assimilation and digestion

Face pimples indicate a consumption of extreme yin foods, such as sugars, fats, tropical fruits, juices, pastries, and candy, in addition to an intake of extreme yang foods, such as meat, eggs, and fish. Yin sweet foods eaten with yang protein foods result in poor protein assimilation; unassimilated proteins are eliminated through the skin as eruptions. Intestinal toxemia, poor quality blood, and constipation are usually present.

Red and white spots or habitual red flushed face indicates heart disease, biliousness, fever, and inflammations caused by extreme yang and yin foods such as animal protein, salt, and sugar and by disorderly eating. Blood becomes too thick to circulate through the body and this results in stagnation and redness.

Orange or yellow skin shows liver, gallbladder, spleen, and pancreas disorders. In vegetarians it indicates an excessive intake of raw vegetables and carrot juice. Sweets are contributing causes.

Green skin indicates liver disease and possible cancer.

Pallor or pale face and cheeks indicate weak glands, congested and inactive liver, and anemia.

Thin, white transparent cheek shows weak glands, stomach, and lungs and lack of energy, as well as a tendency toward melancholy and introversion caused by poor quality food, weak assimilation, lack of oxygen and proper exercise, yin foods (sugar and sweets). It indicates a tendency to consumption and weak intestines.

White patches on face or body show liver and kidney disorders caused by excessive dairy foods, fats, and sugars.

Veins and blood vessels showing at temples indicate heart, liver, and gallbladder disease.

Cheeks with veins showing indicate heart and stomach disorders due to gluttony, alcohol, and disorderly eating.

Dampness, clamminess, and excessive perspiration on face indicates extreme yin and yang food intake and heart and kidney disease.

Yellow, waxy, or pasty face shows liver, stomach, and gallbladder trouble and an edematous condition of the fluid system caused by excessive fat and animal consumption and sugars.

Warts, moles, and beauty marks indicate excessive intake of animal protein, fats, and sugars. Liver and kidney disorders are indicated.

Double chin is a sign of excessive cholesterol and fatty deposits

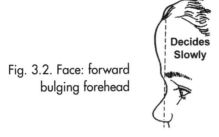

Fig. 3.2. Face: forward
bulging forehead

throughout the system, caused by fats, animal foods, salt, and sugars, and a lack of exercise and natural foods.

A well-developed chin shows a strong heart inheritance, physical strength, and determination to succeed.

A small, narrow, and receding chin denotes less physical endurance/ determination; heart functioning is not as strong as prominent chin, caused by poor quality foods during pregnancy, especially calcium deficiency, resulting in insufficient jaw formation.

Nose Symptoms and Indications

The following symptoms indicate the specific conditions as noted:

Long thin nostrils indicate weak lung power and less physical stamina. They also indicate excessive intake of sugars, fats, dairy, and animal foods during the embryonic period. A person with long thin nostrils requires plenty of exercise, deep breathing, and outside fresh air. To help widen the nostrils, pull them apart and outward; this will open up the breathing channels, help sinus problems, and increase energy. Practice one minute daily.

Wide nostrils indicate strong lung power and good physical vital- ity, strength, and self-confidence. People with wide nostrils make excellent athletes and good orators; they are self reliant and have unlimited energy to achieve success. This is due to their larger lung capacity and ability to take in large quantities of oxygen, which feeds and sharpens the mind and imparts great energy.

Upturned nose with wide nostrils is a sign of a strong yang constitu- tion and physical aggression. People with this type of nose have initiative and a hopeful optimistic attitude. They are cheerful and amiable, with a desire to help others. They are also inquisitive, but they need encouragement to carry out their work.

A long thin bony nose is an indication of yin and people who are more mentally inclined and refined in manners. The voices of thin-nosed people are generally high pitched. They are inquisitive and curious about life, nature, and people. Sharp and quick to perceive, they like details and are sometimes overly analytical and judgmental. To balance this yin personality, more whole grains and cooked vegetables are required. Deep breathing, outside fresh air, and vigorous exercise will strengthen this type of individual.

A red, bulbous, and greasy nose (veins) indicates high blood pressure and heart and liver disorders. Excessive alcohol or sugar, fats, and meat are the main causes. A swollen nose is a sign of an enlarged heart.

A cleft on the tip of the nose indicates heart or circulatory disorders.

A dull ache in the nose indicates blood stagnation and heart trouble from eating rancid oils.

A soft watery nose shows excessive intake of yin foods and a swollen heart.

Sneezing is a discharge of excess yin in the system, coming from sugars, liquids, drugs, and so on.

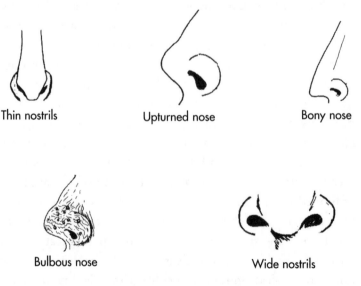

Thin nostrils   Upturned nose   Bony nose

Bulbous nose   Wide nostrils

Fig. 3.3. Nose diagnosis

Mouth and Lips Symptoms and Indications

The mouth and lips are the uppermost part of the digestive system, which ends in the anus. Conditions of the mouth and lips indicate deeper internal problems. Any imbalances in diet cause imbalances in facial features, whether arising from our own eating habits or those of our mother during pregnancy. Extreme yin or yang foods cause internal disease and its symptoms to show up on the mouth and lips. The following symptoms indicate the specific conditions as noted:

> In a normal nose/mouth relationship the mouth is as wide as the outer edges of the nostrils. A balanced mouth shows that the mother ate a balanced diet during the embryonic period. Healthy and strong sex glands and hormones are indicated by a well-defined, long vertical crease from the upper lip to the base of the nose, a wide horizontal area between the base of the nose and upper lip, and even, heart-shaped lips. Heart-shaped lips also indicate a controlled mental and physical nature. These people direct their lives according to discipline and principle. Their eating habits are more balanced and they avoid extremes in living habits. (See fig. 3.4a)
>
> The mouth extended beyond the outer nostrils indicates the mother's consumption of extreme yang and yin foods during pregnancy and the person's consumption of them during early childhood. This condition can be normalized over a period of several years by balancing the diet and avoiding extremes. (See fig. 3.4b)
>
> Mouth extended horizontally and vertically shows weaker internal organs. This is generally a yin or expanded internal condition arising from generations of consumption of yin foods such as tropical fruits and vegetables, fats, sugar, fried foods, and white flour. A return to proper eating will eventually contract (yangize) the internal organs and normalize the exterior features. (See fig. 3.4c)
>
> Lips that are higher vertically indicate a weaker digestive system. Horizontally, the lips are yang, indicating that balanced food was eaten during the mother's pregnancy, but the vertical height shows extreme yin food during childhood. They also show weak sex glands with a lack of the vertical indentation and a short distance between the lips and the nose-base. (See fig. 3.4d)

Thin pale lips denote weak internal glands, hormones, and sexual powers. A horizontal crease between upper lip and nose-base indicates malfunctioning sex glands. (See fig. 3.4e)

Pale or red lips indicate disorders in the stomach and intestines, such as compacted colon, constipation, or indigestion.

Large, loose, open mouth and lips indicate a yin expanded stomach and colon, as a result of extreme yin and yang foods being eaten throughout life. It shows a generally rebellious and uncontrolled nature in mental and physical habits. Can be corrected by natural eating and living habits.

Wrinkles above the lips indicate sexual and hormonal malfunctioning, as well as extreme (yang) dehydration of body, coming from an excessive intake of salt, spices, protein, and insufficient raw foods and liquids.

Cracked corners of the mouth show vitamin B_2 deficiency and digestive and stomach disorders caused by extreme yang and yin foods, such as animal protein, sugar, and fats.

Cleft pallet indicates excessive (yin) sugars during pregnancy.

Sores on lips indicate intestinal and stomach toxemia and general body congestion.

Tight constricted lips show contraction of intestines and vagina.

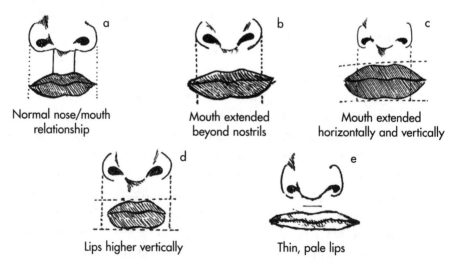

Normal nose/mouth relationship

Mouth extended beyond nostrils

Mouth extended horizontally and vertically

Lips higher vertically

Thin, pale lips

Fig. 3.4. Mouth and lips self-diagnosis

Small mouth shows much yang energy and physical and mental vitality. Constant covering of the mouth shows overeating.

Swollen upper lip denotes stomach disorders and excessive yin food intake.

Expanded protruding lower lip indicates expanded and fallen intestines and constipation; this is a yin condition from excessive sugar, fat, and liquid intake.

Dry, thin, scaly, and mottled appearance of lower lip indicates a disorder of the salivary glands.

Thin, pale, and dry upper lip indicates weakness of reproductive system. If the upper lip is extremely short, it indicates a weak spinal column.

Whiteness around mouth and pale lips indicate anemia, poor circulation, blood stagnation, and lack of expression caused by excessive intake of cheese, ice cream, milk (fats), sugar, and animal protein.

Pink lips (Caucasian) indicate balanced nutrition, good circulation, and health.

Dark lips (Caucasian) show liver, kidney, and gallbladder trouble. Excessive bright red lips show high blood pressure, acute disease or infection, toxic liver, and hemorrhoids.

Pink gums (all races) indicate good health; white gums show poor health and anemia.

Purple lips indicate blood stagnation, diseased heart, and circulatory system.

Corners of mouth turned down show intestinal stasis and stomach disorders caused by dairy foods, fats, and cold food and drinks.

Symptoms and Indications of the Teeth

The following symptoms indicate the specific conditions as noted:

Long front teeth indicate a yin constitution.

Short front teeth and ones that angle inward are yang and indicate an uncontrolled character.

Teeth that angle outward show a passive character.

Pointed teeth, especially the canines, result from excessive eating of meat and other yang foods over generations. The canine teeth will diminish in size as less meat is eaten over generations. Natural and orderly eating results in balanced and normal teeth.

Tooth decay results from excessive intake of sugars, fats, animal foods, protein, liquids, and insufficient calcium from natural whole foods, such as grains, seaweeds, legumes, vegetables, seeds, and fruits. Animal protein and sugar diminish calcium absorption from other foods; calcium deficiency is the end result of tooth decay.

Crowding teeth and extra teeth are caused by extreme yin and yang foods during pregnancy.

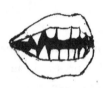

Fig. 3.5. Teeth self-diagnosis

Pointed teeth

Symptoms and Indications of the Tongue

The tongue is an extension of the gastrointestinal track, which terminates in the anal canal. Any problems or disease symptoms on the tongue indicate disorders in the stomach, intestines, and colon. Symptoms in the middle of the tongue indicate disorders of the stomach; symptoms on the sides of tongue indicate disorders of the liver; symptoms on the root of the tongue indicate disorders of the kidneys; symptoms on the tip of the tongue indicate disorders of the heart.

The following symptoms indicate the specific conditions as noted:

White/yellow color and dry coated tongue indicates stomach fermentation, intestinal toxemia, liver and gallbladder disorders, caused by excessive intake of dairy foods, fats, animal foods, and overeating. A short water fast is indicated in this condition.

Green tongue shows liver and kidney disorders.

Blue tongue shows kidney and bladder trouble, arising from disorderly eating. A balanced natural diet will balance the organs.

Violet tongue shows liver and heart disease arising from alcoholism.

Grey or black tongue indicates kidney and heart disease; black at the tongue base shows possible cancer.

Purple tongue denotes sex organ and bladder disease.

Crease down the middle of tongue denotes intestinal disorders and vitamin B complex deficiency, arising from extremes in diet.

Trembling tongue shows a nerve condition and brain weakness.

Sties or growths on tongue indicate excessive intake of animal protein, kidney disease, and a yang heart. Also intestinal toxemia and constipation are generally indicated. Avoid overeating, especially extreme yang foods (meat, eggs, fish, and salt) and extreme yin foods (ice cream, white sugar, pastries, alcohol, and all fats).

Soft, loose tongue shows an expanded gastrointestinal system, resulting from excessive yin foods.

A hard, tense tongue denotes excessive mucus in the system, resulting from animal foods, dairy, sugars, and disorderly eating.

Fig. 3.6. Tongue self-diagnosis

 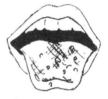

Line on tongue   Sties on tongue

Symptoms and Indications of the Eyes

The eye foretells the truth when all the other features deceive us. When the eye says one thing and the tongue another, the practical person relies on the former. The relationship between the iris and the whites of the eyes is an important indicator of health. *Sanpaku*, meaning "three whites," refers to an iris being so small that it can only cover two-thirds or less of the eye. *Lower sanpaku* means that white is visible on both sides and the bottom. *Upper sanpaku* means that white is visible on both sides and above the iris. A return to whole foods, centered around grains, vegetables, legumes, seeds, and seasonal fruits, along with proper exercise, sufficient sleep, stress-free work, meditation, and harmonious surroundings, can correct and improve one's overall health and center the iris.

Lower sanpaku, when the iris is rolled up, is a poor health sign. It indicates an extreme yin or expanded condition of the brain, nerves, organs, and body. Generally people with this condition are fearful, suspicious, and lacking in physical and mental stamina. The higher the iris rises, the more one is beset with tragedy, usually self-inflicted misfortune, accidents, and problems in relationships with friends or loved ones. Sanpaku denotes a disorderly pattern of eating and living. Excessive amounts of fruits (tropical), juices, alcohol, sugars, ice cream, dairy, and fats, in addition to overworking, overexercising, malnutrition, lack of sleep, and stress conditions, will contribute to and cause sanpaku and its attendant consequences. Many fashion models have varying degrees of sanpaku, due to strict crash weight-loss or starvation diets to maintain the modern skinny look.

A person showing signs of sanpaku is very often difficult to relate to and is skeptical of any help or advice. The criminal mind has also been shown to possess sanpaku. Famous people who possessed sanpaku before dying violently or tragically were: Gandhi, Caesar, the Kennedy brothers, Hitler, Martin Luther King, Elvis Presley, and Freddie Prinze (*Chico and the Man*).

Upper sanpaku is a yang condition, especially of the liver, kidneys, and related internal organs. The rolled-down iris of this condition indicates a cruel nature, physical (yang) aggressiveness, anger, and a fighting character. This is usually caused by an intake of extreme yang foods, such as animal protein. Such a person is easily provoked into anger or fighting, so be agreeable in the presence of someone with upper sanpaku. Being vindictive and merciless, such people often meet violent deaths. An honest person with upper sanpaku is more likely to be a victim of violence than a perpetrator.

In addition to sanpaku, several other eye symptoms are indicate specific conditions:

Excessive blinking is the body's attempt to expel excess yin from the system. The less we blink the better; blinking no more than 2 to 4 times per minute indicates a person of sound health and in control of mind and body. In the animal realm, cats seldom blink; their eyes shine and glow in the dark; they are very independent and in total control of their actions. Humans can accomplish the same, but it may take many years of discipline in diet, health habits, exercise, and meditation to attain superior health and control over your nervous system and bodily functions.

Four white-sided eye is usually accompanied by a bloodshot reddish hue and is uncontrolled. There is usually a psychological problem or conflict in the person's life, accompanied often by a violent temper, outrage, oversensitivity, and assault. The individual's eating habits range from extreme yin to yang, starvation diets to gluttony.

Eyes turned inward toward the nose is a yang or contracted condition, indicating high blood pressure and heart problems, which results from an excessive intake of meat, eggs, and salt by the mother during the embryonic period or by the person during early childhood. Balancing the diet can help to correct this condition.

Eyes turned outward shows a yin or expanded condition of the eyeball, indicating that the liver, stomach, and kidneys are also yin. It is caused by excessive intake of yin foods, such as sugars, sodas, ice cream, fats, tropical fruits, drugs, and alcohol. A person with this condition in the extreme may be prone to chronic disease. A yin and yang balanced diet can help correct this condition in due time.

Normal healthy eyes are centered, with very little eye whites showing on the sides of the iris. The upper and lower eyelids should touch the iris. The eye pupils should function properly in both light and darkness. Healthy eyes do not require glasses or contacts; neither do they squint or function poorly in close and distant vision; the sight is sharp and clear at all times; the eyes sparkle and the eye whites are clear.

Dark eye bags indicate different conditions depending on the color. A dark brown (half-circle) coloring under the eyes indicates weak female organs and constricted (yang) kidneys. Swelling, veins, or dark blue under the eyes denotes kidney stones, gallstones, blood stagnation, and anemia, caused by extreme yin and yang foods. Purple under the eyes denotes adrenal exhaustion. Discolored puffy circles one to two inches below the eyes indicate lung disorders. They are caused by tobacco smoke, sugar, high-fat dairy products (cheese, milk, butter), and a host of other extreme yin and yang junk foods. A person with this condition is generally afflicted with a disease such as lung cancer, tuberculosis, asthma, and other respiratory disorders.

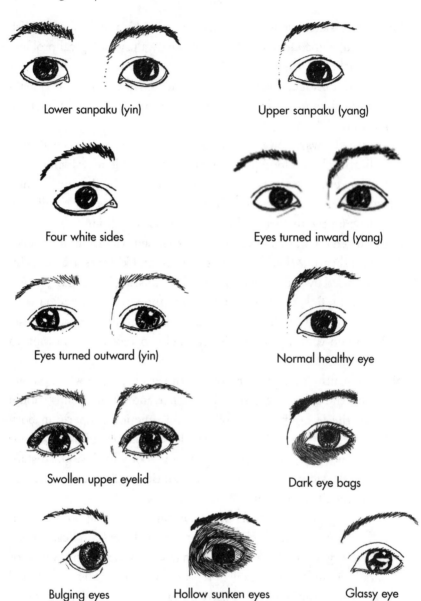

Lower sanpaku (yin)

Upper sanpaku (yang)

Four white sides

Eyes turned inward (yang)

Eyes turned outward (yin)

Normal healthy eye

Swollen upper eyelid

Dark eye bags

Bulging eyes

Hollow sunken eyes

Glassy eye

Fig. 3.7. Eye self-diagnosis

Swollen upper eyelid indicates gallstones and heart and sexual malfunctioning. The swelling usually subsides when the stones pass.
It is caused by sugar, fats, and animal foods eaten to excess.

Bulging eyes indicate lack of iodine in early childhood or embryonic period and thyroid disorder; also a yin/expanded condition of organs, caused by excessive intake of liquids and sugar.

Wide staring eyes indicate poor judgment, credulity, or—if the expression is anxious—fear and apprehension.

Orators and linguists have the full or convex eye. Fullness below the eye indicates verbosity.

Puffiness or bags under the eyes indicates disease from dissipation; it is not the same as fullness.

Dark, hollow, sunken eyes indicate extreme emaciation, deficiency of muscular development, nerve and physical exhaustion. They are caused by extremes in diet, starvation, or malnutrition.

Eyes with light blue indicate internal parasites and kidney trouble.

Scant lower eyelashes indicate deficiencies in sexual glands and hormones.

Scant upper eyelashes denote (yang) mental deficiency.

Itchy eyes indicate liver malfunctioning and lung problems.

Hard yellow spots in eye whites indicate worms in system.

Dry and inflamed eyeballs indicate an extreme yang liver disorder and vitamin A deficiency.

Sties, growths on eyelids, show an excessive intake of protein.

Pale, colorless, white eyelid (upper and lower) denotes anemia; the eyelids should be pink in good health.

Yellow eye whites or yellow deposits in eyes indicate excessive cholesterol in the system and liver and gallbladder blockage caused by excessive intake of fats, oils, fried foods, cheese, ice cream, milk, sugar, and animal protein.

Entire eye is yellow indicates jaundice. A yin and yang balanced diet can correct this situation in due time.

Bloodshot eyes (habitual) indicate an inflamed condition of the intestines and brain, caused by cheese, sugars, drugs, all fats, alcohol, dairy foods, and animal foods. The liver and gallbladder will also be affected and this can lead to chronic disease. Eye strain, poor lighting, constant sun glare, and late night reading can also cause bloodshot eyes.

Dull, lackluster glassy eyes indicate that the nervous system is under strain and pressure. Meat, animal fats, dairy products, sugars, pastries, and oils are causes of nerve disorders and consequently dull glassy eyes. Poor circulation, extremes in diet, hardened arteries, and hardened liver are indicated. A person with glassy eyes requires a complete change in diet and living habits. All drugs, alcohol, cigarettes, marijuana, overwork, excessive sex, stress, and tension must be discontinued if a return to good health is desired.

Excessive large pupils in daylight denote nerve exhaustion and extremes in diet. It is a yin, expanded condition of the kidneys, stomach, spleen, intestines, and bladder, indicating adrenal weakness and brain expansion. It is due to excessive intake of raw food (yin). A balanced diet of grains, vegetables, seeds, and legumes, including seasonal fruit, should normalize the eye pupil in due time.

White ring around the iris indicates excessive intake of table salt, nerve weakness, poor circulation to brain, anemia, and possible senility. Disordered eating and living and extremes in diet are contributing factors.

Symptoms and Indications of the Eyebrows

The following symptoms indicate the specific conditions as noted:

Eyebrows slanting inward indicate yang and aggressive nature caused by generations of animal food consumption.

Eyebrows slanting down and outward show a gentle and compassionate nature caused by vegetarian diet.

Sparse eyebrows indicate a weakening health condition, weak life force, and tendency to chronic disease and degeneration. It is caused by extremes in diet, such as excessive intake of sugars, liquids, fats, tropical fruits, juices, and animal foods.

Connected brows indicate strong life force, vitality, and artistic ability. They also show generations of fatty animal food and dairy intake. The spleen, liver, and pancreas are weakened by these foods.

Thick, separated brows show superb health and long life potential.

High arched brows denote a person with a dramatic and creative flair, with the emphasis on active showmanship and leadership, a person somewhat eccentric in character and mentality.

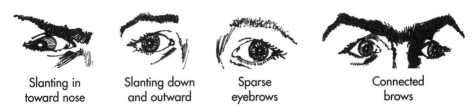

Slanting in
toward nose

Slanting down
and outward

Sparse
eyebrows

Connected
brows

Fig. 3.8. Eyebrow self-diagnosis

Symptoms and Indications of the Ears

The following symptoms indicate the specific conditions as noted:

Large ears and lobes are a sign of health and longevity, indicating a strong inherited constitution, particularly strong kidneys and adrenals. They are caused by generations consuming basically vegetarian foods.

Thickness and height in the outer upper ear shows excellent blood circulation throughout the body and creative mental capacity, as well as the ability to accumulate and successfully handle finances and material possessions.

Large and well-formed inner ear area indicates good digestive and assimilation powers.

Fleshy and thick inner ridge shows nerve force and inner strength.

Creased ear lobe shows heart disorders or diabetes.

Small ears and lobes show a weak inherited constitution, particularly weak adrenals and small kidneys, generally low energy, and little interest in mental pursuits, caused by generations of meat eating. Small-eared people should avoid excessive intake of animal protein, as their kidneys are unable to handle it. Small-eared people

Large ears

Ears protruding

Small ears

Ears close to head

Fig. 3.9. Ear self-diagnosis

should emphasize whole grains, vegetables, soaked seeds and nuts, sprouts, fruits in season, with a minimum intake of protein foods. Cooked legumes should be eaten moderately. Sufficient rest, sleep, and harmonious surroundings are recommended; exercise moderately, but never to exhaustion.

Ears protruding show a yin constitution, leading to impulsive and emotional activity, resulting from too much yin food consumed during mother's pregnancy.

Ears close to head indicate balance in mind and movement. Mother ate a more balanced yin and yang diet during pregnancy.

Ears high on head indicate self-pride, an egotistical nature, base instincts, and material cravings and desires to excess. Mother ate excessively of animal foods and salt during embryonic period.

Ears top level with the eye corners indicate balanced mental and physical development.

Red ears indicate a toxic, overworked kidney (yang), resulting from excessive salt and protein. Spleen disease is indicated if the outer portion of the ear is red. Extreme yang foods should be avoided.

Ear wax is a sign of excessive intake of fats, oils, animal foods, and fried foods. It will not develop if these foods are not eaten.

Symptoms and Indications of the Hair

The following symptoms indicate the specific conditions as noted:

Premature grey or white hair is a sign of an excessive intake of yang animal protein and yin sweet foods. This indicates liver, gallbladder, and kidney malfunction. White-haired people are generally more set in their ways, and it is hard for them to change and be more flexible.

Much body hair denotes a yang inherited constitution and excessive animal protein consumption over generations.

Split hair ends indicate malfunctioning sex glands and hormones in both male and female. Excessive sugars, fats, and animal protein are the main causes of split ends. Poor circulation, overeating, and lack of exercise are other contributing factors.

Dry hair indicates liver, gallbladder, spleen, and pancreatic disorders caused by fats, sugars, and animal protein.

Oily hair is caused by excessive fats and oils in the diet.

Dandruff is caused by excessive animal protein, fats, oils, and sugars and indicates kidney malfunction.

Hair loss indicates internal organic disorders, especially from excessive animal protein, fats, and sugars.

Hair loss at the front of the head is caused by excessive yin liquids, sugars, fruits, and alcohol, which lower kidney and bladder functioning.

Hair loss at the top of the head indicates that the lungs and large intestines are adversely affected; it is caused by excessive animal protein.

Hair loss at the back of the head denotes excessive intake of chemicals, drugs such as marijuana and medicine, which affect the liver and gallbladder.

Hair loss at the temples indicates excessive intake of drugs and sugar foods. The lungs and large intestines are affected.

Fig. 3.10. Hair self-diagnosis

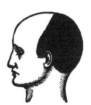

Front of the head
hair loss

Top and side of
the head hair loss

HAND DIAGNOSIS

The entire hand can show past and more recent conditions of the individual, and it can indicate health or disease tendencies in the future or near future. In good health, the hands should be slightly pink and warm, dry and firm, but not hard. The following symptoms indicate the specific conditions as noted:

Swollen knuckles and fingers indicate expanded (yin) kidneys, atherosclerosis, and high blood pressure.

Bluish wrist indicates sex gland weakness.

Reddish palms with white spots show disorderly eating and poor blood circulation, as well as an excessive intake of animal protein and fats.

Bluish palms denote circulatory and heart trouble.

Dark red palm heel indicates bladder and sexual disorders.

Yellow or orange palms indicate pancreas, spleen, and liver disorders. Excessive intake of fats, raw greens, or carrot juice are factors to be considered in causing this problem.

Hot, moist, and red hands indicates yang congested liver and kidneys. Red hands are caused by excess yang foods.

Cold, clammy, and pale hands indicate yin; expanded kidneys, bladder, stomach, and intestines; weak nerves; and anemia. Pale, cold hands are caused by excess yin foods.

Flexible fingers, the ability to bend back ninety degrees to the hand, indicate good health, healthy organs, and normal blood and nerve circulation. They indicate a flexible mental and physical character, able to adapt to outward changing conditions.

Less than ninety degrees of a backward bend indicates calcification or hardening of the bones, nerves, muscles, organs, and reproductive system. The less angle, the more the hardening. Arthritic and painful joints show diseased kidneys. A stubborn and unchangeable character usually accompanies inflexibility and hardening of the joints and muscles, caused by an excessive intake of sugars, salt, fats, oils, cheese, and animal protein. Orderly eating can reverse this condition before terminal degeneration has set in.

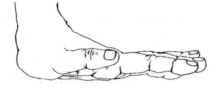

Fig. 3.11. Flexible wrist

Raised blood vessels on the back of the hand indicate an excessive intake of yin foods and a yin kidney.

Trembling fingers indicate weak nerves, nervousness, and heart disorders.

Brown spots on the back of the hands, arms, or body denote liver and gallbladder congestion, caused by excessive intake of animal foods, dairy, fats, and sugars.

Webbed fingers indicate overconsumption of yin foods and liquids during the embryonic period.

Wide palm with firm flesh indicate strong inherited constitution with an active, aggressive nature and robust health (yang).

Narrow hand and long thin fingers indicate sensitivity, intellectual and artistic personality, and delicate health (yin).

Round bulge appearing on the wrist when the palm is pressed above the wrist with the opposite thumb indicates the body is holding excessive liquids or sugar (yin condition); the hands are usually moist.

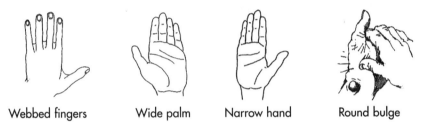

Webbed fingers   Wide palm   Narrow hand   Round bulge

Fig. 3.12. Hand self-diagnosis

Fingers and Nails

The nails are hard or clawlike extensions of the fingers; the fingers, in turn, are extensions of the entire nervous system. The fingers are connected to body organs via nerves and nerve pathways known as meridians. The corresponding reflex finger/organ areas are listed as follows: thumb, Lungs; first phalange, Liver/Large Intestine; second phalange, circulatory system (Heart Governor) and sex glands; third phalange, Kidneys (Triple Heater); fourth phalange, Heart and Small Intestines. If there is a blockage of circulation or stagnation of blood, or an excess of energy in any internal or external area of the body, this deficiency or excess can easily be detected and diagnosed in extremities (hands, nails, fingers, and feet).

A person who is trained in visual diagnosis can detect symptoms before they start to appear. One of the methods to do this is to look at the fingernails, which function like a looking glass or mirror, reflecting inner physiological conditions. Pink nails indicate good blood circulation to the fingertips. Lack of blood flow to the fingertips shows up as clear white nails and is diagnosed as anemia. If the nail thickens noticeably, it is one sign of circulatory weakness, lymph gland malfunction, or blood diseases. When a fingernail has a tendency to become yellow, it may be an early sign of liver disease. Diabetes can be recognized by the gradual disappearance of the pink coloration of the nail. After reading and diagnosing the fingers and nails, proper health measures and corrective eating and living habits can then be recommended to overcome the diagnosed symptoms.

The following symptoms indicate the specific conditions as noted:

Inflamed/reddish finger indicates acute or short-term illness.

Hardened, rigid, and chalky white nails indicate severe and chronic or organic disease.

Wide and short fingers and nails indicate a strong yang constitution and a person who is practical, persistent, physically active, and aggressive.

Long and narrow fingers and nails indicate a yin constitution, and a person who is artistic, sensitive, imaginative, delicate, with a tendency to bronchial disorders.

Extremely narrow fingers and nails denote a delicate inherited constitution and less physical energy.

Lack of half-moons indicates sodium/potassium imbalance, underactive thyroid gland, weak healing power in system, lack of circulation, and low blood pressure. It can also indicate a possible liver disorder. It is usually a yin condition caused by excessive intake of sugars, fats, juices, and raw foods. It can also be caused by an excess of meat and salt. It also indicates little or no physical exercise.

Half-moons more than one quarter of the nail show an overactive thyroid condition, a tendency to excessive physical and mental activity, and nervousness. An excessive intake of high-potassium (yin) foods can cause overdevelopment of the half-moons; however, in time the moons may disappear due to the extreme potassium/sodium imbalance and result in disease or poor health. Excessive half-moons can also mean high blood pressure. On the other hand, an excessive intake of sodium (yang) foods may also cause the half-moons to disappear. Generally a lack of raw fruits and vegetables contribute to a yang system. Regardless of age, the half-moons should always be present; if not, the important healing and beauty mineral element, potassium, will be missing, resulting in deficiency diseases. Yin internal conditions change into yang, and yang ones change into yin (the process of biological transmutation), which is the natural order of Tao.

A healthy half-moon should be no more than one-fourth of the nail, indicating potassium/sodium balance, vital healing power in the system, mental and physical energy, and a balance between activity and rest. The Taoists teach that the normal sized half-moon indicates freedom from chronic disease and good health. The half-moon should show on all nails.

White spots on fingernails indicate zinc, pantothenic acid, and calcium deficiency, poor protein absorption, pancreatic disorders and insulin deficiency, kidney disease, weak stomach acids and possible worms. Sugars and other excessive yin foods (such as dairy products, honey, tropical fruits, sodas, cakes, and candy) and substances (such as drugs, chemicals, marijuana, and alcohol) neutralize stomach acids, causing calcium and mineral deficiencies. Nails take from six to nine months to grow from bottom to top.

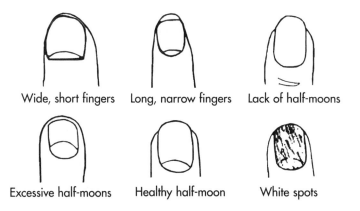

Wide, short fingers   Long, narrow fingers   Lack of half-moons

Excessive half-moons   Healthy half-moon   White spots

Fig. 3.13. Nail self-diagnosis

One can determine, by the location of the white spot, the time of high yin food intake, organ disease, and sugar in the bloodstream.

Nail Color, Shape, and Texture

The following symptoms indicate the specific conditions as noted:

Pale and chalky nails indicate poor circulation, nerve exhaustion, possible stroke, anemia, and poor iron and protein assimilation, caused by extreme yin and yang foods.

Green nails denote improper copper disposal and congenital liver ailment.

Bluish nails indicate lack of oxygen, poor circulation to heart, and heart disorder.

Tiny red dots under the nails indicate possible pinworms.

Transverse white lines across nails denote fever, heart and kidney disease, and malnutrition.

Bitten nails denote intestinal and stomach problems and possible parasites in the body.

Red or purple hemorrhages under the nails indicate an inflamed heart lining.

Excessively shiny nails show an overactive thyroid gland.

Excessively red, dark blue, or purple nails or fingers and swollen hands show heart and circulatory problems.

Triangle shaped nails indicate a weak inherited constitution and a tendency to nerve diseases, such as paralysis or palsy. An individual with this shape nail should watch his or her health, taking care to eat wholesome foods and obtaining proper sleep and exercise.

Short, shrunken, and withered nails denote a hypertensive nervous system, chronic disorders, a critical and fault-finding character, and extreme malnutrition or malabsorption of food, arising from extremes in diet during pregnancy or through early childhood.

Convex or hourglass nails denote lung ailments, scrofula, dyspepsia and a possible yang liver, excessive mucus, and a possible tendency to tuberculosis, arising from a yin lung condition as a result of an excessive intake of yin foods.

Concave or spoon-shaped nails show tendency to infections, chronic anemia, possible hookworms, hyperthyroidism, and malnutrition, arising from extremes in diet.

Vertical ridges denote intestinal, liver, and kidney disorders, circulation and skin impairment, poor protein and calcium absorption.

Deep horizontal ridges indicate severe calcium and protein deficiency, acute illness, nerve exhaustion, anemia, and psoriasis, caused by extreme changes in dietary eating patterns and environment, such as moving from north to south frequently and changing from yang to yin diets, or going from binging on junk foods to yang foods to fruitarian and raw foods or fasting, and repeating the cycle over and over.

Round bulging nails denote lung disorders, possible liver trouble, and hardened arteries; this is a yang sign.

Thick raised cuticle denotes an excessive intake of animal protein, extreme dietary changes, and kidney and liver disorders.

Flat nails indicate a weak lymphatic system, proneness to mumps, tonsils, appendicitis, and other acute disorders; this is a yin condition.

Square nails indicate kidney disorders, excessive intake of animal protein, or malabsorption of food.

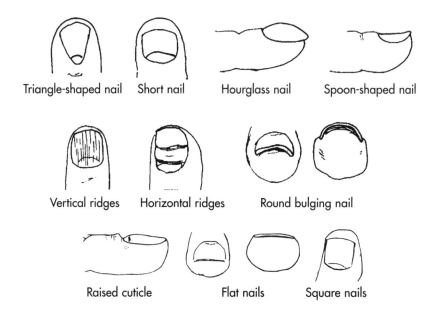

Triangle-shaped nail   Short nail   Hourglass nail   Spoon-shaped nail

Vertical ridges   Horizontal ridges   Round bulging nail

Raised cuticle   Flat nails   Square nails

Fig. 3.14. Nail shape and texture self-diagnosis

Ridges with convex and white chalky nails denote advanced chronic disease, such as stroke, cancer, and hardened arteries.

Cracked and split nails indicate calcium deficiency and weak sex glands.

Red or bleeding cuticle is an extreme condition of kidney and liver disorders caused by excess yin food intake.

Soft nails denote calcium, vitamin, mineral, and protein deficiency from an excess of sugars, dairy, fats, and animal foods in the diet, weak willpower, and general fatigue.

Excessively hard and brittle nails denote anemia and hormonal imbalance.

Anemia Test

One way of detecting anemia is by pressing any fingernail with the thumb. The nail will turn white from the thumb pressure. If the whiteness remains longer than a second after the thumb pressure is released, anemia is indicated. A pink color should show up immediately after thumb pressure is released, indicating good blood circulation and absence of anemia.

FOOT DIAGNOSIS

The feet are a good indicator of health or disease throughout the body. Certain symptoms in the feet signal trouble in the reflex body organs. The following symptoms indicate the specific conditions as noted:

Athlete's foot is a sign of kidney problems caused from excessive animal protein intake.

Fallen arches (yin condition) indicate weak nerves.

Foul-smelling feet are a sign of excess animal protein intake, liver and kidney disease.

Hard calluses on feet or hands denote excessive dairy products and animal protein in the diet.

Cracked nails show liver, kidney, spleen, and pancreatic disease, arising from excessive yin and yang foods.

Symptoms and Indications of the Toes

Each toe is connected to a body organ via nerve pathways (meridians) as follows: big toe, Liver; second toe, Stomach; third toe, Bladder; fourth toe, Gallbladder; fifth toe, Kidneys. Each toe can be massaged or pressed for one or two minutes to help improve the corresponding organ.

The following symptoms indicate the specific conditions as noted:

Hard, withered, and inflexible toes/nails denote organic disorders.
Pain or swelling in a toe or the feet indicates a disorder in the corresponding organ.

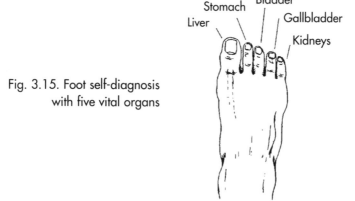

Fig. 3.15. Foot self-diagnosis
with five vital organs

URINE DIAGNOSIS

The following symptoms indicate the specific conditions as noted:

Healthy urine should be straw colored or the color of light beer, which will be 7.0 or balanced on the pH scale. This denotes a balanced yin and yang and acid and alkaline diet.

Dark yellow or brownish urine with a pH under 6.5 denotes constricted (yang) kidneys, a sluggish liver, and bile backed up in the blood, caused by excessive intake of animal protein, fats, chemicals, and sugar.

Light colored or clear urine with a pH over 7.5 denotes an expanded (yin) kidney and liver, caused by excessive intake of yin foods, such as sugars, juices, alcohol, tropical fruits, liquids, and raw foods.

Excessive urination denotes expanded (yin) kidneys caused from an excessive intake of yin foods. Excessive urination with an excessive appetite, a glazed and furrowed tongue, diarrhea, and loss of sexual and mental powers indicates a diabetic condition caused by a diet too high in fats, sugars, animal protein, and empty calories, and excessive intake of extreme yin and yang foods.

VOICE DIAGNOSIS

A healthy voice is enjoyable to hear. It is neither too high or too low, but resonates and vibrates in a clear musical tone. This is the magnetic voice; it soothes and heals those who hear it. Consuming balanced yin and yang foods and correcting the living habits will eventually improve a person's voice.

Many diseases can be diagnosed from the sound and texture of the voice. The sounds of the voice can be designated into yin and yang as follows:

YIN	YANG
Weak voice	Strong voice
High pitch	Low pitch
Slow speech	Fast speech
Softness	Loudness
Wet sound	Dry sound
Looseness	Tenseness
Unclear sound	Distinct sound

The sound of the voice corresponds to inner physiological conditions:

Crackling, hoarse voice always denotes degenerative disease of the sexual glands and hormones.

Watery, loose voice, with slow speech indicates an excessive intake of (yin) liquids, fruits, and sugars. The result is kidney expansion, weakness, and mucus.

Unclear and weak trembling voice (yin) denotes lack of inner energy and vibrant health, and indicates kidney and sex gland disorders. If a person's health is poor, with low energy, the body lacks the force or vitality to express itself in a clear vibrant tone. Very sick people always speak quietly in a trembling tone.

Tense, dry, fast, or high-pitched voice indicates intestinal congestion, sexual degeneration, constipation, high blood pressure, and bladder and circulatory trouble, arising from excessive intake of yang foods, such as meat, eggs, and salt, which contract the sex glands, kidneys, and liver, causing the person to shout or talk in a loud voice.

Fast speech denotes an overactive heart; a yang condition.

Stuttering indicates heart and nervous conditions arising from extremes in diet.

Excessive and confused talking or slow talking indicate extremes in diet and excessive or disorderly eating. If you are not understood, it is because you do not understand yourself due to inner physiological and psychological confusion and dietary imbalances. A healthy person speaks little, says much.

Voice resonating from various sections of the body indicates congestion and mucus in those locations. Healing of a congested section can be aided by making the sound of the associated vowel or letter for a minute or two, while focusing the concentration on the area to be healed. For example, for sinus congestion, the tongue should be placed on the upper palate while the sound "N" is hummed several minutes a day.

Strong, clear voice indicates healthy kidneys, liver, stomach, lungs, and strong sexual power.

Voice Exercise

In order to have a vibrant, pleasant voice, you must speak with an open throat and from deep down in the lower diaphragm-abdominal region. This exercise will aid that.

1. Take a deep breath; open the mouth wide, and make the sound "AH" from the lower abdomen for 5 seconds, then stop. (You may also practice humming with the other body sounds: M, N, E, O, U.)
2. Inhale again and repeat for 10 seconds and stop.

3. Continue in this manner up to 20, 30, 40, or 50 seconds, or as long as comfortable. Always start at the zero second mark and work up in 5-second intervals, that is, 0-5, 0-5-10, 0-5-10-15, and so on.

4. After a few weeks of practice, a minute or two per day, you can be up to 30 or 40 seconds nonstop. The throat will then be opened and relaxed and the voice will be more vibrant and pleasant.

5. If you reach the 60 or 70 second mark while humming "AH" nonstop, you will be on the way to developing a pure magnetic voice, one that others will gladly listen to.

VIBRANT HEALTH AND HUMAN BEAUTY

The idea of the beauty of a person is synonymous with that of health and perfect organization. What an inspiration it is to see a truly robust and healthy man or woman! A radiantly healthy man is always handsome; an energetic healthy woman is always beautiful. Such people possess a magnetic charm that draws attention and compels admiration wherever they go.

Beauty is but the reflection of wholeness, of health. Partial beauty, fading beauty, and decaying beauty are but expressions of partial, fading, or decaying health. An abundantly healthy individual has perfect symmetry and proportion of body. The complexion glows and is free from blemishes, with the red blood shining through at the cheeks, fingers, and toes. The hair sheens, is strong and full of life. The eyes are clear and sparkling, lips are rosy in color, the teeth pearly white, sound, and even. An unmistakable look of confidence, courage, alertness, love, and joy radiates from the countenance of such a person. If you love beauty in body, mind, and spirit, and desire it for yourself and for your offspring, there is only one way to attain it, and that way is to live in harmony with the laws of life.

Perfect health is your natural right. The glossy hair, bright eyes, clear skin, active brain, steady nerves, and happy disposition, together with the strength, vigor, and unlimited energy of a truly healthy human being, are all yours if you want them enough to pay the price. But these things cannot be purchased with money. They are not for sale in any store and cannot be found in boxes or bottles. They can be maintained or regained only one way, and that is by carefully obeying the laws of nature every day.

The qualities of vibrant health:

1. A healthy, normal appetite for natural wholesome foods.
2. Sound undisturbed sleep and a zest for living upon rising in the morning, free from fatigue.
3. Calm nerves, clear thinking, and a steady magnetic gaze.
4. A clear, strong, and musical voice.
5. Hair that is strong, lustrous, plentiful, and shining, without dandruff or dryness.
6. A clear complexion, bright and glowing.
7. A firm, powerful, and flexible grip.
8. A clear, alert mind, with a good memory, without absent-mindedness or forgetfulness.
9. Constructive and happy thoughts about self and others.
10. The attitude is confident, loving, cheerful, and positive; a realist.
11. Perfect eyesight without glasses; eyes clear and sparkling; hearing perfect.
12. The tongue is pink and uncoated; the breath is sweet and clean.
13. No dark circles or puffiness under eyes.
14. A good sense of humor about yourself and others; a calm, peaceful nature.
15. A proper upright posture and carriage, neither bent nor inflexible.
16. Body weight proportionate to height and bone structure; neither thin or fat, but firm.
17. Body joints flexible and free from stiffness and calcium deposits.
18. Taking total responsibility for all your actions and circumstances.
19. Teeth are even and shiny white; gums do not bleed; no cavities and strong bite.
20. Muscles are firm, strong, and smooth; an energetic springing step; athletic ability.
21. Internal organs and glands in their proper place and functioning healthfully.
22. No sensations of pain, pressure, swellings, soreness, tiredness, stress, or indigestion.
23. Neither cold hands nor feet; body temperature and blood pressure normal; pulse not too high or low but even and steady.

24. A grateful and thankful feeling for being alive, with appreciation for the things you now have.
25. You are orderly and precise in thought and action, neither hasty nor plodding.
26. You are an independent thinker, free from dogmas, prejudices, and false notions.
27. You do not follow organizations, groups, teachers, or cults without question, failing to reason and think about the truth of life by your own intelligence and creativity.
28. Your goal in life is to help other people; you are not self-centered.
29. You have plans and goals in life based on your own creativity and individuality.
30. You know who you are, where you are going, and the purpose of your life.

If you possess most of these positive vibrant health qualities, you are living in accordance with natural law; if not, start on a rejuvenation health program today.

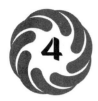

Nutritional Power for Optimum Health

The food question is definitely the most important problem of the present day and, if properly dealt with, must result in the disappearance of the vast bulk of disease, misery, and premature death. Dr. Harvey W. Wiley, who was responsible for our pure food laws, joins Scottish surgeon and health and diet educator Sir Arbuthnot Lane in saying that "I believe I would not be far out of the way if I should say diet may be said to be a factor in every disease to which man is heir."

Natural science teaches us that we must eat for replenishment, drink for replenishment, and breathe for replenishment. Nutritional replenishment means that we must put back into our body and blood what has been used up in the process of living. The ultimate purpose of blood circulation is to feed the hungry cells of your body; this is accomplished by a rich red bloodstream that is built and vitalized through a balanced program of natural foods. This is the great law of life.

Inadequate and incomplete nutrition, along with poor food assimilation and lack of intestinal and muscular tone, cause many individuals to experience hidden hunger pangs or abnormal cravings, which compel them to constantly consume junk food. A well-balanced nutrition, exercise, fitness, and antistress program can help alleviate the problem in a short time. The valuable elements that compose the human body—

vitamins, minerals, trace elements, enzymes, proteins, carbohydrates, and fatty acids—are supplied by natural whole foods in easily available form. The presence of these life-sustaining components in their proper balance determines our state of health, vitality, and length of life. When any one of these natural elements becomes depleted or reduced below the body's requirements, health and vitality begin to diminish in that very instant and will continue to do so until disease appears. If the body's requirements are adequately met in every department, health will be the natural outcome.

Through the power of nutrition, the food we consume daily, we become physically and mentally what we are now and what we will be in the future. Food can build us into dynamos of health, strength, and power or break us down into sick, weak, and powerless individuals. The quality and not the quantity of foods is the determining factor in our overall health and well-being.

Every human being knows that a building cannot be any more perfect than the materials used in its construction. Foods, just as they come from nature's hand, are capable of building perfect human bodies. But when civilized peoples do not use natural foods, and their food is changed from the condition in which nature supplies it, that habit tends toward body degeneration, organic strain, and illness.

CONFUSION ABOUT NUTRITION AND HEALTH

What is a proper diet for human beings? Is there one good diet that is good for everyone, everywhere, which will end all argument on what we should eat? One authority says we should eat only fruits, nuts, and vegetables; another says we should eat only rice and no fruit. Still another advocates eating only fruit. One recommends a high-protein, low-fat diet. One group says that honey, onions, garlic, and grains are taboo. Some say to eat everything, because humans are omnivores. There are diets from each nation around the world, and we can take our pick. One author is against eating breakfast, another says to eat a big breakfast. One says to fast one day a week and another advises fasting forty days at a time.

Here are a few well-known diets advocated by various authorities in the West:

Low-cholesterol diet	High-fiber diet
Policeman's diet	Weight Watcher's diet
Air Force diet	Mucusless diet
Orange diet	Grapefruit diet
Grape diet	High-carb diet
Low-carb diet	High-protein diet
Low-protein diet	Save your life diet
Working man's diet	Drinking man's diet
Rockefeller diet	Mayo diet
Eat all you want diet	No-risk diet
Diet revolution	Inches-off diet
Milk diet	Bran diet
Fruitarian diet	Breatharian diet
Rice diet	

Is the meat diet the answer? What about the all-fruit diet? Or the grain-only diet? It is obvious that confusion and contradiction are rampant in the health and nutrition field. We have personally experimented with many of these diets, including the rice diet, high-protein diet, fruitarian diet, the cooked diet, the raw diet, the juice diet, the water diet, and yes, even the breatharian diet of only pure air. As you will see from the pages of this book, we have discovered that some of these diets can be used without harm for limited period of times in certain conditions, such as to bring about weight loss, lower cholesterol, or for cleansing purposes. However, there are no health or longevity advantages of following any exclusive or extreme dietary fad or program beyond a few days or at most a few weeks. Superior health can only result from a balanced dietary program and proper living habits.

One thing is certain: positive results in health and nutrition are of prime importance, not theories or speculations that look impressive on paper but fail to produce healthy specimens in real life. In order to arrive at a logical and truthful conclusion, we must seek all the facts, clinical and empirical, that produce actual physical healthful results.

No one philosophy has all the answers, but we can learn from them all. We must remain open-minded in our research and study, investigating all sides of the issue before reaching answers or conclusions. The mind is like a parachute: it only functions when open. Unfortunately, all too often, we allow our own subjective egos to obstruct our thinking and reasoning processes. Being human, we tend to hold on to our pet theories and opinions on health, diet, and life, not opening our minds to a higher truth or superior method. When individual consciousness learns how to flow with the universal consciousness or natural law, we can easily discern the proper and true nature of health and life.

The ancient sage Buddha, during his earlier life, attempted to subsist on almost nothing, while fasting and praying in the mountains. One day he became enlightened, fled the mountains, and proclaimed to the masses that fleeing society and depriving oneself of food and other necessities was not the answer to reach heaven or God. He revealed the answer to health, happiness, and long life with one word: moderation. Moderation in all the good and beneficial things of life, moderation in diet, exercise, working, playing, and sleeping, is the answer to living a well-balanced and healthy life. Always keep this important point in mind when studying and practicing health and nutrition.

Improper or one-sided nutrition can cause serious metabolic and chemical disorders that can take years to correct. For example, a heavy meat and protein diet is the cause of kidney disease (contracted), arthritis, gout, premature aging, and cancer tumors. Meat protein is extremely high in phosphorus, which can cause high calcium loss and bone cancer; it is deficient in almost all vitamins, minerals, enzymes, and base elements. Meat can impart strength and power (yang) for a short time, but it is not conducive to a healthy long life. Exclusive meat diets are extremely yang and acid, resulting in very aggressive, hot-tempered, oversexed, and dictatorial characters. Grains, legumes, vegetables, seeds, and fruit are biologically and healthfully superior to meat protein.

A diet exclusively of cooked grains, legumes, and vegetables lacks the elements of sufficient raw fruits, vegetables, and potassium, the beauty mineral. This diet usually leads to extreme underweight conditions or emaciation. Mentally, this diet produces yang temperaments, sometimes uncompromising and arrogant, and organic contraction, resulting in fevers.

The fruitarian diet (watery fruit) is extremism on the alkaline side (yin) and will result in low blood pressure, poor circulation, cold feet and hands, anemia, and nervousness. This last symptom is caused by a lack of sufficient proteins and grains. Mentally, alkaline fruitarians tend to be overcritical. They whine and complain continually, feeling that no one is as moral or as perfect as themselves. They withdraw from society thinking that everyone else is headed for destruction.

If breatharianism were possible, it could be done only through divine intervention (grace) and Taoist practices. The authors advocating diets such as fruitarian, juicearian, breatharian, and mucuslessarian have not been able to live up to their own teachings. They live on the diet for a time, but nature always pulls them back to eat the heavier type of acid foods: protein and carbohydrates.

EAT LOCALLY

The truth underlying the vast subject of health, diet, and nutrition, which must be considered before a specific nutrition plan is advocated for a person, is that there is an affinity between natural foods and the human body. They share the earth as source, and the body fed according to nature's dictates holds energies to be found in no other way.

Nature decides what foods we are to eat, and that decision is made according to the zone or region in which we live. In the cold frigid regions of the far north, fuel foods are required. Fruits, seeds, and grains are very scarce there. Cold (yin) temperatures require heavier and more yang/acid foods, such as cooked grains, legumes, soups, stews, and so on. Generally, those living in a cold climate may consume a higher percentage of natural cooked starches and proteins and a small or moderate amount of raw foods and natural fats. On the other hand, as we travel south to the tropics, we need less fuel foods and more fresh fruits, vegetables, and nuts. A high-meat and -fat diet, eaten in the south, would result in rapid decay and death. Hot weather is yang and requires some summer grains and raw fruits and vegetables. A yin fruit and vegetable diet in Alaska would cause a rapid loss of weight, extreme coldness to the bones, and ultimate sickness.

The temperate zones produce many people with a well-balanced spiritual, mental, and physical nature. Nature provides the greatest variety of foods in these regions. While the tropics grow mostly yin foods and citrus fruits, the temperate zones produce fruits and vegetables tending toward yang elements, such as apples, peaches, cherries, and beets. These yang foods are higher in sodium, which is necessary for the temperate region. Tropical fruits are high in potassium, which is required to cool the body in a hot yang climate.

For optimum health, consume foods grown within a 300-mile radius of where you live. Avoid foods shipped across the country or from other countries. The red pepper (cayenne), which grows so profusely in southern latitudes, is strongly magnetic (yin), and the lemons, limes, oranges, and tropical fruits abound in citric acid; these foods are assimilated and utilized easily by southern inhabitants. In temperate regions, the woods are overflowing with luscious ripe red berries, seeds, and nuts; nature has produced just the right kind of food that the humans and animals inhabiting those regions require.

For those living in climates with a change of seasons and weather throughout the year, the diet must be adjusted to meet the environmental conditions to maintain nutritional balance and optimum health. For instance, during the northern winters of the temperate zone, more yang and heavier foods such as grains, wheat and rye bread, beans, peas, steamed vegetables, and apples are required. Temperate summers require more cooling foods as found in this zone, such as cherries, peaches, plums, grapes, berries, and melons. The spring and fall diets will vary between the winter and summer ones. This is where you must become the final judge in the choice of foods you eat. Listen to the inner voice or feelings as to what the body requires of certain foods on any given day. Age, physical activity, and stress conditions must also be considered as variables in an optimum selection of natural foods.

Be moderate and use supreme judgment. An occasional orange, pineapple juice, or other tropical fruit eaten in the northern zones will do you no harm. Do not become a food fanatic or diet crank. Acid and yang meat eaters can benefit by eating some vegetable and fruit foods to balance their yang characters. Vegetarians, who are mostly yin and alkaline, would do better to eat more of the yang natural foods, such as seeds, peas, grains, beans, miso, cooked vegetables, and so on.

PROTEIN POWER

Proteins are among the most complex organic compounds found in nature. Protein is converted into amino acids, which are the basic building blocks of our body. Like carbohydrates and fats, proteins are composed of carbon, hydrogen, and oxygen, with the addition of nitrogen, sulfur, and phosphorus. Over 50 percent of our body is composed of protein, including skeletal muscles, intestines, skin, ligaments, cartilage, eye, hair, nerve fibers, bones, and blood. Muscle protein is called myosin, connective tissue uses collagen protein, and hair is made up of keratin protein. Protein is necessary for blood clotting and produces hormones and all enzymes. Lack of sufficient protein can cause anemia, skin disorders, constipation, and even death.

However, an excess of protein can also cause health problems. The metabolism of proteins consumed in excess of the actual need results in the accumulation of toxic residues (uric acid and purines) in the tissues, which cause autotoxemia, overacidity, nutritional deficiencies, and intestinal putrefaction. These can contribute to the development of our most common diseases such as arthritis, kidney damage, pyorrhea, schizophrenia, osteoporosis, atherosclerosis, heart disease, and cancer.

To understand this it might be well to know something of the structure of an amino acid. As the name implies, the backbone of every amino acid is an amino (nitrogen) group, NH_2, and an acid (carboxyl) group, COOH, held together by a single carbon atom. To the carbon atom is also attached a chain of organic compounds (usually denoted as R), which give each amino acid its special characteristic. These individualizing chains are made up of carbon, nitrogen, hydrogen, oxygen, and sometimes sulfur. Hence the base of every amino acid looks like this:

$$NH_2 \qquad \begin{matrix} H \\ C \\ R \end{matrix} \qquad COOH$$

Whenever the body cannot use an amino acid, the liver breaks it down into its various parts and uses the oxygen, hydrogen, and carbon atoms to form glucose or saturated fat. The rest, meaning the amino groups and sulfur groups, is discarded as ammonia and sulfuric acid, an excess of which is a set up for all kinds of health disasters.

The ammonia (NH_3) is usually taken care of when it unites with carbon dioxide to form urea, a less nitrogenous substance that can be easily eliminated from the kidneys. However, an excess of ammonia can be converted into uric acid, which has the tendency to accumulate in the system and cause trouble. Sometimes the ammonia just remains as free NH_3. When there is a sufficient supply of minerals in the body, the acids, including sulfuric acid, combine with them and are eliminated as salts. Without enough minerals present, the acids get stuck in the body and clog up the functions of the cells. It is very important, therefore, to make sure that our protein intake meets the body's needs, but no more.

There are eight essential and fourteen nonessential amino acids necessary for growth. All twenty-two amino acids are necessary for health, but the eight essential ones—isoleucine, leucine, lysine, methionine, phenylalanine, tryptophan, threonine, and valine—must be supplied in the diet daily. The fourteen other amino acids are alanine, arginine, asparagine, aspartic acid, cysteine, glutamic acid, glutamine, glycine, histidine, norleucine, proline, selenocysteine, serine, and tyrosine. A good quality complete protein supplies all of the essential eight amino acids for normal growth and health. Incomplete proteins are the ones that lack one or more of the eight essential amino acids and can neither support normal growth nor good health.

Proteins Are Not Fuel Foods

Perhaps the most predominant food fallacy is the high-protein intake usually recommended. Most recent research, worldwide, both scientific and empirical, shows more and more convincingly that our past beliefs in regard to high requirement of protein are outdated and incorrect.

Proteins are used in the body for repair and replacement of worn out cells and tissues, but they are not equally useful as fuel foods. Carbohydrates and starches are our primary energy-supplying foods. The need for protein in the diet can be drastically reduced by including complex carbohydrates such as whole grains, legumes, peas, whole grain breads, whole grain noodles, and so on. These foods also contain an adequate supply of protein in the right proportion, especially when legumes and grains are combined at a meal.

Worldwide Protein Research

Every cell in our body is built of protein, but that is not all we are built of. We are also 70 percent or more water with small amounts of minerals, vitamins, and so on. Proteins are needed for cell building and repair, enzyme and hormone synthesis, mineral metabolism. We need protein. But how much is too much?

Early European investigators advocated from 100 to 150 grams of protein as a daily requirement. These erroneous figures were based on observation of what people were actually eating. Meat consumption was very high during the time of those investigations and it is easy to see how these scientists arrived at their conclusions. Then, in the early nineteenth century, scientific tests conducted on students showed that they could remain in nitrogen balance on less than a third of the amount of protein previously recommended and considered necessary. Even now, we have been made to believe that the more protein we consume, the better. Yet, the most recent worldwide research shows that the actual daily need of protein in human nutrition is far below what has long been considered necessary.

Pritikin Diet Program

The internationally renowned Pritikin nutrition program recommends that we ingest no more than 15 or 16 percent of our total calories in protein. Anything over that amount causes negative mineral balance. In the *Vegetarian Times* article "Pritikin's Program for Vegetarians" (Jan./Feb. 1981), Pritikin states:

> For example, if you drank a quart and a half of milk per day, more calcium would be expelled through your urine than you take in. High-protein diets change the body's metabolism so that it must draw calcium from the bones to neutralize the acid conditions set up by amino acids and high protein, producing increased calcium and mineral excretion through the urine. Vegetarians always ask about getting enough protein. But I do not know any nutrition expert that

can plan a diet of natural foods resulting in a protein deficiency, so long as you are not deficient in calories. You need only 6 percent of total calories in protein to maintain a positive nitrogen balance and it is practically impossible to get below 9 percent in ordinary diets. African Bantu women take in only 350 mg. of calcium per day. They bear nine children during their lifetime and breast feed them for two years. They never have a calcium deficiency, seldom break a bone, rarely lose a tooth. Their children grow up nice and strong. How can they do that on 350 mg. of calcium a day, when the American recommendation is 1200 mg. They are on a low-protein diet that does not kick the calcium out of the body. In our country, those who can afford it are eating 20 percent of total calories in protein, which guarantees negative mineral balance, not only of calcium, but of magnesium, zinc and iron. It is all directly correlated to the amount of protein you eat.

We are in total agreement with the food intake percentages of the Pritikin diet: Fat intake is 5 to 10 percent, protein 10 to 15 percent, and the balance complex carbohydrates, primarily unrefined. If you maintain your calories with whole grains, legumes, seeds, vegetables, and fruits, you will obtain sufficient protein to keep you healthy.

Dr. Paavo Airola on Protein

Dr. Airola reports on a recent American research effort performed under the direction of Dr. Lennart Krook, showing that overeating meat leads to serious mineral imbalance, especially with respect to calcium and phosphorus. Dr. Airola goes on to report on another recent study conducted at the U.S. Army Medical Research and Nutrition Laboratory in Denver, Colorado, demonstrating that a high meat intake results in significant vitamin B_6 losses. He adds that a high-protein diet also causes severe deficiencies in magnesium, calcium, and niacin. Dr. Airola reports further on research conducted in Germany by Dr. Schwarz of Frankfurt University, and studies performed by the famous Swiss biochemist Dr. Ralph Bircher, showing that the aging process is initiated by amyloid, a by-product of protein metabolism, which collects in connective tissues, causing cellular and tissue degeneration. This process carried on throughout an entire organism seems to be the leading cause of premature aging.

Those peoples of the world who show the highest average life expectancy (Hunzas, Bulgarians, Russians, Yucatan Indians) have traditionally subsisted on low-protein diets, whereas those people who show the lowest life expectancy in the world of between thirty and forty years (Eskimos, Laplanders) have traditionally consumed large animal high-protein diets.

Other Protein Studies

Dr. Hindhede, in *Protein and Nutrition*, says:

> A rich protein diet is a cause of various ailments. That luxurious habit, especially overindulgence in meat, can give rise to various stomach, kidney and arthritic complaints, is reported by manifold experience. The office of the liver is to render harmless, by conversion into urea, the ammonium compounds, which arise from the decomposition of animal protein in the intestines; this suggests that the organ performs the same service in regard to various other waste products of metabolism. It is easy to conceive that the liver is to a certain degree composed of these poisonous products, but there are limits to the functional ability of the organ to render these poisons harmless, which may possibly explain some to the maladies from which those who indulge largely in meat suffer.

A series of studies on young adults of both sexes show clearly that, as protein intake is increased, retention of bone calcium decreases. Researchers at the University of Wisconsin found that when the protein intake of young men was raised to 140 grams per day, the subjects proceeded to lose bone calcium at a rate that, if continued, would have left them no bones at all by their early fifties. Not one subject failed to experience rapid bone deterioration, even though they took liberal amounts of calcium and their phosphorus intakes were kept artificially low. Studies with young women show that they too respond to high-protein intake with marked bone erosion. It requires even lower protein intake to effect such losses in women, but this can be explained by their smaller body sizes. Young men had strong bone retention with protein intakes in the range of 50 grams per day. Unfortunately, young American adults are taking on the average as much as 100 grams of protein per day, which suggests that our young may be experiencing rapid bone deterioration.

A build-up in blood urea is associated with kidney failure, whereas doctors in Italy, Hungary, Canada, Russia, and more recently in the U.S. report success in treating kidney patients with low-protein diets. A Quebec physician, Dr. M. G. Bergerson, states that a low-protein diet can be highly beneficial for kidney patients. An Italian researcher reports patients with chronic kidney insufficiency can be rendered symptom-free for years on a diet containing 20 grams of protein per day. A Russian group reports prolonged use of diets containing 18–24 grams of protein per day has netted good results with patients suffering from kidney insufficiency. The Russians have made extensive use of a potato diet for kidney patients and American researchers found plant proteins were far more effective than animal proteins in keeping blood urea levels down.

Dr. Uri Nikolayev is probably the most successful psychiatrist in history; the mentor of Moscow's prestigious Psychiatric Institute has cured thousands of desperately ill schizophrenics. What his technique does is rid the body of protein derivatives and other chemical abnormalities that *Psychiatry Digest* cites as the apparent cause of all forms of schizophrenia. His technique is, of course, fasting. Fasting, it should be noted, is the ultimate in low-protein diets. Low-calorie diets, even protein-free low-calorie diets, sharply curtail the excretion of protein wastes. Only a fast can, in the short run at least, purge the body of the excesses of a lifetime. Dr. Nikolayev's treatment of fasting has received wide acclaim, which it richly deserves. What has escaped attention is the second phase of his treatment, which is the treatment that follows a successful fast. Only with the adoption of a low-protein vegetarian diet are the results lasting, whereas a return to a meat-based diet is a return to emotional stress.

Excess Protein Causes Cancer

High-protein intake is strongly linked to cancer. A Cornell researcher places the blame on ammonia. Ammonia, and possibly other protein wastes, may indeed play roles in cancer, but protein partners with cancer in a number of ways. High-protein intake incites a cancer-like frenzy of activity at the cellular level. It weakens the body's capacity to resist cancer by weakening the liver, it stimulates the production of hormones involved in widespread hormone-dependent cancers, and it promotes the kind of growth on which cancer thrives.

High-protein intake causes sharp increases in the rates of breakdown of existing protein and of synthesis of new protein at the cellular level. In the presence of adequate caloric intake the synthesis of new protein tends to exceed the breakdown of existing protein. The resulting protein build-up causes the cells to grow and divide. Rapid cell growth and rapid cell division are hallmarks of cancer. Tumors are the result of a concentration of frenzied protein synthesis and cell division at the site.

The rapid cell division that accompanies elevated protein intake begins as a general body phenomenon rather than being concentrated in one small region as it would with cancer. And finally, women should find this fact most convincing: high-protein intake leads to increased production of estrogens (female sex hormones) in women; increased estrogen output tends to promote various female cancers.

Meat Eating May Be Hazardous to Your Sexuality

The addition of chemicals and hormones to meat are causing sex gland problems. Experiments by Dr. F. Pottenger Jr. of Monrovia, California, have proven that the physical makeup of men and women is changing. Men are looking and acting like women, and women are looking and acting like men. Hair is growing in abundance on the arms and legs of women. Men are becoming more feminine and weak physically, mentally, and emotionally.

Another experiment was conducted in which a few chosen men and women were lined up facing a wall. Next, a number of doctors were invited to distinguish between the male and female from behind. These doctors had a great deal of trouble distinguishing the difference in gender. The men in this experiment had narrow shoulders and wide hips, which is a female characteristic, while the females had wide shoulders and narrow hips, which is a male characteristic.

Have you ever seen synthetic female hormones at work? Did you know that a cow given a shot of DES (there are eight other lesser-known brand names) will abort her calf? Years ago a rancher found that he could chemically castrate young bulls with a small dosage of this synthetic nonsteroidal estrogen. Any knowledgeable veterinarian will tell you that if a rooster is given DES daily, he eventually will cease to crow and will begin to cluck like a hen. French tests have found that rats fed meat coming from steers fattened with the aid of female hormones were radically affected sexually: impotence and sex reverses were seen among male rats and cancer of the breasts and other female organs was produced in the female rats.

Why, after more than fifty years of flagrant use of synthetic female hormones in the cattle-feeding industry, do we find the chemical companies frantically pushing the new synthetic masculine hormones? Why can't we merely shut off all of these hormones rather than face the long ghastly transition, which seems to be in store for us?

The excessive consumption of hormone-laden meat products, in addition to a large intake of white sugar products, is one of the main causes of reversed sex roles today. This is certainly something each individual must seriously think about, evaluating the effects of their dietary lifestyles.

Protein-Reducing Diets

Most so-called reducing diets are harmful and lead to damaged health. High-protein diets and low- or no-carbohydrate diets are especially harmful. Severe restriction of carbohydrates with no restriction of fats and proteins may take weight off effectively, but it can have the disastrous effect of causing irreparable damage to brain, nervous system, and heart. A high-protein diet, always popular with reducers, will admittedly help to reduce, but always with severe health damage as the result. Over indulgence in proteins is one of the prime causes of such dreaded diseases as arthritis, osteoporosis, heart disease, and cancer.

Mayo Clinic Report

According to nutritionist Dr. R. A. Nelson of the Mayo Medical School, animals fed high-protein diets have increased urea production. Kidney hypertrophy occurs in animals on long-term protein diets; more strikingly, if one kidney is removed, the degree of hypertrophy of the remaining kidney is directly related to the amount of protein ingested. High-protein diets increase albumin and casts in animal urine. Rabbits on high-protein diets develop nephritis, as do rats, if the diet is continued long enough. Trout fed a low-protein diet live twice as long as trout given a high-protein diet.

Scientific Consensus

Perhaps the following fact will convince you more than anything else. The Food and Nutrition Board of the National Academy of Science, in collaboration with the World Health Organization, publishes the Table of Recommended Daily Allowances of various nutrients every four years. In the last two decades, they have lowered the daily recommendation for protein from 120 grams to only 46 grams. This was prompted by world-wide scientific consensus and a growing concern that an excess of protein in the diet, just like an excess of anything else, can be extremely harmful and can contribute to the development of biochemical and metabolic imbalances and diseases.

Important Protein Points

1. Always go outside after eating, especially protein meals. Outdoor oxygen is absolutely necessary for normal protein assimilation and utilization.
2. Eat your protein meals earlier in the day if possible, but never over an hour after sunset. Daytime is for assimilation and digestion of foods. Night hours are for sleep and recuperation.
3. It is best to consume no more than 20 grams of protein at one meal. The body cannot utilize more than this at one time.
4. As a general estimate, the body requires from 30 to 60 grams of protein daily, depending on age, sex, activity, stress, sleep, weather, food quality, and environment.
5. Eat the protein foods that your body can tolerate and easily digest and utilize. Consume only what agrees with your constitution and body intelligence. Meat, dairy, and eggs are not absolutely necessary for protein requirements and health.
6. Legumes can be combined with grains and seeds to form complete and adequate proteins.
7. Junk-food cravings are directly linked to protein deficiencies, incomplete dietary protein, or poor protein utilization.
8. Germinated or soaked (overnight) seeds and nuts liquefied in a blender will increase their quality and net protein utilization. Raw dried seeds and nuts, unsoaked or ungerminated, are inferior foods and do not contain complete proteins.

9. An excess of protein in the diet, especially animal meat protein, including fish and poultry, leaves poisonous residues and uric acid in the system, causing yang disease symptoms, such as constricted (yang) kidneys, high blood pressure, liver congestion, constipation, and cancer.

10. The long-lived people in many sections of the world consume a moderate amount of protein daily, and they remain in vibrant health and vitality past the hundred-year mark. They are able to healthfully sustain themselves on a low-protein diet because of their superior, pure organically grown food, fresh unpolluted air, clean fresh water, little stress, and their joyous attitude. Their meat intake is almost nothing, and they consume mostly raw dairy products (fresh), grains, seeds, nuts, fruits, and vegetables.

11. Americans consume more meat and other proteins than any other nation on earth, and they suffer widely from the most degenerative diseases known to humankind.

12. An excess or lack of protein in the diet can be a quick way to lose beauty, health, and strength; you can develop unsightly facial wrinkles, hair loss, poor sight and hearing, underweight or overweight, premature aging, low blood sugar, and many other disease symptoms. Listen to your inner body (voice) or intelligence for the proper amount you require daily. Only you can be the final judge.

Protein Requirements

The protein requirements for each individual are totally different. Each person has unique nutritional needs, requiring certain foods for his or her own metabolism, glands, and body structure. Hard and fast nutritional rules cannot be applied generally. Each of us must take a close look at ourselves and determine, through self-diagnosis, habits, and heredity, exactly what we require to improve our own health. No book can do this for us; a book can only be a guidepost to teach us universal principles, so that we may apply them to our own individual needs.

Generally, the protein intake need for growing children is higher than for an elderly person. Pregnant women and nursing mothers may need a little extra supply of protein to provide nourishment for two. The supply should only meet the demands of the body, and no more. Weight-lifters and bodybuilders need more grams of good quality protein to compensate for the breakdown and loss of their cells and tissues.

You, as a unique organism, must determine what your protein require-ments are on a day-to-day basis. Some days your inner voice or body intelligence will require that you consume additional amounts of natural protein, other days you will not feel the need for half that much. Stress conditions, exercise, hot and cold weather, sleep and rest, unforeseen envi-ronmental factors, and human physical and psychological variables all play an extremely important role in your daily protein requirements.

The most reliable indicator of protein need is your present overall health. Are you full of pep and energy? How about your skin, nails, hair, and eyes? Also, is your digestion good? Ask questions and experiment on yourself. No authority can decide for you what you need on any given day or hour. You must ultimately depend upon your own body wisdom to determine your own nutritional needs.

Vegetarianism versus Carnivorism

Current methods of food production, especially in the United States, are most uneconomical and wasteful. Nearly half of the harvested land in the United States is planted with crops to feed animals. The United States Department of Agriculture states that the billion people in developed countries use almost as much plant food as feed to produce animal protein as the two billion people in other countries use directly as food. In feed-ing vegetable foods to animals for meat, a 90 to 95 percent waste factor is involved. The cultivation of grains, vegetables, nuts, and fruits can support a population eight times or more than that provided by the present waste-ful system of feeding this food to animals first, then eating the animal.

We must not only provide superior nutrition for human beings, but, most importantly, save the land from exhaustion. Our cosmic spaceship (Earth) is burning and smoldering with chemicals, inorganic fertilizers, fallout, industrial wastes, and destructive poisons too numerous to men-tion. It is time for everyone to take some positive action and to demand that peace be given to our fields, not only to save humans from malnu-trition and disease, but also to improve the diet of the earth itself. Our world leaders are leading us like sheep into mass suicide from the lack of true wisdom and deep insight. We must think of the generations and civilizations to come.

The vegetarian philosophy is appealing to a growing number of people of all ages who desire a peaceful world now and for generations to come all over the globe. Many young people are disillusioned with society. They have witnessed only war, insecurity, economic strife, chaos, and corruption at all levels of government. Many of them are seeking only good and constructive change. The nonviolent plan of eating, if embraced by humankind, would lead to world peace, but it must start with each person. The whole vegetarian ideal will not only improve the individual (the microcosm) but also humanity as a total unit (the macrocosm) and the entire environment.

Scientific and Anatomical Basis of Vegetarianism

A well-selected vegetable diet is capable of producing the highest physical development. This fact was supported by professor E. V. McCollum of Johns Hopkins University in the early 1900s when he stated: "I have not the slightest hesitation in saying that a vegetarian diet is the most satisfactory type of diet that humans can take." Modern physiology also supports the contention that flesh is not an essential part of the diet of human beings.

On the other hand, it is easily demonstrated that animal meat is injurious and that many of the diseases of our civilization are derived exclusively from its use. We will dispose of the meat question with the following incontrovertible scientific facts, which should be sufficient evidence that the practice is an acquired habit and wholly unnatural.

- All animals that are naturally carnivorous are more active at night than in the daytime and are of a nature that makes them positive at night and negative during the day. Man is more active in the daytime than at night by nature, and if he is carnivorous he furnishes an exception to the universal rule. Persons who consume large quantities of meat are rendered sleepy and dull during the day and are sleepless and nervous at night. Heavy meat eating usually accompanies the drinking of alcohol, along with spicy, fattening, and other devitalized foods, during a period of time in which the body requires sleep and recuperation from the daily activities.

- All animals that are naturally carnivorous perspire through the tongue and not through the skin. All naturally vegetarian animals perspire through the skin, as humans do. All carnivores lap liquids with their tongue. We take our liquid through sucking. Meat eaters have a feverish and disagreeable condition of the tongue, causing an unnatural thirst, which vegetarians do not experience.

- Our anatomical structure is not adapted to a meat diet. Our teeth are not adapted to tearing flesh and we have no claws to kill and rend prey. Our tooth structure is designed for biting and chewing grains, legumes, fruits, vegetables, seeds, nuts, and other natural foods, as opposed to the carnivore who kills the animal and eats mostly inner organs, blood, guts, bones, and flesh.

- The perspiration and other forms of excreta thrown off from the bodies of meat eaters is exceedingly offensive, while that from vegetarian eaters is agreeable and less in quantity. Flies and mosquitoes torment meat eaters, while vegetarians are comparatively immune. Vegetarians are seldom constipated, while meat eaters are almost universally so. Humans secrete alkaline saliva, the carnivore secretes acid saliva.

- The carnivore stomach is small and round, as opposed to the oblong stomach of humans, which has convolutions needed for the breakdown of fruits, grains, and sweet tender vegetable foods. The human alimentary canal is twelve times the length of the body. The carnivore canal is only three times the length of its body. The carnivore colon is smooth and short, which is necessary for the quick evacuation of putrefying flesh fare. The human colon is long and convoluted for a more thorough digestion of the food from the plant kingdom.

- The consumption of meat renders the individual more ferocious and disagreeable in manner, less considerate of others, and more inclined to acts of brutality and selfishness than to acts of kindness. In many cases, it produces the effect of continued irritation, nervousness, and sometimes results directly in insanity.

- When humans consume meat they literally poison themselves. Flesh foods begin to putrefy about one-fourth of the way down the intestinal canal, causing uric acid poisoning, ptomaines, chemicals, deadly hormones, and the waste products from the animal's metabolism at the time of slaughter. Meat products in the human system overstimulate the heart, causing it to beat up to 50 percent more than average, which leads to high blood pressure.

- Carnivores have large livers to handle the heavy meat consumption. The human liver is small and not developed to handle a flesh diet. Flesh-eating animals secrete ten times the hydrochloric acid into their stomachs; it is required for the breakdown of meat, bone, organs, sinews, feathers, and so on. Carnivorous animals eat mostly the inner organs of their prey in a raw state. Vultures, hyenas, and other scavengers feast only on the left over muscle meat, after the tiger or lion has finished feasting on the best inner parts. When humans consume aged, bacteria-ridden, and cooked flesh, they fall into the scavenger category. Muscle meat is highly deficient in vitamins and minerals and contains an excessive amount of phosphorus, which, if eaten to excess, throws off the calcium balance within the body. Phosphorus thus robs the bones and teeth of valuable calcium and generates uric acid crystals throughout the body joints, causing stiffness, pain, and disease.

    The gorilla, elephant, oxen, and horse are all tremendously strong, with great endurance, and they subsist solely on vegetarian fare. Repeated experiments have proven that vegetarians can equal or excel meat eaters in tests of endurance and strength, both physical and mental. Meat is not needed for heavy work. Prof. Voit of Munich discovered that "heat and energy are almost exclusively created by carbohydrates."

- Fruits, vegetables, grains, and seeds repair and replenish the cells and tissues, whereas meat overstimulates and tears them down. Flesh food often causes a ravenous appetite, which nothing but more flesh can satisfy. Meat, being an extreme yang substance, causes an internal craving for extreme yin substances, that is, sugar, alcohol, drugs, and sodas. Extremes in diet cause extreme conditions or chronic diseases such as cancer.

- Meat contains a high proportion of cholesterol (an important causative factor in thrombosis and high blood pressure) with no lecithin (nature's antidote) to balance it. All vegetable proteins, on the other hand, contain lecithin to naturally counterbalance it.

Sources of Protein for Long Life

Where do you get your protein if you do not eat meat? How many times have vegetarians been asked this question throughout the history of nutrition? Why not ask how a cow produces milk and attains great size on vegetable matter, or where elephants, gorillas, and rhinoceroses obtain their protein?

Consider Mr. Elephant, with huge tusks and teeth and bones. Or the ox, the bullock, or the camel: where do they get the protein with which to build their powerful muscles? They are all total vegetarians. The vegetable kingdom is, in point of fact, the only natural firsthand source of all the protein on this planet. Not one animal creates protein but by eating protein foods; none can synthesize calcium or other elements within the body; every one depends on the vegetable kingdom for the raw materials to restructure into its own particular type of makeup. No two types of animals have the same general protein type. But all vegetarian creatures can obtain their essential ammo acids (the building blocks of all proteins) from the vegetable proteins that are so abundantly and widely distributed in the world of plants.

Even the fang-and-claw predators, such as the dog and cat families, must obtain their protein from plants ultimately, though they get it secondhand by eating vegetarian animals. However, they pay a price in parasitic diseases and other problems associated with flesh-eating, even as humans do if they become dietary copycats and try to eat like a tiger or jackal. Truly man is the king of beasts, for his brutality exceeds them. Leonardo da Vinci stated, "We live by the death of others. We are burial places. I have since an early age abjured the use of meat, and the time will come when men will look upon the murder of animals as they now look upon the murder of men."

Rather than asking where cows and elephants get their protein, it would be better to ask the vegetarian centenarians, worldwide, about their sources of protein. There are people living in the mountains of Russia, Turkey, India, Northern Hunza, Iran, and Poland who live over a hundred years in good health. Their main diet consists of whole unprocessed grains (such as rye, wheat, oats, millet, buckwheat, and rice), seeds, nuts, locally grown fruits, vegetables, and raw cultured milk products. Their diet is basically high in natural complex carbohydrates and not in protein.

Their approximate protein intake ranges from 25 to 40 grams daily. These centenarians work all day long in the fields and never experience fatigue as we know it. They are not protein deficient. They know nothing of high-protein or other fad diets. They exist healthfully and happily, and they are not skinny or fat but firm, muscled, robust, and energetic. We have personally observed these tireless people subsist on a bowl of rice, beans, and vegetables daily, using meat mainly as a condiment in soups and vegetable stir fries. They simply radiate beauty and tranquility. They possess well-formed physiques, and they maintain the same body weight throughout a long healthy life.

These are empirical (derived from observation without reliance on theory) facts, not personal opinions. These dietary patterns have been tried and tested for centuries. One only has to observe how the long-lived people live and eat and gently follow in their footsteps. The nutritional skeptics of the West should take an example from these wise and healthy old people. Their diets, habits, and cultures have been around long before America was discovered and long before books and magazines were published on health and nutrition. We must remember that supermarkets, processed foods, drug companies, and trendy diets are all modern inventions, not more than sixty to eighty years old, mere seconds in the history of the world.

The longest-lived and healthiest people in the world live chiefly on the natural whole foods grown in their own region and climate. The Bulgarian diet, for example, consists largely of whole rye and barley bread, sunflower seeds, vegetable soups, and fermented foods such as yogurt, sauerkraut, sourdough bread, and soured milk. They are mostly lacto-vegetarians who seldom eat meat. They consume goat or sheep milk and fresh raw honey.

The Himalayan Hunzas consume a similar diet, with the addition of apricots, millet, buckwheat, mulberries, buttermilk, soups, fruits, and vegetables. They work outside most of the day, getting sufficient exercise and oxygen to digest their food properly. They drink the highly mineralized water coming down from the majestic glaciers. They maintain a positive, happy attitude and youthful condition well into advanced age. Many Hunzas reach the age of one hundred years and beyond.

Long-lived Mexicans, on the other hand, utilize the foods grown near them, such as papayas, pineapple, corn, cornbread, beans, limes, lemons, oranges, red peppers, bananas, avocados, various vegetables, and many herbs, including damiana and sarsaparilla. The Russians who live to a healthy advanced age consume an abundance of garlic, onions, honey, pollen, buckwheat, sunflower seeds and oil, and fermented lactic acid foods such as soured milks, sauerkraut, sourdough bread, and pickles. Their foods are unprocessed. They eat very little meat and live an outdoor life.

Common Characteristics of Centenarians

1. Eating pure, whole, organic foods grown on humus-rich black soil.
2. Consuming clabbered goat milk products, fruits, vegetables, seeds, nuts, and grains, and very little or no meat.
3. Eating when hungry and only when hungry; drinking only when thirsty.
4. Eating and living in moderation.
5. Getting daily exercise outdoors, such as walking, running, farming, gardening.
6. Maintaining a positive mental attitude.
7. Having a strong belief in a supreme guiding force: praying often, fasting occasionally, living without fear, and being serene and loving.
8. Developing and maintaining perfect bodily posture, which is necessary for good circulation, nerve flow, and superb health.
9. Living in almost perfect environments: altitude of about 4,000 feet (perfect for the heart, metabolism, and thyroid); where sunshine and rain are abundant throughout the year; where food grows continuously; with an atmosphere that is brisk, bracing, energizing, and pure; where it is never too cold or hot, but just right.
10. Making their work their play and their play their work. They do what they enjoy and they love what they do.
11. They are never in a hurry or under stress, which is the greatest killer and life-shortener of modern humans.
12. Not smoking or drinking alcohol.

13. Living by the cycles of the earth: early to bed when the sky darkens and up with the sun at the crack of dawn.
14. Marrying one or more times; having grandchildren and great grandchildren and enjoying being around young people.
15. Often climbing up and down steep inclines as a part of life at high altitudes, which ensures good body circulation from the leg muscles to all parts of the body and brain.
16. Obtaining an abundance of ultraviolet light from the sun daily, which controls calcium, found in the long bones of the body that produce new rich red blood cells.
17. Drinking pure mountain glacier water and consuming a variety of herb teas, such as ginseng, peppermint, and alfalfa.
18. The greatest secret of centenarians is living a well-balanced life, mentally, physically, emotionally, and spiritually.

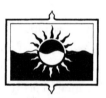

Fig. 4.1. We squander health in search of wealth,
we scheme and toil and save;
then squander wealth in search of health.
And all we get is a grave.
We live and boast of what we own;
we die and only get a stone.

Vegetable Protein Superior

The animal cannot exist without the vegetal. The human body cannot digest inorganic substances or manufacture them from proteins, carbohydrates, vitamins, or minerals. The synthesizing and vitalizing of inorganic elements is a vegetal function, called autotrophism. Only the vegetable kingdom can perform this phenomenon. Vegetables absorb inorganic elements and convert them into organic foods, which are very complicated in their composition and construction. This is a veritable miracle produced by the interworking of the forces of nature.

Biologically speaking, we are children of the vegetal mother. Without vegetable life, no animal on the earth would survive. Our hemoglobin is derived from chlorophyll. All vegetal foods are virgin materials for the purpose of maintaining or constructing our body. Neither meat nor animal products are pure virgin material for us. We must eat vegetables and their direct products. This is the biological principle and fundamental law: vegetables are the superior food.

Why the Vegetarian Diet Is Superior

1. Vegetarian food can feed the world ten times over and better.
2. Vegetarian food is free from hormones, antibiotics, drugs, chemicals, and cancer-causing agents.
3. Vegetarian food is free from trichina worms, parasites, food-poisoning bacteria, and uric acid.
4. Vegetarian food is high in vitamins, minerals, enzymes, and other fresh food factors.
5. Vegetarian food supplies adequate proteins with complete amino acids for growth and health.
6. Vegetarian food maintains the arteries, internal organs, heart, and body in a youthful condition.
7. Vegetarian food does not require the killing of animals for food and is free from animal diseases.
8. Vegetarian food makes you kinder, more peaceful, gentle, and loving to both animals and humans.
9. Vegetarian food is more economical individually and on a worldwide basis.
10. Vegetarian food gives you more endurance, strength, health, and longevity.

Meat: Unnatural Substitute Food

When thinking about vegetarianism people quite naturally ask what they can use in place of the various animal-source foods. It should be clearly understood that every one of these animal-source foods is already a substitute food: a perversion of the natural diet that is ideally suited for the normal human body.

Milk, eggs, and meat are all mere substitutes for our natural vegan foods. If we bear this in mind we will not be so concerned with searching for substitutes for substitutes: for items that look, smell, or taste like the barnyard/slaughterhouse products we are so used to. There are many vegetable-source replacements for the various animal products, but these are more in the nature of a dietary crutch to help in a transition period rather than a nutritional necessity. We should really learn what our natural foods are and go on to build our diet from these.

The protein contained in seeds and nuts (soaked overnight or germinated), all grains, all legumes, vegetables, sprouts, and fruits, supplemented with nutritional yeast, soybean, tofu, soy powder, miso, and seaweed products, is biologically superior and pound for pound much cheaper than meat, eggs, or dairy.

GRAMS OF PROTEIN IN VARIOUS FOODS

FOOD	QUANTITY	GRAMS OF PROTEIN
Seeds and Nuts		
Filberts	½ cup	6
Almonds, raw	½ cup	13
Brazil nuts	½ cup	10
Cashews, unsalted	½ cup	12
Pecans	½ cup	5
Sesame seeds	½ cup	9
Sunflower seeds	½ cup	12
Walnuts	½ cup	7
Pumpkin seeds	½ cup	14
Grains, Fruits, and Vegetables		
Barley, whole	½ cup	13
Buckwheat, whole	¾ cup	12
Lima beans, cooked	1 cup	16
Kidney beans	1 cup	15
Broccoli, steamed	1 cup	6
Cauliflower	1 cup	3
Corn, steamed	1 ear	3
Kale	1 cup	4

FOOD	QUANTITY	GRAMS OF PROTEIN
Lentils	1 cup	15
Peas, steamed	1 cup	5
Peas, split	½ cup	8
Potatoes, baked	1 med	2
Squash, winter	1 cup	4
Avocado	½	2
Apricots, soaked	½ cup	4
Blackberries	1 cup	2
Dates, soaked	1 cup	4
Prunes, soaked	1 cup	3
Raisins, soaked	½ cup	2
Wheat bread	1 slice	2
Cornbread	1 slice	3
Soy flour, powder	1 cup	39
Oatmeal	1 cup	5
Rice, brown	1 cup	15
Rice polish	½ cup	6
Wheat germ	1 cup	17
Bean soups	1 cup	8
Creamed veg. soups	1 cup	7
Nutritional yeast	¼ cup	13
Soy powder, concentrate	1 T	12
Dairy and Other Animal Products*		
Raw goat milk	1 cup	8
Buttermilk	1 cup	9
Yogurt (low-fat)	1 cup	8
Skim milk	1 cup	8
Cottage cheese	1 cup	35
Swiss cheese	1 oz.	7
Egg	1	6
Skim milk cheese	1 oz.	8
Flesh	4 oz.	20

*Use these foods sparingly. Listed for clarity and information.

Protein versus Complex Carbohydrates

In an article entitled "Carbohydrates—No Villain," which appeared in *Iron Man* magazine, Vince Gironda, bodybuilding champion and exercise and nutrition researcher, makes a clear case for the body's needs for carbohydrates. Even though the article appeared in 1978, his message is still timely:

> I advocate a relatively low protein intake, about 45 grams per day. Too much protein creates a negative nitrogen balance, which in turn leads to gout, sluggishness, and liver and kidney problems. The body cannot digest more than 20 grams per meal, and anything beyond that leads to problems. At least one meal per day should be carbohydrates in the form of vegetables or grains, thereby giving the body a protein break. Furthermore, it has been demonstrated repeatedly that protein combustion is not higher during heavy exercise than under resting conditions, while on the other hand the body uses carbohydrates stored first before it turns to other sources. Even after depleting the carbohydrate deposits, continued exercise does not hike protein needs significantly. According to my research, athletes performing strenuous, endurance tasks such as bodybuilding, and burning up 9,000 calories per day, show no noticeable increase in protein needs. If this all is not enough to turn your heads, Dr. Per-Olaf Astrand, a famous exercise physiologist in Sweden, performed a study which concluded that endurance tends to decrease as protein intake is elevated. He discovered that a high-protein diet lowered endurance as well as reduced buildups in muscle carbohydrate, more than high-carbohydrate diet. Experiments by Christensen and Hansen found that in heavy work such as powerlifting or bodybuilding, the major participant toward endurance was, once again, carbohydrates. Also, the subjects were able to perform three times longer on a carbohydrate diet than a protein or fat diet.
>
> Probably the most asked question now is, if bodybuilding essentially is the tearing down and building up again of muscle tissue, then is not increased protein necessary for that process? The answer is no. A high-protein intake even after a sustained injury,

does not prevent a transient rise in nitrogen losses. Dr. Doris Callaway and a team of researchers found that animals fed three times as much protein as normal recovered no better than those on normal amount of protein. Now let us get one thing straight before we go any further. There is a quality difference between carbohydrates. Do not go out and load yourself up with candy and that type of junk carbohydrates. Carbohydrate loading with sugar is a mistake. Carbohydrates replace glycogen, which the body stores and uses for energy. Sugar in any form leaches the stored glycogen from the liver and produces nervousness, irritability, fears, doubts, and various psychic changes in the personality. The major sources of carbohydrates should be from, as stated earlier, grains, and vegetables.

Muscleman Advocates Low Protein

Vegetarian world champion bodybuilder Bill Pearl (Mr. America, Mr. Universe) states quite emphatically that a growing bodybuilder simply does not need 300–400 grams of protein to reach his potential, and that there is absolutely no question that it is possible to build a high-class physique and be a vegetarian at the same time. Mr. Pearl believes that one can build health, strength, and muscles on 50 to 70 grams of protein per day on a well-balanced vegetarian diet. Pearl has been a vegetarian since he was thirty-nine and has been pumping iron for more than fifty years. He is now over eighty years old and weighs well over 200 pounds of solid muscle with Herculean strength to match.

Pearl further says that vegetarian eating has had numerous positive effects on his body. His cholesterol gradually dropped down to a normal level of 198, and blood pressure lowered. His pulse rate and other physiological processes improved. One of the most dramatic changes was in his uric acid level. Previously it was so sky high that every joint in his body ached, he could hardly move his hands, and he actually thought he was getting arthritis. Now it has dropped down to zero. His energy levels are incredible, and he feels like a million dollars all of the time.

The biggest change has been in his attitude toward himself and his fellow man. He is not as aggressive as he was in the past. Vegetarianism has definitely had a mellowing effect on him. He is a firm believer in sticking to convictions and says that once he began eating as a vegetarian, he could not be swayed away from it by anyone: even if someone offered him $50,000 to eat a steak, he would tell him to stick it in his pocket.

Choosing Your Own Diet

The question of whether to eat flesh products or not is strictly an individual matter. It depends on how far you desire to progress on the path to health and well-being. It has been scientifically proven that an excessive consumption of meat can easily lead to arthritis, gout, and stomach, colon, and bone cancer. We contend that overeating of any food item, either natural or unnatural, can cause a host of physical and mental diseases, from colds to cancer.

Certainly we are not claiming that if you consume a very moderate and limited amount of meat per week or day that you will immediately drop dead from doing so. Almost everyone has eaten their share of meat before becoming a vegetarian. Our aim is not to coerce people into giving up meat against their will. Each individual must accomplish this transition when he or she is physically and mentally ready.

Our main purpose here is to present the facts and scientific data as it is revealed to us. You can choose not to partake of meat products for the following reasons: health, economic, spiritual, moral, ethical, ecological, aesthetic, scientific, and humanitarian. Likewise, this decision should be based upon your own deep study, contemplation, and overall commitment to higher ideals: physically, mentally, and spiritually. You must make that choice for yourself and be given the freedom and love to do so.

CARBOHYDRATES AND SUGARS

Carbohydrates are composed of carbon, hydrogen, and oxygen. They are foods that provide fuel, heat, and energy. The main sources of carbohydrates are grains, fruits, vegetables, seeds, nuts, legumes, potatoes, and so on.

Digestion of starch foods begins in the alkaline saliva of the mouth and is completed in the small intestine. For this reason, starches should be thoroughly masticated and salivated in the mouth before swallowing. Starches are converted into dextrines and sugars, then into dextrose and glucose, before entering the bloodstream, where they are readily utilized and produce animal heat.

Cooked starch is acted upon by saliva and pancreatic juice very quickly; raw starch is not. Raw starch granules are surrounded by an envelope of cellulose, which the saliva and pancreatic juice penetrate very slowly. Therefore, the digestibility of starch (grains, legumes, potatoes) depends upon the cooking. Improperly cooked or imperfectly chewed starch foods pass mostly undigested into the feces. This is also true of poorly baked bread.

Glycogen, like starch, is insoluble. Hence it is stored in the liver until needed for use; it is also stored in the muscles. Every cell in the body contains a small amount of glycogen. When fuel is needed, the glycogen is again transformed into sugar (dextrose), which nourishes the body. The body maintains its heat by the burning of glycogen. Muscular work is supported by the energy set free by the burning of glycogen, just as the work of a steam engine is performed through the energy obtained from coal. When glycogen becomes exhausted, the bodily forces fail. The heart consumes glycogen with every beat. Without glycogen the heart could not beat and no muscle in the body could contract. The body contains about 4 percent glycogen. The greatest source of glycogen is found in natural foodstuffs, that is, grains, vegetables, fruits, seeds, nuts, and legumes.

When no starches or carbohydrates are eaten, the body makes glycogen by splitting the protein molecule. By this means, about half the weight of protein may be converted into glycogen. The other half of the protein is converted first into ammonia then into urea. The fuel value of protein is then only half its face value, and the body is taxed in the disposal of the large amount of poisonous waste. Consequently, protein is a very poor fuel food, while carbohydrates are protein-sparing: instead of the body converting protein into glucose for energy, they provide the heat, energy, and fuel so that protein may be used for tissue building. Proteins are utilized more fully for tissue repair if some form of natural carbohydrate food is consumed at the same meal.

Starch, after being swallowed, is converted into glucose in the intestines, absorbed and carried by the bloodstream to the liver, where it is converted into glycogen. When a muscle contracts it needs fuel, so the glycogen is carried by a blood vessel from the liver to the muscle, converted again into glucose, mixed with oxygen from the lungs, and fired by insulin from the pancreas, producing energy.

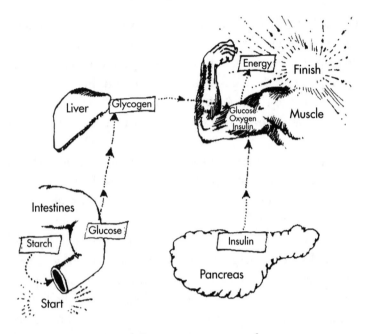

Fig. 4.2. Where our energy comes from

Tea and coffee, both of which contain considerable amounts of tannic acid, prevent the action of saliva upon starch foods. Tea and coffee drinkers experience much gastric acidity and poor digestion and health.

Fruit Sugars

Natural fruit sugars are digested and absorbed into the bloodstream within thirty to sixty minutes. The natural sugars contained in all fruits, dried fruits, honey, and maple syrup contain fructose, grape sugar, and levulose. Honey contains equal amounts of dextrose and levulose. Milk sugar contains lactose. Refined white sugar, commercial sugars, brown sugar, saccharine (made from coal tar products), chemically treated sweets, ice cream, candy, cakes, pies, and sodas are all devoid of vitamin and mineral elements, create calcium loss, and cause conditions from anemia to schizophrenia. If you value your health, avoid these junk-food refined sugars. Natural sugars from fruit eaten in season (moderately) will satisfy your sweet tooth and give the body wholesome minerals, vitamins, and natural fiber/bulk for intestinal health.

FATS

Fats are called hydrocarbons because they produce oil when heated. Fats are used in the body as heat, energy, and fuel. They are found in butter, cream, seeds, nuts, avocado, cheese, milk, egg yolks, and all oils. Fats are digested slowly and remain in the liver and stomach longer, delaying hunger for quite some time. Fats differ from other foods in that they are stored in the body in almost unlimited amounts. Fat is somewhat of a reserve fuel that the body draws upon when the sugar stores are greatly reduced. A normal amount of fat is stored in the body to maintain body heat, protect and lubricate internal vital organs, and give a graceful contour and shape to muscles and skin. An overconsumption of fatty foods will congest the liver and weaken the digestive organs. Fats are needed more in cold weather than hot to keep the body warm.

Cholesterol is a chemical component of oils and fats. The body forms fat from starch and sugar foods. If no natural fats are included in the diet, the body will produce fats from starch and sugar foods. It is best to take fat in small quantities; this gives the body a chance to manufacture its own fat. If our diet is adequate in B vitamins, fresh fruits, grains, vegetables, seeds, nuts, and soy products, we can produce all the lecithin and anticholesterol agents our body needs.

An excessive consumption of eggs, meat, and cheese can contribute to a rise in body cholesterol. Other cholesterol-forming foods are: hydrogenated oils, margarine, butter, white flour, white sugar, and salt. A small amount of natural fats eaten daily will maintain the body in good health and vitality. Remember, the body will produce its own fat if the diet is deficient in it.

Although they are natural, certain foods with a high fat content, such as avocados, nuts, and soybeans, should not be used excessively; they are not staple foods and should be eaten very sparingly.

The greatest cause of cholesterol build-up is a combination of two things: first, fatty foods, sugar foods, white flour, and salt; second, a lack of daily exercise and fresh outdoor oxygen, as well as stressful conditions. To help overcome this, consume a low-fat, low-protein, and high-natural-carbohydrate diet, including: whole grains, low-fat dairy, legumes, peas, seeds, fruits, vegetables. Eventually this diet will balance the internal organs and stabilize the mind and emotions. Obtain sufficient daily

FAT PERCENTAGES OF SELECTED FOODS

FOOD	PERCENT FAT
Butter	90% to 100%
Vegetable oil	80% to 90%
Ice cream	70% to 90%
Regular cheese	60% to 80%
Nuts	40% to 70%
Meat	40% to 50%
Avocados	25% to 40%
Cream	25% to 40%
Ripe olives	25% to 40%
Soybeans	20% to 30%
Eggs	10% to 20%

exercise, fresh air, sunshine, and sleep. Exercise helps keep the bloodstream flowing freely and the arteries free of cholesterol deposits. The body weight will normalize itself, along with blood pressure, pulse rate, and cholesterol levels.

Free Fats Are Harmful

All extracted or refined oils, whether animal or vegetable, are referred to as free fats or triglycerides; all of the bulk, fiber, vitamins, enzymes, and minerals are removed from the food, and it is no longer a water soluble food. Even pure vegetable or nut oils are harmful, if taken to excess, especially if eaten in hot weather. A small amount (1 teaspoon per day) may be used in cold weather for body warmth. The body can obtain its fatty acids from whole foods such as legumes, grains, and germinated seeds and nuts. The human system cannot properly handle extracted or fractionated free fatty oils in any form. These include: butter, cream, sour cream, nut butters, egg yolks, mayonnaise, margarine, lard, seed/nut oils, and vegetable oils. Pure vegetable oils are the least harmful, but they should also be used sparingly.

Polyunsaturated fats can cause disease as well as saturated ones. Polyunsaturates do lower serum cholesterol levels in the blood, however, the cholesterol moves out of the blood and into the cells and tissues. These free fats then clog and block the oxygen-carrying red blood cell from entering the tissues. Oxygen is thus reduced to the brain and body cells, which causes many internal disorders. All fats, both animal and vegetable, if eaten beyond the needs of the body, can cause the following diseases: gallstones, diabetes, tumors, skin diseases, liver disorders, obesity, colitis, cancer, heart disease, and lung disorders.

Human requirements for fatty foods are very low. We do not need an extra abundance of free fats in our diet; this only leads to ill health. Obtain your fats from whole foods in their natural state, and watch your health improve tremendously. When you realize that each body cell is a small battery, needing constant recharging through the food you eat, you will really begin to think about diet.

Your food shall be your medicine, and your medicine shall be your food. Eat sparingly and defy the physician. The human is the most helpless creature on the face of the earth. When we come into existence we have to be taught everything, which forms our habits. But this is our salvation. If we are creatures of habit, why not make our habits good ones? We can reeducate ourselves and take control of our own destiny. Love does not dominate; it cultivates.

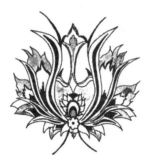

Fig. 4.3. Life starts with nature and blooms with life.

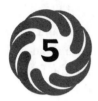

Increasing Life Force

How to eat, when to eat, what to eat, and where to eat are some of the basic questions people ask when starting a program of natural eating. We all should eat to live, not live to eat. An old Chinese proverb says, "When feasts are spread the doctor rolls his pills. In fifty dishes lie a hundred ills." Most people today live to eat, and they end up with enormous medical bills for all of their ills.

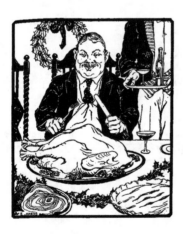

Fig. 5.1. When feasts are spread the doctor rolls his pills. In fifty dishes lie a hundred ills.

TWELVE KEYS TO GOOD HEALTH

The three vital functions of food are to rebuild the living tissues, to supply energy, and to preserve a proper medium in which the biochemical processes of the body can take place. To ensure that these vital functions take place, it is important to follow twelve rules of healthful eating.

1. Eat only when hungry and stop before you are full.
2. Maintain proper balance of acid and alkaline and yin and yang.
3. Chew your food well and mix thoroughly with saliva.
4. Refrain from eating when emotionally upset or physically exhausted.
5. Eat food at room temperature.
6. Eat fresh natural organic raw and cooked foods daily.
7. Fast or follow an eliminative diet when necessary.
8. Combine food properly.
9. Refrain from close eye work or intense brain work before, during, or after meals.
10. Eat your last meal at least three to four hours before bedtime.
11. Be cheerful and calm at mealtime.
12. Follow the law of moderation.

1. Eat Only When Hungry and Stop Before You Are Full

Overeating causes malnutrition. Do not eat unless you have absolute hunger. True hunger is a mouth and throat sensation. The mouth waters when true hunger is present. True hunger is not stomach pangs or that empty feeling at the pit of the stomach. These symptoms are a form of addiction to highly seasoned and stimulating foods, such as meat products, coffee, salt, spices, and alcohol. When these foods are eaten, they create withdrawal symptoms and the body again craves them with a burning desire. True hunger leaves the body in a relaxed state with no morbid cravings for junk foods. Eat only to satisfy hunger, no more. Hunger is the true spice of eating.

A completely full furnace smokes and will not readily burn. The stomach acts in the same manner; when completely full, it will not digest the excess load of food but instead will ferment and putrefy, poisoning the body and causing toxemia. A furnace not quite full will burn beautifully. The stomach, not quite full, will also burn (digest) beautifully. If you are not hungry at a mealtime or in the morning, skip that meal and you will fully enjoy your next meal. Eating three full meals a day, in most cases, overworks the digestion and internal organs.

Listen to that small inner voice within you. It will tell you what to eat, how much to eat, and when to eat, and you will seldom go wrong. Never eat between meals. Eat a meal, then do not eat again until you experience true hunger. Your stomach will thank you. To lengthen your life, lessen your meals. Surveys of individuals living past the age of one hundred reveal that they are always moderate eaters. The glutton will never reach the age of one hundred. Who is strong? One who can conquer bad habits.

2. Maintain Proper Balance of Acid and Alkaline and Yin and Yang

As we have seen, all watery type fruits, vegetables, and their juices are classified as alkaline quality foods. Acid quality foods are all proteins, starches, fats, and sugars; that is, all nuts, seeds, cheeses, bread, potatoes, rice, oils, and dried and sweet fruit, like dates, raisins, figs, and bananas. All heavy type foods are acid-forming.

To achieve yin and yang balance, consume the foods grown near or in the climate in which you live and in season. Use more cooked grains, legumes, vegetable stews, and soups in the winter, and eat more raw food during the summer months. Listen to your inner bodily needs; you may require more or less of the acid foods at different times. Also, eat sparingly of fats and sugary type foods, such as honey and dried fruits. Please refer to chapter 7 for extensive guidance on achieving the correct balance of yin and yang, acid and alkaline.

3. Chew Your Food Well and Mix Thoroughly with Saliva

Indigestion is a universal malady. One of the main causes of stomach ailments is bolting food in a hurry. Nothing ages a person faster than this pernicious habit. The stomach has no teeth to break up large particles of food. Nature has endowed us with a set of teeth to break down food into fine, almost liquid particles, so that the digestive enzymes and juices may easily mix with it. Adequate chewing and salivation of all food, including liquids, ensures healthy and thorough digestion and assimilation, allowing us to eat less and to utilize food better. Mastication allows us to enjoy and taste our food to the highest degree. Eating should be a pleasurable experience. Hurried eating never allows full enjoyment of a meal.

4. Refrain from Eating When Emotionally Upset or Physically Exhausted

Eating food when upset or under physical strain will cause faulty digestion and the result is toxemia. Working under mental or physical strain will similarly retard or suspend digestion. Eating under these adverse conditions slows down and impedes the peristaltic action of the stomach and its juices. We should follow the example of animals, who will not eat if wounded, sick, excited, frightened, or maddened. Never eat during a fever, as it will only feed the fires. The rule is: when sick or in distress, stop eating until normal hunger returns. Rest and a short fast should be the only remedies.

5. Eat Food at Room Temperature

It is best to allow food and drink to reach room temperature before consuming it, as cold and hot food suspend digestion for some time. A great amount of body energy is wasted by consuming food and drink at extreme temperatures. In China one of the causes for failing to achieve longevity is considered to be the use of ice in food and drink.

6. Eat Fresh Natural Organic Raw and Cooked Foods Daily

Eat according to season, climate, and weather variations. The best way to accomplish this is to eat foods locally grown on organic farms, including a mix of raw foods and cooked foods. A temperate diet arms the body against all external accidents, so that it is not so easily hurt by heat, cold, or labor.

7. Fast or Follow an Eliminative Diet When Necessary

A fast or an eliminative diet, when needed, is an excellent way to cleanse the body. Fast three to five days on distilled water with plenty of rest and fresh air, followed by a day of fruit. The eliminative diet of three days on watery fruits or vegetables or juices will also bring superb health results. Refer to chapter 9 for more detailed information on fasting and eliminative diets.

8. Combine Food Properly

"You are what you eat" is an old health saying that is only partly true. More importantly, you are what you digest, assimilate, absorb, and utilize. Our total health depends not only on what we eat but how efficient our digestive and assimilative powers are. Understanding proper food combining can make a tremendous difference in our overall health and well-being. It can even extend our lives far beyond the average and slow down the aging process.

Most people consume food indiscriminately, that is, without regard to what happens to the incompatible food mixtures when they reach the stomach—flatulence and indigestion. It is not necessary to get bogged down in strict, unbending food combining rules in order to achieve good health. One need only apply a few important principles, as outlined below, to obtain excellent health benefits.

9. Refrain from Close Eye Work
or Intense Brain Work Before, During, or After Meals

This is so important that observing it will add many years to your life. Oxygen is necessary to properly digest and assimilate the food eaten. Performing close work or reading or staying indoors after eating will hinder digestion and result in poor eyesight and other ills, because close work diverts the blood out of the stomach and into the head and brain area, causing a lack of blood for proper food digestion. After meals, go out into the open air and look into the distance. This will relax the entire nervous system, resulting in improved digestion, assimilation, and better health. Never lie down after eating, because the digestive juices do not flow freely in this position, and it results in fermentation and gas. Too many people (even those devoted to health) are wearing glasses and weakening their eyes, because of not resting the brain and not getting fresh air after eating.

10. Eat Your Last Meal
at Least Three to Four Hours before Bedtime

The body has the least amount of energy and vitality at night, which prevents the proper digestion and assimilation of foods eaten at a late hour.

Good sound sleep is necessary for the repair of the cells, tissues, and organs of the body. Eating a heavy meal at night before going to bed prevents the body from repairing and replenishing itself after the daily activities.

By evening, the body's energy has been mostly expended. Because of this low energy flow, the food consumed in the evening hours should be relatively light and easy to digest. After sunset, the ionic charge of the atmosphere drops, and the later one eats, the more likely the food is to be improperly digested. The last meal of the day should be taken at or before sunset. If you are hungry later in the evening, eat an apple or pear, or a few grapes and berries. Heavy food eaten before bedtime causes muscle twitching and cramps. Yellow and bilious skin can be attributed to this practice, as well as anemia and poor circulation.

This faulty habit weakens the vital organs and uses up a large amount of energy, causing a lack of good sound sleep. The best time to eat the heavier foods is earlier in the day, when the body has the vital energy to digest and assimilate the food properly. The average person does just the opposite: eats a big meal just before bedtime. No wonder there are so few magnetically healthy people around today.

11. Be Cheerful and Calm at Mealtime

Anger, hate, anxiety, and worry stop digestion. At mealtime keep calm and think about the lovely and beautiful things in life. Above all, enjoy your meal, and do not become a hypochondriac over your health or natural eating. Learn the rules, practice them always, make them your habit, and then take up a worthwhile hobby or profession with the zest for living and doing.

Of all the functions that affect the body and soul together, laughter is the healthiest. Gloom and depression of spirits will produce dyspepsia and indigestion, while laughter aids digestion, circulation, sweating, and has a refreshing effect on the strength of all organs. Cheerfulness and gladness are not only of value in preserving health, but they are of equal service as a remedy in disease. A calm, happy, and positive attitude lifts the soul and body and inspires all who come in view of such a person.

12. Follow the Law of Moderation

The human body requires just the right amount of proteins, starches, sugars, fats, minerals, vitamins, and liquids. An excess or deficiency of any one food element, over a period of time, can cause acute, chronic, or deficiency diseases, such as diabetes, cancer, obesity, high and low blood pressure, emaciation, hypoglycemia, and schizophrenia. A balanced and moderate amount of all food elements, coupled with physical fitness, is the master key to good health, nutrition, and longevity.

For example, too much protein damages the kidneys, ages the cells and tissues, and pollutes the bloodstream with uric acid and toxins. A deficiency of protein atrophies the kidneys and causes anemia, falling hair, emaciation, fatigue, and mental depression. An excess of starch injures the liver, causes nerve depletion, constipation, skin eruptions, and mental fatigue. A deficiency of starch causes cold hands and feet, weight loss, a nervous and irritable condition, loss of energy, and lack of body heat during cold weather.

All sugars eaten to excess impair the pancreas and kidneys and cause poor eyesight, falling hair, tooth decay, impotence, schizophrenia, paranoia, and premature aging. An excess of fat overworks the gallbladder and liver and, together with refined sugar, raises the blood cholesterol. Fat is difficult to digest if eaten in excess of bodily needs and causes anemia, skin problems, and obesity. A deficiency or an excess causes nerve disorders, falling hair, poor eyesight, lack of body heat, and general fatigue.

Vitamins and minerals also are essential in preventing various deficiencies and diseases. Lack of adequate vitamins and minerals can cause beriberi, pellagra, rickets, scurvy, and other deficiency diseases. Severe mineral and vitamin depletion can be fatal. Likewise, an excess of vitamin and mineral supplements in megadoses can be dangerous. Consult a competent health doctor of nutrition to advise you on their use.

Learn to listen to your inner bodily cravings for the proper amount of proteins, starches, sugars, fats, vitamins, and minerals; this will lead you to health and longevity.

Moderation in all of the healthy activities and functions of life is the key to attaining good health and spiritual development. Overdoing anything in life tends to weaken our vitality and physical powers. Excessive sleeping can make us sluggish, lazy, and dull; the proper amount of sleep revitalizes and rejuvenates the body for daily activity. Excessive exercise, work, or mental activity can lead to nerve and adrenal exhaustion and the consequent loss of personal magnetism, vitality, and health. If we live within these magnetic margins (of moderation) we can build a reserve energy supply to cope with any stress or heavy physical or mental emergency situation.

Sleep, activity, and proper eating habits are the three most essential functions of life. When any one of these essentials is out of balance in some degree, we suffer the consequences. Natural law cannot be violated with impunity; the rich and poor are equal in respect to the yin and yang laws that govern physical life. We learn through experience, and if we have suffered enough and learned our lessons well, we may alleviate our sickness and self-induced misery.

Remember These Suggestions on Moderation

Eat only when hungry and stop before full.
Drink pure liquids when thirsty.
Rest or sleep when fatigued or exhausted.
Exercise daily, with moderation.
Cultivate cleanliness of body and mind.
Study and read when alert and willing.
Maintain a poised, confident, cheerful, and thankful attitude.

These little secrets may not seem like a big deal, and you may want to neglect them, but we can assure you they are very important for the maintenance and preservation of your health and happiness.

FOOD COMBINING MADE EASY

The food we eat is as important as the most potent medicine, or even more so, for what we eat becomes part of us, part of our blood, our heart, our brain. The following is a list of food classifications and food combining groups, to be used at your own discretion, according to your individual needs and requirements.

FOOD COMBINING GROUPS

GROUP A: PROTEINS

All meat	Eggs
Beans and peas	Nuts and seeds
Dairy	

GROUP B: STARCHES

All grains	Chestnuts
All nuts	Legumes
Bananas	Parsnips
Beets	Potatoes
Bread	Pumpkin
Carrots	Rutabaga
Cauliflower	Turnips

GROUP C: FATS

All oils	Fat meats
Avocado	Margarine
Butter	Milk
Cheese	Nuts
Cream	Olives

GROUP D: ACID FRUITS

Grapefruit	Sour apple
Lemon	Sour grape
Lime	Sour plum
Orange	Strawberry
Pineapple	Tangerine
Pomegranate	Tomato

GROUP E: SUB-ACID FRUITS

Apple	Mango
Apricot	Nectarine
Blackberry	Papaya
Blueberry	Peach
Fig	Pear
Grape	Plum
Guava	Quince
Huckleberry	Raspberry

GROUP F: SWEET FRUITS

Fresh, Raw	Dried Fruit	
All melons	Apple	Pear
Banana	Apricot	Pineapple
Persimmons	Date	Prune
	Fig	Raisin
	Peach	

GROUP G: NONSTARCHY VEGETABLES

Alfalfa	Chard	Lettuce	Sprouts
Artichoke	Chicory	Mushrooms	Squash
Asparagus	Cucumber	Okra	String beans
Bamboo shoots	Eggplant	Onions	Sweet pepper
Broccoli	Escarole	Parsley	Water chestnut
Brussels sprouts	Fresh peas	Radish	Watercress
Cabbage	Kale	Sorrel	Zucchini
Celery	Leeks	Spinach	

HOW TO COMBINE THE GROUPS

A + B = Fair	A + G = Good	B + G = Good
A + C = Fair	B + C = Fair	C + G = Good
A + D = Fair	B + D = Poor	D + E = Good
A + E = Fair	B + E = Poor	D + F = Poor
A + F = Poor	B + F = Poor	E + F = Good

Eight Food Combining Principles

1. Salads should not be eaten before protein or starch (beans, grains) but always with or after these foods. Protein and yang foods require plenty of stomach hydrochloric acid for proper digestion. If yin salads, fruits, or other light carbohydrate foods, for which hydrochloric acid is not needed, are eaten first and protein/yang foods are eaten last, the yin foods will interfere with protein/yang food digestion because of diminished hydrochloric acid in the stomach. Therefore, when eating a grain/bean dish, cheese, or yogurt, eat them before or with the vegetable salad, never after. You can alleviate much gas and indigestion by eating in this manner. The body secretes enzymes and hormones at all times on a healthy and well-balanced diet, so there is no need to eat salads first in the meal to supply any missing enzymes to digest protein or yang foods.

2. Many foods, such as grains and beans, contain both protein and starch. Eaten in moderation, protein and starch foods are not incompatible, as some erroneously believe. Nature produces a variety of protein and starch mixed foods, such as wheat, peas, beans, corn, buckwheat, potatoes, seeds, nuts, rye, and all other grains, and generations of healthy people have eaten protein and starch foods at the same meal. Complex carbohydrates, like grains, beans, and root vegetables are energy- and heat-producers. If an insufficient amount of these are eaten with a protein, the protein is then used as a secondary source of energy and heat, which requires extensive energy conversion and deprives protein of its main function: hormone building and tissue repair.

3. Acid and sub-acid fruits combine reasonably well with pure protein foods, such as yogurt, cottage cheese, buttermilk, raw milk, and eggs. Milk always curdles as soon as it is mixed with the gastric juice, and this helps rather than hinders digestion, as it would leave the stomach too quickly if it remained in the fluid state. Fruit acids are mild compared to gastric secretions; therefore, they will not interfere with the digestion of a pure protein food eaten in moderation. This mixture can be eaten more in hot weather or tropical climates.

4. This is the most important food combining principle to follow! The worst combination of all is mixing acid or sub-acid fruits with starch foods, such as beans, bread, and grains. The acids in the fruit impede starch digestion considerably, causing fermentation and gas. It is best to eat fruit alone. Stewed or baked fruit with a starch meal, however, will not cause any problems. Cooking fruits diminishes their acids, so they can be eaten occasionally with grains or other starch foods.

5. Avoid combining protein and sweet fruit or any other sweets, such as honey, sugar, and corn syrup. Sweets inhibit stomach secretions (hydrochloric acid) and result in poor protein assimilation and digestion, along with fermentation and gas. Sweet fruits, such as melons, bananas, and dates, should be eaten on an empty stomach. You may eat fruit or melons in the morning, at least one-half hour before a protein or yang food meal. Fruit for breakfast gives the stomach natural bulk and acts as an intestinal cleaner and eliminator.

6. Foods rich in fat, especially high-fat cheeses, meats, nuts, milk, oils, and butter, inhibit the flow of gastric secretions, slow down digestion, and delay the emptying of the stomach by several hours. If an excess of fatty foods are eaten at one meal, there will be digestive problems.

7. Avoid sulfur foods, such as onions, garlic, and leeks, at the same meals with sweet foods, such as fruits or honey. Stomach pains, gas, fermentation, and indigestion can easily result from this poor combination.

8. The three most important points to remember are to: a) never overeat at mealtimes; b) eat only when truly hungry; and c) limit the combination and variety of foods at a meal—three or four items per meal are sufficient for health and nourishment. Generally, the more foods that are mixed at one meal, the more digestive trouble one will have. Those with very weak digestive systems will benefit greatly by eating only one or two foods at a meal, thus lessening the burden on the entire digestive process. If you are sick, eat only one meal per day until your digestion is back to normal; it usually takes about one week to get back your normal digestion. The one meal per day plan can include

cooked grains and vegetables in winter and a sub-acid fruit with the seed/nut milk or fruit alone; or cultured raw dairy products alone. Keep your meals simple, but delicious and nutritious.

Avoid Becoming a Food-Combining Crank

Try to follow these simple food-combining principles as much as possible, but do not become a fanatic over the subject of food combining and nutrition. When visiting friends, relatives, or restaurants, do not become a food-combining crank by lecturing others on dietetics. Do not give advice unless asked, and then give just a little. Listen more and talk less: no one likes a know-it-all. Extend the freedom to others to do as they wish. Living by example is a far better teacher than excessive talking or preaching. Be careful of giving advice; wise people do not need it, and fools will not heed it anyway.

ENZYME POWER

All growing and living things, including the foods we eat, contain enzymes. Where we find minerals, vitamins, and protein, we also find enzymes. Enzymes are tiny, almost invisible ferments, which cannot even be seen by the strongest microscopes. They help us digest our food and keep the fires of metabolism alive in our system. Without sufficient enzymes, vitamins, minerals, and hormones cannot carry on their activity. Biochemist and enzyme researcher Dr. Edward Howell states: "Enzymes are substances which make life possible. They are needed for every chemical reaction that occurs in our body. Enzymes may be the key factor in preventing chronic disease and extending the human lifespan."

The body produces only two enzymes, amylase and protease, which digest carbohydrates and proteins. Enzymes are contained in proteins and some vitamins. Enzymes require a protein carrier to charge us with health and vitality. In fact, if we eat raw food exclusively, that is, raw fruits and vegetables, our enzyme activity will decrease. The body needs a certain amount of all natural elements to function properly and increase the enzymes in our system. If enzyme activity is increased in the system, our health and longevity improve. When enzyme activity slows down, we age and slowly die. Enzyme levels are generally low in cases of chronic disease.

Foods that lower enzyme activity are fats, ungerminated seeds and nuts, nut butters, excess oils, alcohol, eggs, sugar, white flour, and excess fruits. Overeating, which causes constipation and obesity, also reduces internal enzymes. Foods and habits that increase enzyme activity are germinated or sprouted seeds, nuts, and grains, fermented seeds, miso, tofu, tempeh, tamari, and cultured products. These foods contain aspergillus plant enzymes, the highest source of enzymes as yet discovered. Fasting when not hungry and obtaining sufficient exercise, sunshine, and fresh air also aid our enzyme production.

MILLION DOLLAR MINERALS

Are you timid and shy? Are you easily discouraged? Do you constantly worry and show fear? Why is fear unknown to others? Do you bite your nails? Are you anemic, weak, underweight (or overweight)? Are you a negative thinker? Is your memory poor? Why are some people serene, dynamic, and vital? What makes certain women kissable at any age? Why can some people sell snowballs in Alaska while others cannot sell water in a desert? Why can some men and women entice the fortunes of life to themselves? What is it? What is the secret of super health, youth, and vitality?

The answer to these often-asked questions lies in the powerful mineral elements that compose our bodies: sixteen primary minerals, plus over thirty other trace minerals needed in small quantities by the body. It is important to learn all about these miraculous vital elements and how to use them. Then you will be able to harness them, direct them, and transform your life with their life-giving power.

Sixteen Primary Mineral Elements

Calcium	Hydrogen	Manganese	Potassium
Carbon	Iodine	Nitrogen	Silicon
Chlorine	Iron	Oxygen	Sodium
Fluorine	Magnesium	Phosphorus	Sulfur

Charm your world with sulfur and iodine. Master your world with calcium and fluorine. Laugh with your world with silicon and potassium. Prosper in your world with manganese, iodine, calcium, and phosphorus. Entertain and fascinate your world with sodium, magnesium, iodine, and chlorine. Love your world with iron, copper, phosphorous, and potassium. Be self-confident in your world with all the powerful minerals that regulate our social, mental, health, business, and aesthetic life.

Many business executives have conquered their nerves and fatigue as well as other serious deficiencies by using all twelve of the body minerals. Some perpetually tired people may be hungry for iodine, sulfur, phosphorus, and manganese to reinforce their vital system. Arthritic sufferers are hungry for sodium, chlorine, iodine, and sulfur. Diabetics need sodium. Fearful, timid people need calcium, fluorine, iodine, and oxygen, attracted to the body by the use of potassium. Those low in muscular power need potassium, sodium, and chlorine, along with vitamin C. Sad, melancholy, and easily infected types need silicon, fluorine, and iodine. Most of us who study, work, and read are hungry for these tiny units of power, the sixteen mineral elements, and just a little lack brings disastrous consequences.

A tiny amount of copper is like an electric dynamo, charging complexion, hair, bloodstream, and even the intestinal tract with an essence that enables other minerals to provide their benefits. Copper, manganese, and iron are an unbreakable corporation in the financial affairs of body chemistry. They are needed by fatigued mental workers who are low in drive and energy.

Hunger for phosphorus, calcium, silicon, and fluorine is found in tuberculosis. Fluorine starvation means erratic characteristics, infections, premature aging, and graying. Potassium hunger is found in those with no resilience and those who suffer with intestinal agony. Sodium, chlorine, and potassium assist assimilation and elimination. Sulfur is the queen of enthusiasm, beauty, and golden nerves, yet if it is taken without balance, it becomes a Vesuvius of drying, scorching irritation. Magnesium and silicon, diplomats of optimism and poise, never let one down. Iodine, the confidence artist, the clever, original life-enjoyment chemical, turns back the clock toward youthful appearance and ambitions, and combines with any of the other minerals to accelerate assimilation.

Though very small amounts of these precious elements are contained in the normal body, they are vitally important to our health and well-being. They have very individual and distinct physiological functions to perform. They are necessary to the life processes of plants, animals, and humans. These precious little minerals preserve our life and repair our tissues and bony structures. They impart firmness, form, and grace to our body. Without them, our glands—which maintain metabolism, secretions, digestion, mental activity, and all physiological functions— would stop functioning. The body fails to rebuild, repair, and regenerate without an adequate supply of these dynamic little wonder-workers.

Minerals give us vital electricity and magnetic power; they are cease- lessly working to recharge physical and mental batteries, and they carry life-sustaining oxygen to all parts of the body. They are powerful neutral- izers of toxins and wastes, purifying the blood and casting uric acid and other poisons out of the system. They are the natural healers and give the body vital resistance and immunity against so-called germs of disease.

Our cells are constantly being used up and repaired daily, and this repair comes from within. Minerals and vitamins supply the body through the bloodstream and must be daily replenished. Wholesome, organic, and natural foods adequately supply the body with minerals. However, if mostly unnatural and devitalized foods are eaten, only a small fraction of the requirements are supplied, resulting in severe min- eral starvation and depletion, leading to ill-health, depression, fatigue, and common symptoms of low energy.

Nature placed these elements in the soil and not upon the drug shelf. More powerful than drugs in lasting nourishment, they provide the spark of life, the immunity against disease, the enthusiasm of youth, the endurance of health, the enchantment of well-being and calmness. To neglect them in our diet is to turn our face from nature's bountiful sup- ply. Raw fruit and vegetable juices contain the organic minerals the body can use, which are stored in the chlorophyll found in the green coloring matter of plants. These vital mineral elements aid the body in producing and sustaining the supply of internal hormones, enzymes, and secretions to keep us youthful and zestfully alive. They are necessary for the proper digestion and assimilation of proteins, starches, and fats.

Iron (Blood Builder Mineral)

Iron is an oxygen carrier in the blood and is found in the hemoglobin of the red blood corpuscles. Anemia cannot be present when the blood has a good supply of iron flowing through it. Iron in the blood allows you to utilize the oxygen out of the air. The thyroid is considered the oxygen gland and iron helps the thyroid gland, along with the oxygen, to eliminate the cellular wastes, use them up, and make the foods you consume ready for blood assimilation. Iron imparts strength, vitality, courage, warmth, creativity, and mental power. It gives you ambition to succeed and to be a go-getter.

Inorganic iron, as found in drugs, irritates the kidneys and cannot be assimilated by the body. Organic iron, as found in natural foods, builds rich red blood. Anemic, pale, thin, depressed, and sick people need large quantities of iron from quality organic products. The lack of iron brings on sleeplessness, irritability, neurasthenia, starvation, disease, and unhappiness. If you want success, happiness, and love to be a part of your life, eat organic iron-rich foods.

Food Sources of Iron: Spinach, sorrel, lettuce, cherries, grapes, raw egg yolks, sunflower seeds, strawberries, asparagus, cucumbers, rye, goat cheese, blackberries, blueberries, apricots, lentils, currants, pomegranates, prunes, carrots, walnuts, figs, apples, wheat, pumpkins, tomatoes, radishes, cabbage, onions, and chard.

Silicon (Optimism Mineral)

Silicon makes you happy, joyful, and zippy. It builds the bones, hair, teeth, eyes, nails, and eyesight, improves the complexion, and is needed in the structural system, membranes, and arterial walls. It brings beauty and firmness to the cells and tissues. Silicon is a good antiseptic, alkaline in composition. It is a great body toner and builds up body resistance. People plagued with sexual weakness, tumors, bad circulation, liver problems, and constipation are in need of silicon. Skins of fruits and vegetables and the outer coats of whole grain cereals are high in silicon.

Food Sources of Silicon: Whole wheat, seeds, oats, barley, figs, strawberries, apples, grapes, cherries, peaches, carrots, greens, walnuts, almonds, rye, onions, spinach, egg yolk, asparagus, and lettuce.

Calcium (Willpower Mineral)

Calcium gives strength and durability and maintains the bone structure. It builds teeth and nails and steadies the nerves. It adds strength and firmness to the arteries and pulse. Calcium imparts endurance, willpower, good memory, strong bones and teeth. It heals wounds and neutralizes toxic acids in the system. It is needed for concentration and strengthens the heart and courage. Calcium is destroyed in the body by white flour products, white sugar, candy, and so on. It extends life and prolongs youth. Pregnant women need calcium to produce healthy children and to maintain health. The infant will draw the calcium from the mother's bones if she has a lack of it in her diet. Lack of calcium brings on rotten teeth, rickets, anemia, weak and soft bones, and diseased bodies. Calcium requires vitamin D for proper assimilation.

Food Sources of Calcium: Goat milk, egg yolk, Canadian wheat, kale, Swiss cheese, buttermilk, green vegetables and juices, garlic, oats, lemons, oranges, berries, cabbage, dates, prunes, apricots, sesame and sunflower seeds, and cauliflower.

Phosphorus (Brain and Nerve Building Mineral)

Phosphorus stimulates powerful mental thought and brain activity. It helps promote digestion and better metabolism of carbohydrates and fats. Phosphorus works along with calcium as a bone builder, assisted by vitamin D. The diet should consist of a ratio of 2.5 calcium to 1 phosphorus to maintain a healthy ratio within the body. People eat too much phosphorus and consequently need to increase their intake of calcium. Lack of this magic mineral will make you look old, but it maintains your youth if eaten daily. Lack of phosphorus can cause nerve and brain disorders, fatigue, weakness, and poor elimination.

Food Sources of Phosphorus: Almonds, rye, egg yolk, wheat bran, rice bran, goat cheese, turnips, soy beans, oats, barley, seeds, nuts, peas, beans, lentils, buckwheat, asparagus, yellow corn, parsnips, whey, cauliflower, and kale.

Sulfur (Sex Appeal Mineral)

Sulfur cleans, tones, and purifies the system, feeds the nerves, and fosters vitality and beauty and an abundant growth of hair. Sulfur is associated with insulin, the hormone secreted by the pancreatic gland to properly digest carbohydrates. It throws out body impurities and promotes bile secretions, enabling the liver to utilize all food minerals. It promotes better bowel action and helps manufacture hormones for the generative system. It increases feelings and emotions. Lack of sulfur produces dull brains, poor blood, lusterless hair, impotence, nervousness.

Food Sources of Sulfur: Cabbage, onions, garlic, radishes, raw egg yolk, asparagus, almonds, chestnuts, cauliflower, kale, brussels sprouts, pecans, mustard greens, broccoli, leeks, horseradish, string beans, endive, thyme, and figs.

Sodium (Youth Mineral)

Sodium cleanses and sweetens the body. It builds the glands, ligaments, and blood. Sodium neutralizes acidosis, helps digestion, overcomes fermentation, and prevents hardening of the arteries and joints. High-strung people need this mineral in abundance. It improves good nature in the personality. Lack of sodium results in catarrh and congestion and slows the mental processes. Depressed, discontented, and downhearted people are usually deficient in it. Increase your sodium intake and watch yourself become optimistic and contented.

Food Sources of Sodium: Celery, carrots, asparagus, seeds, beets, pumpkin, squash, apples, cherries, egg yolk, berries, turnips, spinach, rice, goat cheese, black figs, string beans, oats, dandelions, whey, radishes, and goat milk.

Magnesium (Nerve Relaxer Mineral)

This wonderful mineral calms and steadies the nerves, calms irritability and hot tempers, relieves mental fatigue, and enhances sleep. Magnesium has recently been found to activate about thirty enzymes within the body; it also helps to metabolize protein, starch, and fat, and to promote vitamin and hormone activity. It helps overcome constipation and toxemia. It also protects against strontium 90 fallout in the air. Lack of magnesium leads to hysteria, nerve disorders, insanity, constipation, and fainting spells. City tap water (high in fluorides) will immobilize the usable magnesium in the body, so drink pure distilled water and be safe.

Food Sources of Magnesium: Nuts, seeds, whole grain foods, greens, peas, beans, almonds, apples, brown rice, goat milk, raw egg yolk, whole barley, black figs, walnuts, apricots, wheat, dandelion, garbanzos, pomegranates, and corn.

Chlorine (Body Cleanser Mineral)

Chlorine purifies, cleanses, and cleans out body waste. It disinfects, freshens, and sweetens the entire system, promotes joint agility and flexibility, cuts down fat and autointoxication. Lack of chlorine may cause mucus, fear, anemia, depression, kidney problems, indigestion, and no ambition to succeed.

Food Sources of Chlorine: Beets, red cabbage, cucumbers, spinach, radishes, sea salt, goat cheese and milk, carrots, egg yolk, lettuce, olives, and pears.

Iodine (Thyroid Regulator Mineral)

Iodine normalizes the metabolism and protects the brain and nervous system from body toxins. It is a natural germicide, protecting, balancing, and immunizing the internal system. Iodine normalizes the body weight through the function of the thyroid gland. The thyroid produces a hormone called thyroxin, which is 65 percent iodine. Thyroxin controls the glandular secretions and the heat and energy production in the body. It helps digestion and assimilation. It slows aging and prolongs life. Iodine detoxifies the cells and tissues and regulates the cellular structures and the heart and circulatory system. It prevents goiter, loss of hair, brain fatigue, shyness, glandular problems, excitability, and irregular pulse rate.

Food Sources of Iodine: Sea kelp, dulse, Irish moss, pineapple, brown rice, garlic, apples, raw egg yolk, strawberries, potato skin, watercress, sea foods, carrots, onions, tomatoes, and artichokes.

Plate 1. The Professor's Ambrosia: Food of the Gods Morning Cereal

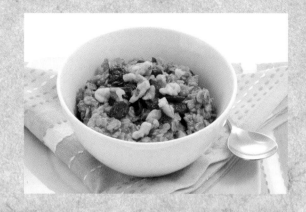

Plate 2. Tao Garden Fruit Compote (builds digestive fire)

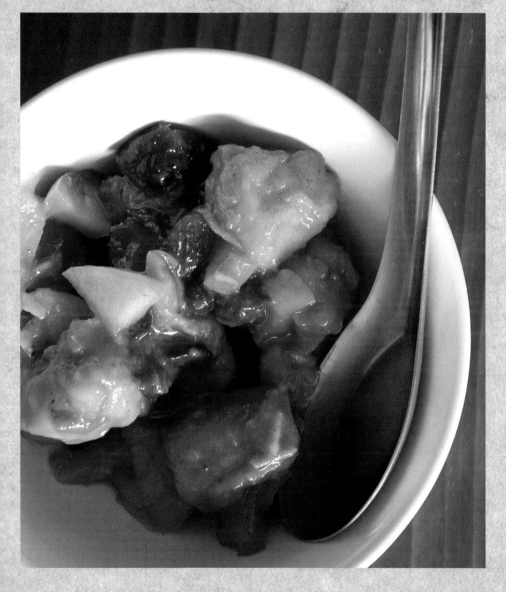

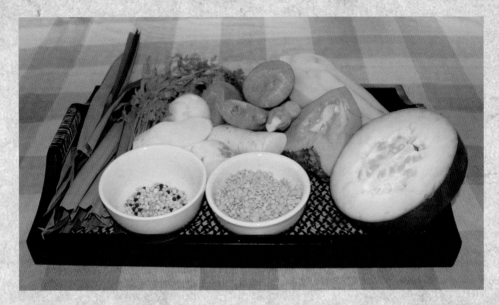

Plate 3. Tao Garden Vegetable Broth (mineralizing and alkalizing)

Plate 4. Tao Garden Brown Rice Soup (Kao Tom Tan Ya Peut)

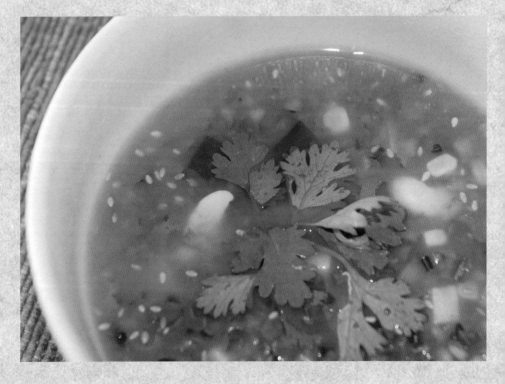

Plate 5. Tao Garden Goat's Milk
Yogurt (cooling and probiotic)

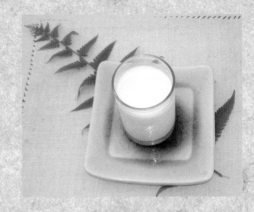

Plate 6. Tao Garden Broccoli Soup
(calming and moves stagnant chi)

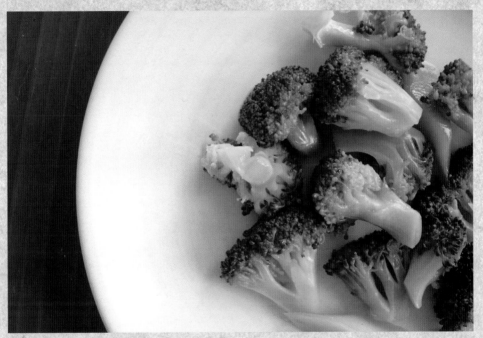

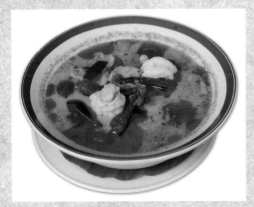

Plate 7. Tao Garden Tom Yam Soup
(stimulates stagnant chi)

Plate 8. Tao Garden Pumpkin Soup (builds digestive fire)

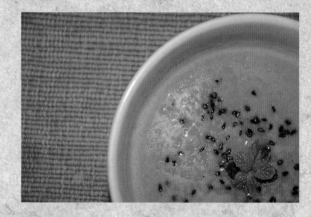

Plate 9. Tao Garden Green Papaya Salad (antiparasite remedy)

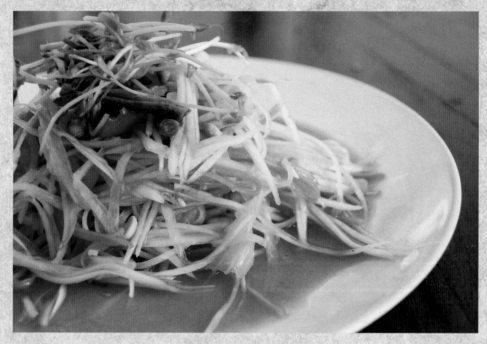

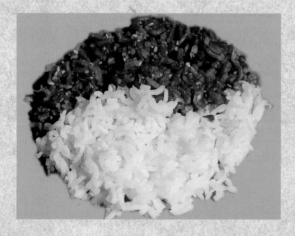

Plate 10. Tao Garden Rice (balancing)

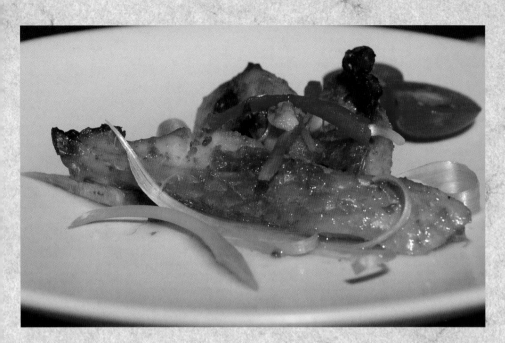

Plate 11. Tao Garden Baked Fish
(with turmeric, anti-inflammatory)

Plate 12. Tao Garden Curried
Chicken with String Beans (warming)

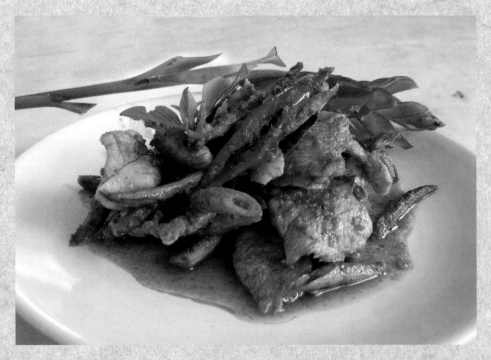

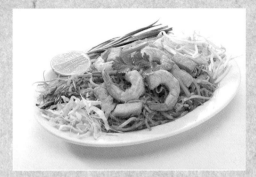

Plate 13. Tao Garden Fried Noodles
(Pad Thai) (cell builder)

Plate 14. Healthful salad (cleansing)

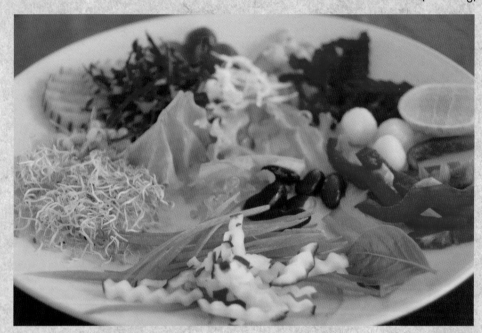

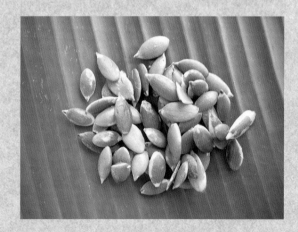

Plate 15. Pumpkin seeds

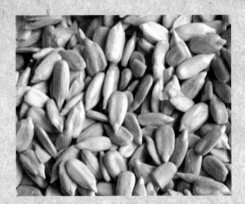

Plate 16. Sunflower seeds

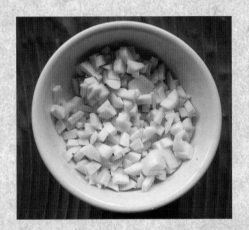

Plate 17. Garlic

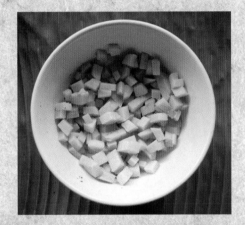

Plate 18. Ginger

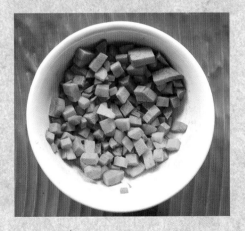

Plate 19. Turmeric root

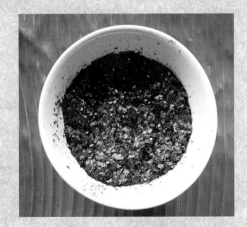

Plate 20. Dried seaweed
and sesame seeds

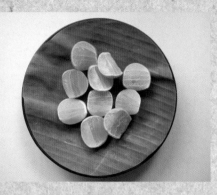

Plate 21. Limes

Plate 22. Tao Garden Mung Beans
(Thua Khiaw Tom Nam Taan)

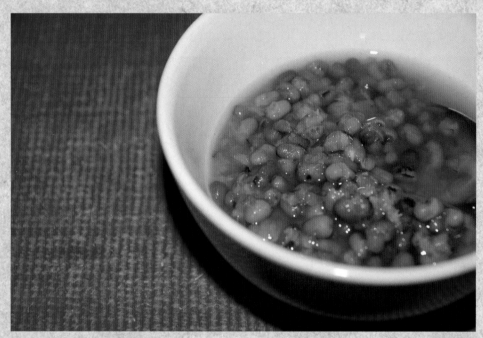

Plate 23. Tao Garden
Rice Balls in Coconut
Milk (Bualoi)

Manganese (Nerve Controller Mineral)

A thought coordinator, manganese increases mental and nerve force, aids quick recuperation, and improves memory. It feeds the brain and nerves and increases resistance to disease. It is the mineral that controls the emotions and affections, giving social poise, confidence, and steady nerves. It also imparts to the body elasticity and fast recuperative ability. Lack of manganese causes confusion and scatterbrained activity in work, studies, and love. It can lead to nerve disorders if deficient too long.

Food Sources of Manganese: Almonds, walnuts, endive, wintergreen, raw egg yolk, prunes, peppermint tea, parsley, pine nuts, rye meal, sun-dried fruits, and greens.

Potassium (Strengthener Mineral)

Potassium nourishes, giving health, strength, and quick recuperative powers. It puts fire and zip into the body. It reduces pain and regulates the brain and body. It promotes elastic and supple muscles and creates grace, beauty, and good disposition. It helps to prevent constipation. It activates the liver and is alkaline to the body. It aids the tissues and internal secretions. Stress depletes the potassium in the body and this leads to an acid condition. People on the go need potassium. It helps to control temper. Get your share of this magic mineral daily.

Food Sources of Potassium: Potato skin, almonds, parsley, watercress, carrots, berries, cherries, figs, grapes, lemons, olives, alfalfa, cucumber, dandelion, sage, dill, lettuce, peaches, oranges, and tropical fruits.

Fluorine (Beautifier and Youth Mineral)

Fluorine protects against sickness, knits bones, aids teeth enamel, and strengthens tendons. As the youth element, it gives you strong mental powers and keeps you elastic. It works with calcium to build strong tooth enamel, bone structure, hair, and elastic tissues. Fluorine is the rejuvenation mineral and helps to keep you young. It improves the eyes, hair, and nails. The lack of fluorine causes premature old age, fear, hair loss, brain and body fatigue, tuberculosis, paralysis, and a run down condition.

Food Sources of Fluorine: Raw goat milk and cheese, spinach, cress, garlic, oats, greens, beets, wheat, brussels sprouts, cabbage, and cauliflower.

Oxygen (Life-Giving Mineral)

Oxygen is primarily found in the air. Mountain and ocean air is the purest type available. City air is polluted and its oxygen is full of chemicals. Pure oxygen gives us brain and body stimulation. Oxygen comprises over half our body weight. Normal breathing is not enough. We must get out into the fresh air, exercise, and expand our chest to its fullest capacity with the life-giving oxygen. Fresh oxygen helps to digest our food. It purifies the bloodstream and cleans out the lungs. It is necessary for the metabolism and all processes of the body. Oxygen makes us happy, buoyant, and fresh. Lack of it causes depression, anemia, low energy, and a hopeless outlook on life.

Food Sources of Oxygen: Pure water, all fresh fruits, vegetables, juices, and pure outside air.

Carbon (Body Heater Mineral)

One fifth of the body is composed of carbon. Only so much carbon is needed by the body. Too much can break down the liver and cause disease. Carbon is the fuel and heater for the body. Carbon is mostly found in fats, which yield 4,040 calories per pound, while carbohydrates furnish only 1,820 calories per pound. Fats are composed of about 76 percent carbon, 12 percent hydrogen, and 12 percent oxygen. After digestion, fats are absorbed and then oxidized to produce energy, carbon dioxide, and water. Eaten to excess, fats may be stored as body fat or converted into carbohydrates and stored as glycogen. Lack of carbon may cause coldness, forgetfulness, laziness, fear, brain deficiency, and overall lack of energy. White flour products, white sugar, lard, fatty animal foods, and fried foods are dangerous to life and health.

Food Sources of Carbon: Rice bran, oats, corn, millet, cheese, butter, egg yolk, goat milk, avocado, pure vegetable oils, nuts, rye, wheat bran, barley, pecans, brazil nuts, walnuts, peanuts, and coconuts.

Nitrogen (Muscle Builder Mineral)

Nitrogen is mainly found in the form of protein, which is composed of carbon, oxygen, hydrogen, sulfur, and nitrogen. Nitrogen furnishes building material to keep the cells and tissues together. In the construction of the protein molecules of plants, nitrogen is absorbed from the soil in soluble forms, as compounds of nitrates and ammonium salts, which are converted first into amino acids and then into protein. The body takes up this protein and converts it into amino acids for the promotion of growth, life, health, and vitality. This is known as the nitrogen cycle, and all plant and animal life is dependent upon it for existence. The atmosphere is 75 percent nitrogen, with oxygen, carbon, and hydrogen composing the balance. We could not breathe or live on 100 percent pure oxygen without the other three elements. Nitrogen keeps the oxygen from burning up in the body.

Food Sources of Nitrogen: Nuts, seeds, legumes, milk, eggs, whole grains, cheese, and all other foods high in protein.

Hydrogen (Cooling Mineral)

Hydrogen maintains body coolness and body temperature. It is the youth mineral that helps to overcome inflammation and pain. It also flushes the inner organs of toxins and waste matter. It is involved in the nitrogen cycle of plants and animals. It is located in the atmosphere and fresh foods.

Food Sources of Hydrogen: Fresh fruits and vegetables, lettuce, tomatoes, celery, juices, cucumber, water, and all foods with a liquid content.

Trace Minerals

Copper, zinc, cobalt, selenium, and over twenty-eight other trace minerals are found in the body. Even though they are found in very small quantities, they are vitally important and as necessary to your health and well-being as the sixteen primary magic minerals. These trace elements are found in all plant life.

Zinc

Zinc is found in the hair, nails, bones, liver, skin, glands, kidneys, and the prostate gland. It increases blood production in weak areas. Wounds heal faster with zinc, and it can act as an antidote to certain poisons. Zinc deficiencies cause diabetes, retardation, schizophrenia, fatigue, infection, and poor skin. If you have white spots on your fingernails, you have a zinc deficiency.

Food Sources of Zinc: Apricots, nutritional yeast, nuts, pumpkin and sunflower seeds, wheat germ, egg yolk, soybeans, spinach, and mushrooms.

Copper

Copper assists in forming rich red blood cells. It prevents anemia, builds the bones and circulatory system, heals the body, and improves the hair and skin. Lack of copper causes weakness, skin trouble, poor respiration, baldness, and fatigue.

Food Sources of Copper: Nuts, raisins, molasses, soybeans, legumes, apricots, dark fruits and juices.

Cobalt

Cobalt is needed in small amounts only. It assists the absorption of vitamin B_{12} in the body. It is contained in a variety of natural foods listed under the other minerals.

Selenium

Small amounts of selenium are needed. It functions similar to vitamin E in the system. It is located in small traces in seawater and is contained in all natural foods.

VITAMINS FOR VITALITY

Vitamins were discovered by Dr. Casmir Funk about one hundred years ago. The word *vitamin* comes from the Latin word *vita*, which means "life," and *amines* refers to "amino acids" (because vitamins were originally thought to contain amino acids). Vitamins are those atomically small sparks of food energy that carry on the process of metabolism:

the activation, assimilation, and utilization of minerals, fats, carbohydrates, trace elements, and other nutritional factors in our food. They seem to offer the kick to the minerals that enter our bodies. They are little invisible helpers ready to right every wrong that may come about in the complicated processes of building and maintaining a perfect body.

Vitamins keep the fires of life aglow. They secretly control the internal chemical process, converting food into blood, tissue, and dynamic energy. The body needs vitamins from outside sources and they must be eaten daily, for it cannot store them.

All earthly life forms are created and sustained by the process of photosynthesis (involving air, light, and water). Through this process nature manufactures the organic vitamins, mineral salts, and enzymes in plant life (in the form of fruits, vegetables, seeds, nuts, and sea vegetation). Plant life is the number one source of nutriment for all beings and creatures on this planet. Natural foods contain all the vitamins that have been discovered and will be discovered. Scurvy, pellagra, beriberi, rickets, and similar diseases are caused by vitamin deficiencies. Cheat the body of vitamin-rich food and you are on a disease-producing diet.

Nature makes no artificial substitutes for vitamins and minerals. No other substances can take their place in human and animal chemistry. We need them in abundance daily, in whole food form and in natural food supplement form, to assure adequate and complete nutrition. The difference between synthetic and natural vitamins may be the difference between disease and health. Synthetic vitamins and minerals are inorganic chemical substances and cannot be utilized by the cells and tissues of the body. The chemist will never produce a single blade of grass, yet the body can assimilate and utilize that blade of grass, while rejecting the chemist's synthetic formula.

Vitamins are classified by the materials in which they will dissolve: either water or fats. Fat-soluble vitamins are absorbed into the bloodstream through the intestinal tract with the help of lipids (fats). Excesses of these vitamins are stored in the body. Because they are stored, they are not needed every day in the diet. Water-soluble vitamins dissolve easily in water and, in general, are readily excreted from the body. Because they are not readily stored, we need a continuous supply of them in our diets.

Vitamin A (Fat-Soluble)

Vitamin A is necessary for night vision and builds resistance to colds, especially lung and sinus trouble. It helps conditions of acne, colds, allergies, eczema, diabetes, stress, and arthritis. It increases growth and blood quality with the help of B complex, vitamins C, D, E, F, calcium, phosphorus, and zinc. Lack of this vitamin may cause night blindness, poor eyesight, rough skin, infections, dry hair, and fatigue. Stress and strain will quickly use up vitamin A. It is destroyed by high heat in the presence of oxygen. The recommended daily allowance (RDA) is 5,000 to 25,000 International Units (IU) daily. A glass of fresh carrot juice contains 9,000 to 12,000 units.

Food Sources of Vitamin A: Alfalfa, green vegetables, carrots, tomatoes, apricots, cherries, egg yolk, papaya.

Vitamin B Complex (Water-Soluble)

The B complex family consists of the following B vitamins: B_1 (thiamine), B_2 (riboflavin), B_6 (pyridoxine), B_{12} (cobalamin), biotin, choline, folic acid, inositol, B_3 (niacin or niacinamide), pantothenic acid, para-aminobenzoic acid and pangamic acid. The first three of these vitamins are the most important: they are active in enzyme production; they calm the nervous system; they improve the digestive tract, skin, nerves, eyes, and liver, as well as the absorption of food. Together the B vitamins help metabolize fats, starches, and proteins; reduce blood cholesterol; increase appetite; increase cell life; build rich red blood; prevent gray hair; promote sex hormone production; control weight; maintain the sodium-potassium balance of the body and nerves; aid circulation of blood and lymph; improve friendly bacteria activity in the digestive tract; and help depression, insomnia, fatigue, heart disease, and gland and nerve disorders. They also overcome anemia, skin disorders, acne, dizziness, irritability, learning disabilities, weakness, and hair loss. Under stress conditions and anemic conditions the body needs extra amounts of the entire B complex of vitamins. For a calm disposition and steady nerves, grains, fruits, vegetables, seeds, and nuts will provide the essential nutrients to overcome stress.

Food Sources of Vitamin B Complex: Nutritional yeast, wheat germ, whole grains, egg yolks, brown rice, sunflower, pumpkin and sesame seeds, mushrooms, brown rice polishings, beans, buckwheat, lentils, peas, spinach, walnuts, goat milk, asparagus, tomatoes, green juices, berries, rye, wheat, almonds. These foods eaten in moderate daily quantities will supply all the B complex required.

Vitamin C (Water-Soluble)

This vitamin is essential for tissue respiration, improves appetite, builds capillary walls and connective tissue, gums, heart, skin, teeth, and bones. It is good for colds, shock, infection, and tooth decay. It improves anemia, bleeding gums, cavities, poor digestion, and tissue damage. Vitamin C works best with all vitamins and minerals, particularly calcium, magnesium, and bioflavonoids. It is destroyed by high heat, antibiotics, aspirin, tobacco, fever, stress, cortisone, and other drugs.

Food Sources of Vitamin C: Citrus fruits, all berries, green peppers, tomatoes, currants, cress, cabbage, apples, green vegetable juices, papaya, melons, lettuce, peas, and pineapple. It is not stored in the body and must be supplied daily. Fruits and vegetables eaten in season and grown locally will meet your daily vitamin C requirements. Rosehip powder can be used to supplement your diet with extra C.

Vitamin D (Fat-Soluble)

Vitamin D helps the absorption of calcium and phosphorus and is a good bone builder. It controls mineral metabolism. It favors good posture, bone growth, and tooth development, and fights fatigue, caries, nerve disorder, infections, poor skin tone, rickets, and constipation. Heat or oxidation does not affect this vitamin. A limited amount of vitamin D is stored in the body. The greatest source is from the sun. When the skin is exposed to sunlight, the ultraviolet rays change the ergosterol in the skin into small amounts of vitamin D.

Food Sources of Vitamin D: Fruit and vegetables grown in the sunshine and their juices, butter, chlorophyll, goat milk, and plenty of solar light. Crude mineral oil destroys vitamin D in the body. Daily amount should be from 500 to 1,000 IU.

Vitamin E (Tocopherol, Fat-Soluble)

An adequate supply of vitamin E helps to retard aging, controls blood cholesterol, tones muscles and nerves, keeps the blood from clotting, protects the lungs from pollution, increases male and female fertility and potency, and strengthens blood vessels, arteries, and veins. It fosters healthy skin and reduces abnormal hair growth on women. It is good for lactation, menstrual disorders, miscarriage, and reproduction. Deficiencies of vitamin E can cause sterility, loss of vitality and virility, lack of courage, pessimism, and impaired mentation. It improves blood vessel and heart function. It builds the nerves and promotes pituitary gland activity. It is not affected by heat or oxidation. The body stores a limited supply of vitamin E.

Food Sources of Vitamin E: All whole grain foods, green vegetables, wheat germ, olive oil, corn, most fruits, cottage cheese, goat milk, soybeans, tomatoes, egg yolks, and oats. Vitamin E oil can be used topically for burns, wounds, warts, and scars with good results. Vitamin E is destroyed by birth control pills, tap water, crude mineral oil, and hard fat.

Vitamin F (Unsaturated Fatty Acids, Fat-Soluble)

Vitamin F prevents stiff joints and hardened arteries. It controls blood cholesterol and improves blood pressure and glandular activity. It helps functioning of adrenal and thyroid glands. It calms the nerves and beautifies the skin. Lack of vitamin F causes acne, gallstones, diarrhea, allergies, poor nails and hair, underweight, and varicose veins; it results in stunted growth, poor sexual development, and loss of appetite. Excessive heat destroys vitamin F. Radiation and x-rays harm this vitamin in the body.

Food Sources of Vitamin F: Nutritional yeast, spinach, fruits, all seeds and nuts, egg yolks, wheat germ, olive oil, sunflower oil, whole grains, orange juice, and root vegetables. An adequate supply from these foods should be eaten in moderation.

Vitamin K (Menadione, Fat-Soluble)

Vitamin K improves the blood-clotting system and can be used for hemorrhages, menstrual problems, and bruising. Lack of vitamin K causes nosebleeds, diarrhea, tendency to hemorrhage, and possible miscarriages. X-rays, radiation, drugs, hard oils, and fats destroy this vitamin.

Food Sources of Vitamin K: Blackstrap molasses, yogurt, safflower oil, green juices and vegetables, oats, tomatoes, green peas, carrots, cauliflower, and spinach. One to two milligrams per day are enough.

Vitamin P (Bioflavonoids, Water-Soluble)

Bioflavonoids build and maintain the blood, connective tissues, skin, gums, bones, teeth, and capillary walls. Good for cold sores, colds, and the flu.

Food Sources of Vitamin P: Cherries, apricots, grapes, grapefruit, lemons, plums, and the inner skins of most fruits.

WHOLE FOOD SUPPLEMENTS

Our first obligation to ourselves and our families should be to obtain the highest quality food grown locally, prepared in a nutritionally healthful manner, and also, if conditions permit, to grow as many organic foods as possible in our own backyard garden. If we all had our own gardens on well-mineralized fertile soil, food supplements might not be needed. If we ate foods that were not overprocessed and overmilled, the capsule might never have been invented.

Under ideal conditions, food supplements would not be needed. But what are those ideal conditions? They are: 1) all foods are grown in rich, natural, organically fertilized soils year round; 2) these organically grown foods are available and raised in your locality; and 3) you are living in a totally stress-free, natural, and unpolluted environment. Are you living in this naturally perfect environment? Are you obtaining all your food from such organically rich soil? Are you eating the organic food grown in your locality, not shipped from across the country? Are you living and working outdoors daily in natural light, and without stress conditions? Do you spend hours each day in the outdoor atmosphere? Do you obtain sufficient exercise? The majority of individuals cannot answer yes to most of these questions. If you are one of them, you can tremendously benefit from the daily use of natural whole food supplements and organic food concentrates, which furnish the missing organic minerals, vitamins, and trace elements required by every cell of the body.

There are those who would have the Western public believe that present-day foods are adequate in their vitamin and mineral content and that vitamin deficiency diseases and subclinical deficiencies are too rare to be a threat to public health. However, most Americans are poorly nourished and consume nutritionally poor food. If sixty times as much mineral values were not taken each year from the soil as are restored to it in fertilizer, and if in some households up to 77 percent of the mineral values were not lost or destroyed by heat and oxidation, we would not require the use of food supplements. In addition, hereditary factors also play an important part in your overall health and nutritional needs. If your parents were in poor health and consumed mineral-deficient foods, you may require more food supplements than a person who had parents with strong and healthy constitutions and ate mineral-rich and nutrition-ally superior organic foods.

We each must judge our own nutritional needs and eat the whole foods and food supplements that fulfill the requirements of our totally individual body. If you constantly crave junk foods, a dietary deficiency may be present and you may be severely in need of a balanced dietary program, plus whole food supplements. Nutrition-rich food concentrates can help you to overcome the junk-food syndrome and protect against any possible deficiencies from the use of commercially grown foods that are poor in minerals.

Food supplements should not be taken with the erroneous idea that they will give you super health while you continue living on a diet of conventional calamity foods. They will, however, add some improvement to the conventional Western diet. The following food supplements are some of the best-known health aids to assure us of obtaining complete nutrition for superior health.

Alfalfa (Liquid, Tablets, or Powder)

This amazing plant travels twenty-four feet into the soil and picks up the trace minerals so lacking in the average person. Alfalfa grown on organic soil and made into liquid, tablet, powder, or tea can be used with great benefit by all persons, healthy or sick. The ancients knew its value, yet the ancient learning was forgotten. For centuries sick farmers watched their cattle grow sleek and robust on alfalfa without the glimmer of an idea that this remarkable plant might help them. Even today, when food scientists cite the countless cases of benefits achieved by the use of alfalfa, the uninformed raise skeptical eyebrows.

It may be a generation before most of our physicians and the general public wake up and grasp the truth about the place of alfalfa in human nutrition. The same opinion was voiced by C. H. Burgess of the Michigan State Agricultural College, who said: "Rich in medicinal properties beneficial to the human race, the real value of alfalfa is but little known." But evidence now shows beyond dispute that alfalfa has more total food minerals and trace elements than any other known plant that grows on land. The famed farmer-writer Louis Bromfield spoke of alfalfa's unique ability to tap the deep mineral richness of soil and to bring that richness upward to the sunlight and the air.

Alfalfa closely approximates the blood hemoglobin and is one of the most highly potent vitamin and mineral foods. It is rich in protein and contains every essential amino acid. It also contains eight essential enzymes, which help in the buildup of the internal bodily enzymes.

Lipase is the fat-splitting enzyme.
Amylase acts upon starches.
Coagulase coagulates milk and clots the blood.
Emulsin acts upon sugar.
Invertase converts cane sugar into dextrose.
Peroxidase has an oxidizing effect on the blood.
Pectinase forms a vegetable jelly from a pectin substance.
Protase digests protein.

Alfalfa contains vitamin U, an element that is an aid for peptic ulcers. It improves digestion and a lagging appetite and is a good diuretic and excellent regulator of the bowels. It has sufficient vitamin D and phosphorus to build strong bones and teeth. Alfalfa has vitamin K, flavones, growth and antistiffness factors. This remarkable product helps to prevent fatigue and provides a perfect calcium-phosphorus ratio (2:1). The pure vegetarian or vegan who uses no dairy products will be happy to know that alfalfa has 0.3 mg of vitamin B_{12} per 100 grams.

Nutritional Yeast

The ancient Egyptians are said to have used yeast, and it has been used for baking, brewing, and other uses throughout history. "Yeast is the smallest of all cultivated plants, about 1/4000th of an inch in diameter or about the size of a human blood corpuscle," notes *The Complete Book of Food and Nutrition*, edited by J. I. Rodale. Rodale continues:

> The yeast plant stores enormous quantities of vitamins for its own use. These are then utilized as a food supplement by human beings, after the yeast plant is dried. Brewer's Yeast contains all the elements of the Vitamin B complex. It is also a rich source of complete protein. Brewer's Yeast contains 16 of the 20 amino acids forms of protein that are essential for the proper functioning of our bodies for longevity, for resistance to disease, for rebuilding tissues.

Many years ago, yeast as a supplement was available only as a by-product of the beer vat, but today "Brewer's Yeast" from beer breweries is a thing of the past. The correct name for what is now available is "primary grown nutritional yeast." Yeast is a miniature sprout of high nutritional value, and it is dried in such a manner as to preserve its wealth of nutrients. The yeast cell is a terrifically small unit of living matter, similar to the cells of the human body. Nutritional yeast, which is grown without soil, has a very pleasant taste and is higher in nutritional value than the old time Brewer's Yeast. (However, yeast cakes used for baking bread should not be eaten raw, as they rob the body of B vitamins.)

Many health authorities state that yeast contains more nutritional power than any other single food factor. A recent science writer once called the tiny yeast cell a terrific chemical factory for the manufacture of all the vitamins of the B complex. Nutritional yeast is reported to contain the nucleic acids RNA and DNA, antiaging and youth-sustaining elements. Laboratory tests have shown that RNA and DNA protect mice and rats against lethal radiation doses. Yeast also contains the amino acids lysine and tryptophan, which may be missing from certain cereal and grain foods.

Due to its high natural B complex factors and minerals, nutritional yeast helps to build strong nerves and calmness under stress and other difficult living conditions. A lack of the essential B vitamins results in nerve disorders, irritability, depression, fatigue, skin problems, muscular weakness, and underweight conditions. Nutritional yeast can put an end to the junk-food syndrome once and for all. It is rich in essential super food factors necessary for complete nutrition.

Nutritional yeast can be used in soups, salads, and other dishes to improve the nutritional value of foods. It is available in various concentrated forms in powder, flakes, or tablets. Some people prefer to take yeast mixed in a glass of their favorite juice on an empty stomach, assuring quicker assimilation and no digestive interference with other foods. If yeast causes you gas when eaten with other foods, try this method.

Kelp and Other Seaweed

Scientific tests have shown that seaweed contains over thirty vital mineral elements and life-sustaining organic substances that are absolutely necessary for a high state of health. The body loses these essential minerals daily, and they must be replaced by organic mineral-rich foods such as found in seaweed products. Kelp and dulse are sea plants high in iron and copper, even more so than 1 pound of spinach or 7½ pounds of tomatoes. Kelp contains more phosphorus than 1½ pounds of carrots.

Iodine is necessary for the proper functioning of the thyroid gland, which affects body growth, metabolism, and overall health. Our soils are almost totally lacking in this very essential element. This is why certain sections of the country are known as goiter belts. Kelp is a great source of iodine, even more so than oysters.

Here are a few of the major minerals and trace elements found in kelp:

Nitrogen helps to build and repair the body.
Iodine provides prevention against goiters.

Iron is the blood builder.

Copper together with iron builds the blood and helps the body to absorb oxygen.

Silicon helps to give beautiful sheen to the hair, nails, and skin, prevents wrinkles and sagging skin.

Sodium helps to digest food, purifies the blood, and prevents acidosis.

Sulfur builds the body cells.

Manganese builds the reproductive organs and is necessary for bone formation. It is a protective agent, especially for the heart, blood vessels, brain, and urinary passages.

Zinc helps prevent diabetes and prostate problems.

Kelp, dulse, or other seaweed foods such as hijiki and nori can be purchased in dried, powdered, or liquid form. You can eat them whole, chew the tablets, add the liquid to soups, or sprinkle the powder over your favorite vegetable salads and grain meals. Kelp is a yang food and can be consumed year around. Be sure to include kelp in your daily diet for better health and long life.

Spirulina Plankton

Spirulina plankton is a microalgae, like hijiki, nori, and wakame. It grows in lakes and salt water, but the best spirulina is said to come from fresh water ponds. The Aztecs ate spirulina with corn and millet more than four hundred years ago. Spirulina plankton is the most basic food in the whole food chain. It is a simple hydrocarbon made directly from photosynthesis, the interaction of sunlight and water.

Spirulina is the most concentrated form of any known organic food: a complete protein containing eighteen of the twenty-two known amino acids (the building blocks for living cells), including the eight essential amino acids. Spirulina is twenty times as high in protein as soybeans, forty times as high as corn, four times as high as beef. Spirulina has incredibly long strings of amino acids of several kinds. The proteins of spirulina are 80 to 85 percent assimilated compared to 20 percent for beef protein. Spirulina contains the biologically active sugar rhamnose.

Spirulina contains the highest natural known source of vitamin B_{12}, as well as many other vitamins, and all the cell salts and enzymes essential for body metabolism. The nutrients in spirulina are up to 95 percent digestible. Spirulina is also helpful in removing radioactive agents and other pollutive metals from the body. As spirulina is low in the amino acid methionine, so other grains, beans, and seeds should be eaten at the same meal or during the day to make up the loss. One tablespoon of spirulina contains:

6 to 7 grams of protein
35% of the RDA for vitamin B_1; 25% of B_2; 6% of B_3
90% of carotene (provitamin A)
10% of vitamin E
29% of iron
Small % of trace vitamins, minerals, and enzymes

Spirulina is mass-produced in two locations: Lake Texcoco in Mexico and Thailand. Spirulina can be purchased in tablet, powder, or liquid form. There is a new pasta on the market made with spirulina—pastalina—a combination of wheat, soybeans, and spirulina. It is delicious and highly nutritious.

Calcium (Carrot)

Calcium builds strong teeth, bones, hair, connective tissue, and organic structures. It is one of the most important but difficult to obtain foods in the diet. Calcium is missing from almost all processed, canned, and packaged supermarket foods. A calcium supplement is available, however, which is made from pure fresh raw carrot juice, from carrots grown in highly mineralized soil and then dehydrated into a pure powdered concentrate, which is easily assimilable. One level teaspoonful of carrot calcium supplies 1,000 mg of pure calcium. The body requires from 800–1,000 mg of this important element each day.

Vitamins and Mineral Food Supplements

In addition to the food sources of minerals and vitamins listed above, the following supplements derived from natural foods are also good sources:

1. Alfalfa liquid, powder, or tablets: 2 teaspoonfuls or 3–5 tablets daily.
2. Nutritional yeast (B complex and protein source): 2–4 tablespoons daily.
3. Wheat germ oil or flakes (vitamin E, protein, B complex, minerals): 2–4 tablespoons daily of flakes. Must be fresh.
4. Sea kelp or dulse (high in iodine, trace minerals): 3–5 tablets or 1 teaspoon daily. Use in salads and cooking.
5. Pure rosehip powder (high in vitamin C, bioflavonoids, and enzymes): 1 teaspoon.
6. Pure cold-pressed vegetable oils, such as sesame, sunflower, or safflower (high in unsaturated fatty acids): no more than 1 tablespoon in summer and 2 in winter.
7. Rice polishings (high in B complex and minerals): 2 teaspoons daily.
8. Fresh squeezed vegetable juices (vitamins, minerals, and enzymes): 4–8 ounces in summer; less in winter.
9. Spirulina plankton (high in vitamins, minerals, enzymes, and protein): 2–4 tablets, or 2 teaspoons daily. Protects against radioactive agents.
10. Powdered carrot calcium (Dr. Bronner) (high in calcium and minerals): 1 teaspoon daily.

Miso

Miso is a dark paste made from fermented soybeans and other grains. Miso broth aids digestion and food absorption, it helps to alkalize the system, and balances the metabolism. Miso is also a protein source. It can be sipped slowly on cold winter days to keep one warm and cozy on the inside. Miso is a healthful salt substitute, which can be used in soups, bean and grain dishes, casseroles, and wherever a salty flavor is required in cooking. Miso is one of the best sources of iron and vitamin B_{12}. Due to its fermented quality, miso builds up the intestinal flora and helps to overcome anemia.

The three types of miso are: *kome*, made from soybeans and rice; *mugi*, made of barley and soybeans; and *hacho*, made with soybeans only. Miso is aged in wooden barrels from three to eighteen months, depending on the type. Hacho miso should be used more in winter due to its yang quality. Mugi or kome miso can be used moderately in the summer.

Soy Sauce

Soy sauce is a close kin to miso; it is also fermented and made from soybeans with the addition of sea salt, wheat, and water. It contains easily absorbed proteins, vitamins, and minerals. Soy sauce can be used in soups, vegetables, and grain dishes.

Tofu

Tofu is a soybean product with a consistency of farmer's or pot cheese. It is a very delicious, nutritious, protein-packed food. It contains all of the amino acids necessary for healthy growth. Tofu can be used in soups, salads, sandwich spreads, grain dishes, and bean and vegetable stews. It contains vitamin B_{12} and builds friendly intestinal bacteria, due to its fermented quality.

Beet Juice (Tablets or Powder)

Beets are a powerful blood builder, with a high and easily assimilable iron content. Beets contain several digestive enzymes. They are used in diabetic disorders. Beets should be used only in small amounts because they may overwork the liver if overeaten.

Garlic

Garlic has been used successfully for high blood pressure, intestinal problems, colds, flu, and lung disorders. Garlic is also a powerful internal germicide and bactericide, which keeps the system free from pathogenic or cancer-causing agents. Garlic is used by all of the long-lived people throughout the world. However, garlic should not be used excessively every day, as the body will begin to emit a garlic odor in public, and one may chase away more than colds. Also, Chinese herbalists caution against the use of garlic and sweets at the same time, as this mixture can cause nausea and indigestion.

Balanced Mineral Salt

Balanced mineral salt is a seasoning vegetable powder to be used in place of salt. It contains a balanced proportion of minerals and trace elements, such as powdered soybeans, anise seed, calcium-magnesium phosphate, dulse, parsley, lecithin, vitamin C, rosehips, thyme, and other dried vegetable ingredients. It can be used on all main dishes, grains, beans, vegetable stews, and soups. It is very delicious and nutritious.

Umeboshi (Salted) Plum

Umeboshi plums are pickled in salt for about two years, by an acid bacterial method. They have been used for centuries in Japan as a mainstay in cooking. They are used in main dishes and dressings and take the place of vinegar. They are especially delicious with rice and other grains. They help to alkalize the system. They are used as remedies for stomach trouble, headaches, and internal acidity, as they aid the digestion and assimilation of food. They also help in cases of dysentery and fatigue.

HERBS: ELIXIRS OF LIFE

Herbs have been used as life-givers and healers since the beginning of time. The ancient Egyptians, Greeks, Lemurians, and Chinese studied herbs systematically, and they respected the powerful rejuvenating qualities of nature's healing plants. Moses taught the Israelites to subsist on

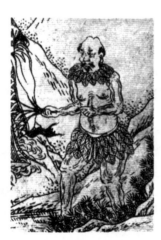

Fig. 5.2. Red Emperor Shen-Neng, patron saint of Chinese herbalism

natural simple foods and to use the herbs of the field for disease. Paul recommended the consumption of herbs for fatigue and sickness. The best biblical argument for the use of natural foods and herbs is found in Genesis 1:29, which states: "And God said, Behold, I have given you every herb bearing seed, which is upon the face of all the earth, and every tree in which is the fruit of a tree yielding seed; to you it shall be for meat."

The early Native Americans were well-versed in the use of herbs and plants. They were seldom sick, always full of vitality, stamina, endurance, and fighting force. Our first colonists learned many things from the Native Americans, including the use of herbs in the treatment of disease and maintaining vigorous health.

Hippocrates, who lived some 2,500 years ago, was known as the Father of Medicine. He taught moderation in all things. Hippocrates said: "The body has within itself the power to heal," and he used the constructive properties of herbs to facilitate the healing. He had a working knowledge of more than four hundred various herbs. He was a true physician. Interestingly, the word *physician* is derived from *physics*, a Greek word for "nature." So, Hippocrates was a "doctor of nature."

About 1500 CE, Philippus von Hohenheim (Paracelsus) began using inorganic chemicals to treat disease. He and the medical men that followed him believed that the body could be healed and purified chemically. They wanted full power over the lives of sick people, to administer chemicals in place of herbs. They burned the books of Hippocrates and Galen in public, for they wanted no competition from the natural methods of healing. Hohenheim was the first practitioner to give mercury as a medicine. He who for an ordinary cause resigns the fate of his patient to mercury is a vile enemy to the sick. The true successors and pupils of Galen and Hippocrates are the herbal doctors of Great Britain, whereas Hohenheim's successors are today's modern medical profession.

Dr. Otto Mausert states that: "Chemistry of today has accomplished wonderful results in many ways, but all the laboratories in the world will never be able to supplant the remarkably fine process which takes place in the living cell. They will never successfully imitate the wonderful methods that Nature uses in performing its work in the plant, as well as in the human body." The great American inventor Thomas A. Edison once wrote: "Until man duplicates a blade of grass, Nature can laugh at his so-called scientific knowledge."

Drugs versus Plant Herbs

The list of drug-induced diseases is growing every year. About 20 percent of the drugs in vogue twenty years ago are now listed as harmful, yet many were considered wonder-drug discoveries. The AMA admits there is always a great risk in drugging a person. Chloromycetin, for example, is toxic to the blood-producing system. Modern medical drugs are powerful chemical agents; most of them are yin/expanding in action, while a few are yang/contractive in quality. The yin drugs expand the brain and body cells, causing the patient to lose sight of reality, that is, to experience grogginess, loss of will, and unclear thinking and perception. Hospitals and clinics are full of pickled brains and bodies.

The average person takes very good care of a new car. It must be perfect in every respect. The owner has it checked every few months to ensure that it runs like new. He would not think of putting sand or water in the gas tank! The best grade of gas and oil must go into that car, and it must have the best possible maintenance and care available at all costs. And the auto mechanic must fix it right, or the owner does not pay him. Yet the average person blindly accepts, without a word of objection, a dose of some medicine, tablet, or drug, without thinking of what it might do to his or her body. Or harmful serums and vaccines are injected into the bloodstream without a whimper or question from the person as to what the substance is or what value or harm it will do.

Herbs, on the other hand, are natural remedies found in all parts of the world. Their use has become a lost art, but, fortunately, they are again gaining in popularity and usage by intelligent and advanced-thinking physicians. Herb teas assist nature in purifying the body, while chemical medicines squelch the symptoms and drive the disease deeper into the body. Herbs and natural foods are more beneficial in the long run to restore and maintain health indefinitely. Even modern medicines that are alkaloid chemicals taken from plants do not contain the same health-building and restoring properties as herb teas made from the original plant. In addition, iatrogenic diseases (drug induced) side-effects are often far more harmful than the original sickness. This is the result of direct drug interference with the body's own natural healing powers.

HEALTH AID GUIDE

FOODS TO AVOID	REPLACEMENTS
Tea, coffee, alcohol, sodas, tap water	Herbal teas
Chocolate, candy, artificial sweets	Dried or fresh fruit, honey
Gelatin	Agar
Canned bouillon, meat broths	Vegetable broth, miso
Cold drinks, sodas, sugared beverages	Fresh fruit and vegetable juice
Tap water	Spring, distilled, or pure water
Devitalized commercial sugared cereals	Whole grain cereals
White commercial crackers and snacks	Whole grain rye, corn, and wheat snacks
White bread	100% whole wheat, rye breads
Lard, margarine, butter	Sesame, tahini sauce, seed butters
White vinegar, wine vinegar	Lemon juice, apple cider vinegar
Commercial vegetable oils	Cold pressed olive and sunflower oils
White rice, white flour noodles	Whole brown rice, noodles, and pasta
Pasteurized cow's milk and cheeses and other dairy foods	Raw cow's or goat's milk, yogurt, tofu, soy milk, seed and nut milks
Salted, roasted seeds and nuts	Raw soaked seeds and nuts
White flour pastries	Whole grain baked pastries
Meat, fish, fowl, eggs	Seeds, grains, legumes, nuts
Common salt, pepper, condiments	Kelp, dulse, thyme, parsley, ginger
Spices, mustard	Vegetable seasoning, tamari, sea salt
Baking powder	Nutritional yeast, wheat germ
Food thickening agents (eggs, gelatin)	Arrowroot, agar, seaweed

In his book *Herb Growing for Health,* Dr. Donald Law writes:

The whole theory of botanic medicine is based upon the logical and simple practice of building up the human body to strengthen all the natural eliminating and healing processes . . . Botanic medicine does not seek to cure you by "killing off germs," it strengthens your natural functions of phagocyte production (the little cells that eat up alien organisms invading your body); it strengthens your liver and kidneys to do their clearing out functions better, and it makes defecation and perspiration function efficiently so as to expel the toxic matter you have acquired.

Another intelligent author, Dr. Otto Mausert, writing in his book *Herbs for Health,* states: "Herbs contain the vital elements, vitamins and organic minerals that are deficient or lacking in the diseased body. They contain them in such a finely distributed and prepared state that they may be readily assimilated by the system and conveyed to the blood. Herbs also promote the elimination of waste matter and poisons from the system by simple, natural means. When correctly used, they support nature in the fight against disease."

It is the opinion of those who best understand the physical system that if the physical laws were strictly observed from generation to generation, there would be an end to the frightful diseases that cut life short, and make life a torment or a trial. The more you know the less you know but the more you become.

Health Wisdom of Benjamin Franklin

- To lengthen your life, lessen your meals.
- I saw few die of hunger; of eating, 100,000.
- Eat to live, and not live to eat.
- A full belly makes a dull brain.
- Hold your council before dinner; the full belly hates thinking as well as acting.
- He that never eats too much will never be lazy.
- Eat few suppers, and you will need few medicines.
- Many dishes, many diseases; many medicines, few cures.

- Hunger is the best pickle.
- To live long it is necessary to live slowly.
- Wish not so much to live long, as to live well.
- Keep out of the sight of feasts and banquets as much as possible.
- If a man casually exceeds (overeats), let him fast the next meal, and all may be well again.
- A temperate diet frees from diseases and illnesses.
- Early to bed and early to rise, makes a man healthy, wealthy, and wise.
- A sober diet makes a man vigorous; it preserves the memory and helps the understanding; it makes the body a fit tabernacle of the Lord to dwell in.
- Drink does not drown care but waters it and makes it grow faster.
- He is the best physician that knows the worthlessness of most medicines.
- Health is not lost by accident, nor can it be repurchased at the drug store. It is lost by physiological errors and can be regained only by erring no more.
- Disease is nature's protest against a gross violation of her laws. The reward for service is more service.

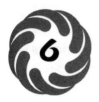

The Five Elements of Life

The cycles of yin and yang that evolve from the eternal Tao or creative force of the universe produce the five elements—wood, fire, earth, metal (air), and water, which in turn produce all other physical phenomena. The five elements are not only expressed as physical reality but are more intimately associated with the energy they express in their formation. The universe is the macrocosm of which humans are the microcosm; we are made up of these five elements, and we are subject to the interplay

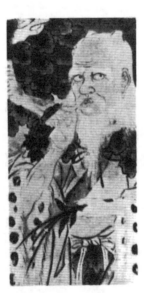

Fig. 6.1. Huang-Ti, the Yellow Emperor

of these five ancient forces, which operate according to natural rhythms, such as seasonal changes, the moon's phases, and astrological changes. They result in variable nutritional needs and psychological patterns, daily, monthly, and yearly.

A theory derived from a deep study of these complex transformations is presented in the *Nei Ching*, attributed to Huang-Ti, the Yellow Emperor, who is respectfully known as the father of Chinese medicine. Subsequent Chinese philosophers and physicians have since contributed material to the *Nei Ching*, which now contains twenty-four books.

The five elements are related to each other both as part of a creation cycle and a destruction or subjugation cycle. The relationships in the five-element creation cycle are as follows:

Wood burns to create fire.
Fire leaves behind ashes and decomposes into earth.
Earth is mined and becomes metal.
Metal when heated and melted becomes molten like water.
Water produces and nourishes trees, plants, and wood.

In the five element destruction (subjugation) cycle:

Wood is cut and felled by metal.
Fire is extinguished by water.
Earth is penetrated by wood.
Metal is dissolved or melted by fire.
Water is halted, absorbed, and obstructed by earth.

Each of the five elements is also associated with a season and a direction and with specific emotions. Each element is associated with a specific organ (which is also linked to a corresponding organ) and each gives birth to a food flavor: wood creates sour, fire creates bitter, earth creates sweet, metal creates a hot (pungent) taste, and water creates a salty flavor. We can live a healthy and harmonious life by applying these universal principles to our everyday needs, whether they are to plant crops, measure our everyday nutritional requirements, use observational diagnostic procedures, or overcome a disease. The figure on the following page diagrams the various energy relationships. These energy transformations

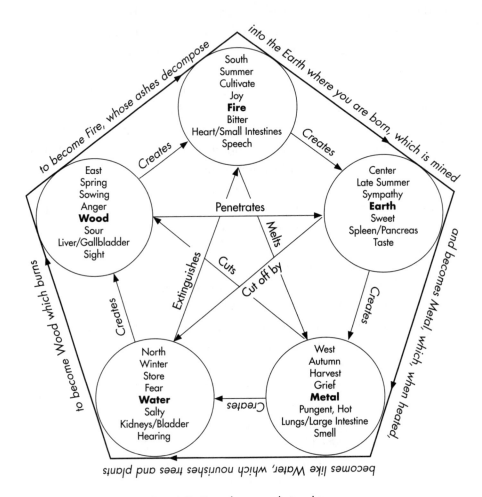

Fig. 6.2. Five-element relationships

are used in Oriental diagnosis, massage, acupuncture, shiatsu, exercise therapy, and dietary considerations.

The *Nei Ching* describes the five elements involved in various relationships, such as the secretions and spiritual resources connected with the internal organs and the effect of climate upon the organs. The five fluid secretions of the body are connected with the major internal organs as follows:

Perspiration is connected with the heart.

Mucus is connected with the lungs.
Tears are connected with the liver.
Saliva is connected with the spleen.
Spittle is connected with the kidneys.

The five major organs have specific interrelationships. Each major organ controls, nourishes, and strengthens other aspects of the body's anatomy, rules over another major organ, and governs its related sensory organ.

Organ-Body Relationships

Heart controls the pulse and rules over the kidneys.
Lungs control the skin and rule over the heart.
Liver controls the muscles and rules over the lungs.
Spleen controls the flesh and rules over the liver.
Kidneys control the bones and rule over the spleen.

Nourishing Organ Body Relationships

The liver nourishes the muscles; the muscles strengthen the heart; the liver governs the eyes.
The heart nourishes the blood; the blood strengthens the stomach; the heart governs the tongue.
The stomach nourishes the flesh; the flesh strengthens the lungs; the stomach governs the mouth.
The lungs nourish the skin and the hair; the skin and the hair strengthen the kidneys; the lungs govern the nose.
The kidneys nourish the bones and the marrow; the bones and the marrow strengthen the liver; the kidneys govern the ears.

The five spiritual resources are controlled by the internal organs.

Liver controls the soul.
Heart controls the spirit.
Spleen controls the ideas.
Lungs control the animal spirit.
Kidneys control the willpower.

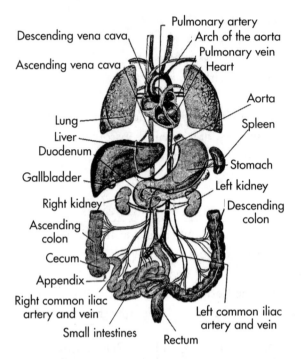

Fig. 6.3. This diagram shows the general position of the five major organs of the trunk in relation to each other. The method by which veins and arteries maintain circulation of the blood is shown also.

The five seasonal climates affect the internal organs as follows:

Heat injures the heart.   Cold/dry injures the lungs.

Wind injures the liver.   Humidity injures the spleen.

Dryness/cold injures the kidneys.

The injuries caused by the climate of one season also impact the body in the following season.

Injuries caused by the cold of winter cause a recurrence of the illness in spring.

Injuries caused by the wind of spring make people unable to retain food in summer.

Injuries caused by the heat of summer cause intermittent fever in fall.

Injuries caused by the humidity of fall cause cough in winter.

The organs are also related to the emotions and moods.

Five Emotions to Organs Relationships

Anger is injurious to liver, but grief counteracts anger.

Excess joy is injurious to heart, but fear counteracts joy.

Excess sympathy is injurious to stomach, but anger counteracts sympathy.

Extreme grief is injurious to lungs, but joy counteracts grief.

Extreme fear is injurious to kidneys, but sympathy overcomes fear.

Five Moods in Relation to the Organs and Daily Time Cycles

People troubled with liver disorders appear mentally alert during the morning hours, are active and bright toward sundown, and of quiet mind at midnight.

People troubled with heart disorders are mentally alert at noontime, active and bright at midnight, and quiet in the early morning.

People troubled with spleen disorders are mentally alert just after sundown, active and bright at sunrise, and are quiet during the afternoon.

People troubled with lung/respiratory disorders are mentally alert just before sundown, active and bright at noon, and are quiet at midnight.

People troubled with kidney disorders are mentally alert at midnight, active and bright during the last days of the four seasons, and are most quiet before sundown.

The five flavors of food to which the five elements give birth have specific effects on the body, which are influenced by the seasons.

Effects of the Five Flavors upon the Body

Excess of salty flavor injures the heart, causes high blood pressure, hardened pulse, and weak bones; tears make their appearance and the complexion changes. It is balanced by a moderate amount of sweet food.

Excess of bitter flavor injures the lungs, withers the skin, and causes body hair to fall out and the stomach to become congested. It is balanced by a moderate amount of salty food.

Excess of pungent flavor injures the liver, knots the muscles, slows the pulse, and causes fingernails and toenails to wither and decay. It is balanced by a moderate amount of bitter food.

CLASSIFICATION OF THE FIVE ELEMENTS
AND TRANSFORMATIONS

	More Yang	Less Yang	Center Yin/Yang	Less Yin	More Yin
Five Elements	Wood	Fire	Earth	Air	Water
Yang Organs	Liver	Heart	Spleen/Pancreas	Lungs	Kidneys
Yin Organs	Gallbladder	Sm. Intestines	Stomach	Lg. Intestine	Bladder
Inner Anatomy	Muscles	Blood Vessels	Flesh	Skin	Bones
Outer Anatomy	Nails	Complexion	Breast/Lips	Hair/Breath	Head Hair
Sense Organ	Eyes	Tongue	Mouth	Nose	Ears
Five Senses	Sight	Speech	Taste	Smell	Hearing
Body Fluids	Tears	Sweat	Saliva	Mucus	Urine
Direction	East	South	Center/Earth	West	North
Climate	Windy	Hot	Humid	Dry	Cold
Seasons	Spring	Summer	Late Summer	Autumn	Winter
Five Sounds	Shouting	Laughing	Singing	Weeping	Groaning
Five Emotions	Anger	Joy	Worry	Depression	Fear
Body Changes	Control	Anxious	Sobbing/Belch	Coughing	Trembling
Creation	Inspiration	Aspiration	Intellect	Dominance	Will
Five Functions	Color	Odor	Taste	Voice	Fluid
Skin Color	Blue/Grey	Red	Yellow/Milky	Pale	Black/Dark
Daily Periods	Morning	Noon	Afternoon	Evening	Night
Weather	Crisp/Dry	Fog/Mist	Mellow	Snow	Ice/Frost
Planet	Jupiter	Mars	Earth/Saturn	Venus	Mercury
Monthly Cycle	(+)Half-Moon	Full Moon	Hidden Moon	(–)Half-Moon	New Moon
Number	8	7	5	9	6
Color	Green	Red	Yellow	White	Black
Controller	Spiritual	Soul	Mind	Ambition	Body Strength
Movement	Upward	Active	Downward	Solidified	Floating
Energy State	Gas	Plasma	Condensation	Solid	Liquid
Manifestation	Tree	Heat	Soil	Metal	Water
Five Tastes	Sour	Bitter	Sweet	Pungent	Salty
Grains	Wheat	Red Millet	Yellow Millet	Rice	Legumes
Fruits	Apple/Plum	Berries	Dates/Olives	Melon	Citrus
Vegetables	Leeks	Shallots	Mallow	Onions	Greens
Foods to Avoid	Rancid, Oily	Burnt	Fragrant	Rotten	Putrid
Disease Areas	Nerves	Viscera	Tongue	Upper Back	Cavities
Modalities	Prayer	Healthy Habits	Herbals	Acupuncture	Heat Therapy

Excess of sour flavor injures the spleen and stomach, toughens the flesh, and causes the skin to become wrinkled and slack. It is balanced by a moderate amount of pungent food.

Excess of sweet flavor injures the kidneys and causes hair loss and aching bones. It is balanced by a moderate amount of sour food.

All five tastes must be balanced daily more or less according to the seasons, climate, and region of residence.

Seasonal Effects of the Five Flavors

Pungent flavor has a dispersing effect required in fall.

Sour flavor has a gathering effect required in spring.

Sweet flavor has a retarding effect required at all times.

Bitter flavor has a strengthening effect, required in summer.

Salty flavor has a softening effect, required in winter.

OTHER CORRESPONDENCES WITH THE FIVE ELEMENTS

	Metal	Water	Wood	Fire	Earth
Tissues	Skin	Bones	Nerves	Blood	Muscles
Bodies	Emotional	Dream	Mental	Spiritual	Physical
Mental	Sensitivity	Creativity	Thinking	Intuition	Spontaneity
	Nonjudgmental	Concept	Planning	Communication	Judgment
	Discrimination	Willpower	Strategy	Consciousness	Cleverness
Function	Detoxification	Creation	Elimination	Circulation	Digestion
Kingdom	Jester	Queen	General	King	Prime Minister

Controlling Cycle (Ko Cycle)

Fire Forges Metal

Metal Cuts Wood

Wood Roots Earth

Earth Dams Water

Water Puts Out Fire

Wood Covers Earth

Fire Melts Metal

Earth Contains Water

Metal Cuts Wood

Water Puts Out Fire

LIVER AND GALLBLADDER CONDITIONS

SIGNS OF MALFUNCTIONING YIN OR YANG

Blockage of the tear ducts or excessive tears	Poor vision and light sensitivity
Bloodshot eyes	Shouting and anger
Fuzzy thinking	Soft ridged nails
Liver pain (under right rib cage)	Weak knees and muscles

SYMPTOMS OF YANG (CONTRACTED)   SYMPTOMS OF YIN (EXPANDED)

Aversion to heat	Impaired hearing	Nearsightedness
Cataracts	Insomnia	Nausea
Dizziness	Irritability	Poor appetite
Farsightedness	Nosebleed	Depression
Headaches	Red eyes	Apprehension

LIVER AND GALLBLADDER ARE WEAKENED BY AN EXCESS OF

All chemicals	Alcohol	Fats, butter, dairy	Overeating
All drugs	Cold drinks/foods	Nuts and nut butters	Sweets
All rancid fats and oils	Eggs and vinegar	Outdoor wind	

SOUR FOODS THAT STRENGTHEN

Grains

Rye
Wheat

Fruits

Apples	Cherries
Berries	Plums

Vegetables

Artichoke	Cabbage	Parsley
Beets	Celery	Watercress
Burdock	Leeks	

HERBS (IN SMALL AMOUNTS) THAT DISCHARGE TOXINS   FOODS THAT DISCHARGE TOXINS

Burdock	Holy thistle	Lettuce	Potatoes
Dandelion	Raspberry leaf	Mushrooms	Radishes
Goldenseal			

YIN HERBS THAT BALANCE YANG SYMPTOMS   YANG HERBS THAT BALANCE YIN SYMPTOMS

Garlic	Marsh mallow	Slippery elm	Chaparral	Sage
Licorice	Nettle	Watercress	Echinacea root	Wild yam
			Oregon grape	

NOTES FOR A HEALTHY LIVER AND GALLBLADDER

1. Excessive or lack of sour food injures the liver and gallbladder.
2. Eat more steamed food during spring to strengthen the liver and gallbladder.
3. Anger is injurious to the liver and gallbladder.
4. Excessive running or walking injures the liver and gallbladder.
5. Excessive blowing wind injures the liver and gallbladder.
6. A malfunctioning liver and gallbladder cause anger and irritability.
7. Signs of a healthy liver and gallbladder include an agreeable personality and disposition, confidence to achieve success, and the ability to make good decisions and plans.
8. A healthy liver and gallbladder instill peacefulness and calmness.

HEART AND SMALL INTESTINES CONDITIONS

SIGNS OF MALFUNCTIONING YIN OR YANG

Cleft in nose
Excessive sweating or not at all
Swollen nose and hands

Emotional ups and downs
Excessive joy
Excessive laughing

SYMPTOMS OF YANG (CONTRACTED)		SYMPTOMS OF YIN (EXPANDED)	
Back pain	Excess perspiration	Facial pallor	Shortness of breath
Chest constriction	Laughing fits	Rambling talk	Sorrowful and listless
Dizziness	Little talk	Sciatic and lumbar	
Dry palate	Stroke	pains	

HEART AND SMALL INTESTINES ARE WEAKENED BY AN EXCESS OF

Burnt food
Excess salt and spice

Hot drinks and food
Overdressing (hot clothing)

SOUR FOODS THAT STRENGTHEN

Grains	Seeds and Nuts	Fruits	Vegetables		
Corn	Most notably	Apricots	All greens	Garlic	Scallions
Red millet	almonds	Cherries	Burdock	Oils	Seaweed
		Strawberries	Chickpeas	Pumpkin	White beans

HERBS (IN SMALL AMOUNTS) THAT DISCHARGE TOXINS		FOODS THAT DISCHARGE TOXINS
Bayberry	Mint	Beans, most notably white beans
Cayenne	Motherwort	Seaweed
		Vegetable oils

YIN HERBS THAT BALANCE YANG SYMPTOMS		YANG HERBS THAT BALANCE YIN SYMPTOMS
Borage	Ginseng	Black cohosh
Comfrey root	Hawthorn berry	Caraway seed

NOTES FOR A HEALTHY HEART AND SMALL INTESTINES

1. Excessive or lack of bitter foods injure the heart and small intestines.
2. Eat more raw food during summer to strengthen heart and small intestines.
3. Excessive joy and excitement are injurious to the heart and small intestines.
4. Excessive eye focusing, reading, and close work weaken heart and eyesight.
5. Excessive heat injures the heart and small intestines.
6. A malfunctioning heart and small intestine causes hysteria.
7. Signs of a healthy heart and small intestines include honesty and integrity, an optimistic personality, someone who is poised in mind and body and extends love to family and humanity.
8. A healthy heart and small intestines instills happiness.

STOMACH, SPLEEN, AND PANCREAS CONDITIONS

SIGNS OF MALFUNCTIONING YIN OR YANG

Abdominal pains	Heavy limbs	Obsession
Drooling	Intestinal problems	Overweight
Excess or diminished saliva	Lack of taste	A sing-song voice
Excessive worry	Low energy	Ulcers
Fatigue	Mental depression	Vomiting

SYMPTOMS OF YANG (CONTRACTED)   SYMPTOMS OF YIN (EXPANDED)

Constipation	Quarrelsome moods	Diarrhea	Heaviness
Flatulent stomach	Sweet/greasy mouth taste	Emaciation	Indigestion
Light-headedness	Watery stools	Gastric cramps	Nausea

STOMACH, SPLEEN, AND PANCREAS ARE WEAKENED BY AN EXCESS OF

Damp clothing	Eating too fast and too much	Lack of mastication
Damp ground	Hot food	Sweets

SOUR FOODS THAT STRENGTHEN

Grains	Fruits	Vegetables	
Yellow millet	Dates	Dark greens	Squash
	Olives	Parsnips	

HERBS (IN SMALL AMOUNTS) THAT DISCHARGE TOXINS   FOODS THAT DISCHARGE TOXINS

Gentian	Goldenseal	Vervain	Dark greens
Ginger	Juniper berry		Spices

YIN HERBS THAT BALANCE YANG SYMPTOMS   YANG HERBS THAT BALANCE YIN SYMPTOMS

Fennel	Licorice	Basil	Fennel
Ginseng	Orange peel	Catnip	Lobelia

NOTES FOR A HEALTHY STOMACH, SPLEEN, AND PANCREAS

1. Excessive or lack of sweet food injures the stomach, spleen, and pancreas.
2. Eat more stewed food during late summer to strengthen the stomach, spleen, and pancreas.
3. Extreme sympathy, moodiness, and worry are injurious to the stomach, spleen, and pancreas.
4. Prolonged sitting weakens the stomach, spleen, and pancreas.
5. Excessive humidity (moisture) injures the stomach, spleen, and pancreas.
6. Malfunctioning of the stomach, spleen, and pancreas causes suspicion and mistrust.
7. Signs of a healthy stomach, spleen, and pancreas include a calm disposition and satisfaction, constructive thinking and action, sound ideas and an excellent memory, a sympathetic nature, and a balanced critical faculty.
8. A healthy stomach, spleen, and pancreas instills trust.

LUNGS AND LARGE INTESTINES CONDITIONS

SIGNS OF MALFUNCTIONING YIN OR YANG

Anguish and helplessness	Chest congestion	Sinus and mucus problems
Bowel difficulties	Hemorrhoids	Whimpering and sorrow

SYMPTOMS OF YANG (CONTRACTED)   SYMPTOMS OF YIN (EXPANDED)

Chest pain	Nonproductive	Cold hands and feet	Loose stools
Cracked lips	cough	Cramps	Never thirsty
Dry rough	Rapid and deep	Drowsiness	Shallow respiration
skin	breath	Emaciation	Shortness of breath

LUNGS AND LARGE INTESTINES ARE WEAKENED BY AN EXCESS OF

All cold drinks	Excess dairy	Oils
All cold foods	Excess fats	Underdressing in cold weather

SOUR FOODS THAT STRENGTHEN

Grains	**Fruits**	**Vegetables**	
Barley	Lemon	Cider vinegar	Hot pepper
Oats	Melons	Comfrey	Onion
Rice	Peaches	Garlic	Radish
		Green pea	Tomato

HERBS (IN SMALL AMOUNTS) THAT DISCHARGE TOXINS   FOODS THAT DISCHARGE TOXINS

Elecampane	Slippery Elm	Cider vinegar	Lemon
Goldenseal	Wild Cherry Bark	Green peas	Radish
Horehound			

YIN HERBS THAT BALANCE YANG SYMPTOMS   YANG HERBS THAT BALANCE YIN SYMPTOMS

Cayenne	Osha root	Coltsfoot	Ginger	Myrrh
Comfrey	Yarrow	Eucalyptus	Lobelia	Pleurisy Root
		Garlic	Mullein	

NOTES FOR HEALTHY LUNGS AND LARGE INTESTINES

1. Excessive or lack of pungent food injures the lungs and large intestines.
2. Eat more baked foods during the fall season to strengthen the lungs and large intestines.
3. Extreme grief is injurious to the lungs and large intestines.
4. Excessive lying down or sleeping weakens the lungs and large intestines.
5. Excessive dryness (extreme low humidity) injures the lungs and large intestines.
6. Malfunctioning lungs and large intestines cause depression.
7. Signs of healthy lungs and large intestines include buoyant health and vitality, good mind and body rhythm, harmonious personality and intuition, and physical strength and endurance.
8. Healthy lungs and large intestines instill positivity and confidence.

KIDNEYS AND BLADDER CONDITIONS

SIGNS OF MALFUNCTIONING YIN OR YANG

Arthritis	Frequent urination	Moaning sound	Scant urination
Backache	General fatigue	Painful joints	Sex problems
Dandruff	Hair loss	Poor hearing	Weak ankles

SYMPTOMS OF YANG (CONTRACTED)

Cold diseases	Nymphomania
Dry mouth	Painful swelling
Excess mucus	Perspiration after eating
Fevers	Restlessness

SYMPTOMS OF YIN (EXPANDED)

Chills/coldness	Poor memory
Fatigue	Soft speech
Headaches	Swollen legs
Impotence	Ulcers
Indecisiveness	Weak joints

KIDNEYS AND BLADDER ARE WEAKENED BY AN EXCESS OF

Alcohol/drugs/chemicals	Excess sweets/liquid	Scalding hot drinks
Excess protein and vinegar	Hot clothing (Overdressing)	Scalding hot food

SOUR FOODS THAT STRENGTHEN

Grains	**Fruits**		**Vegetables**	
Buckwheat	Grapefruit	Adzuki beans	Cauliflower	Parsley
	Grapes	Black beans	Green vegetables	Seaweed
	Oranges	Cabbage	Miso	Sea salt

HERBS (IN SMALL AMOUNTS) THAT DISCHARGE TOXINS

Berries	Plantain leaf
Cleavers	Raspberry leaf
Nettles	Saw palmetto

FOODS THAT DISCHARGE TOXINS

Adzuki beans	Citrus fruit
Black beans	Oils (vegetable)
Cider vinegar	

YIN HERBS THAT BALANCE YANG SYMPTOMS

Horsetail
Marsh mallow root
Oat straw

YANG HERBS THAT BALANCE YIN SYMPTOMS

Asparagus root	Juniper berry
Dandelion	Myrrh
Gravel root	Parsley leaf

NOTES FOR HEALTHY KIDNEYS AND BLADDER

1. Excessive or lack of salty food injures the kidneys and bladder.
2. Eat more sautéed food during winter to strengthen the kidneys and bladder.
3. Extreme fear and moaning is injurious to the kidneys and bladder.
4. Prolonged standing is harmful to the kidneys and bladder.
5. Excessive cold temperature injures the kidneys and bladder.
6. Malfunctioning kidneys and bladder cause fear and depression.
7. Signs of healthy kidneys and bladder include a clear beautiful voice, excellent concentration, strong sex glands and personal magnetism, and tenacious willpower.
8. Healthy kidneys and bladder instill courage and fortitude.

USING HERBS ACCORDING TO FIVE ELEMENTS

Herbs do not cure; the body cures or heals itself. Herbs are used only for remedial measures. For specific disease conditions, herbs always remedy, correct, and balance the system with optimum results when the cause or causes of disease (improper food, overeating, poor health habits, and so on) are eliminated and rational, healthful living and eating habits are adopted.

If you wish to use herbs, you should use only the specific herbs designated for a particular symptom or condition, as shown in the tables on the preceding pages. Use one or two herbs from the discharge toxins category and one or two herbs from either the yin or yang category necessary for your specific symptoms or condition. Herbs should not be used indiscriminately without regard for their yin or yang qualities, as is commonly practiced by most American herbalists. The Chinese yin/yang herbal system is far more accurate and scientific in the diagnosis, treatment, and use of herbs. Yin herbal teas are used for yang conditions and ailments, for those who are heavy meat, egg, and salt consumers. Yang herbal teas are used for yin conditions, such as those who have been on a strict (yin) raw food or fruitarian diet, or those eating excessively of fats and sugars, such as ice cream, cheese, sweets, donuts, and soft drinks.

Herbal teas are best utilized and assimilated on an empty stomach, in the morning, or before a meal. However, a small amount of tea may be used after a meal to help to assimilate fat eaten in the meal and aid digestion; no more than 2 to 4 ounces may be taken after meals, sipped slowly.

Herbal teas should be limited to 1 or 2 cups per day. Most herbs and herb teas should be used only to balance diseased conditions or symptoms and their use should be discontinued after the health problem is overcome. The Chinese herbalists teach that an herb, taken in excess, can cause the very same condition or problem that it can cure. For example, if you attempt to correct or balance yang (contracted) constipation with a yin herb such as senna leaf (a laxative), without removing the initial cause (overeating, white flour, salt, meat, dairy products), the tea will help temporarily, for a few days or weeks, but the constipation will still remain a problem. If larger doses of senna leaf tea are then taken, they will compound the problem by further weakening the intestines. The continuous use of laxative teas in large doses poisons and irritates the system.

Or, for example, if you suffer from frequent or excessive urination, a yin (expanded kidney/bladder) condition caused by an excessive consumption of liquids, fruits, juices, tropical fruits, melons, and sugar, 1 or 2 cups per day of corn silk tea will help to constrict and strengthen the kidneys and bladder and eventually correct the yin condition, provided the above-mentioned causes of the disorder are removed. However, many herbalists recommend drinking large quantities of water, and using yin herbs such as parsley and yin foods such as cucumber and watermelon for kidney and bladder problems, without regard to whether the disorder is a yin or yang condition. If yin herbs and yin foods are used for yin (expanded) kidneys and bladder, it will further weaken and expand them. Moderation in herbs as well as foods is the key to superior health.

Herbal teas should be used for short periods of time only (two to four months); discontinue their use, or change to different herbs for your condition. Herbs are strong agents and should not be used for too long a time, as the body will not respond or heal as quickly if they are used continually. However, some herbs, such as alfalfa, dandelion, bancha, cinnamon, chicory, and grain beverages, can be consumed in small amounts (1 or 2 cups) daily for better health and enjoyment.

Dr. Chang and His Long Life Tea

Dr. Chang, trained in both Chinese and Western medicine, herbology, and acupuncture, has created a delicious herb tea recipe using peppermint, honeysuckle, licorice, ginseng, cinnamon, poria, and chrysanthemum. He says this about herbs:

> Herbs, like the regular foods, work by adjusting the flow of vital energy in the entire body of the human being. This is accomplished by increasing the energy where it is too low and lessening the energy where it is too high. When herbs are assimilated by the body, their vitality is absorbed too. The herb's vitality passes through the pathways of energy (meridians) to reach the internal organs and to support and adjust them to their optimal functioning. The most useful purpose of herbs is the prevention of illness, rejuvenation, and longevity. Everyone, whether sick or healthy, can benefit from herbs. A complete diet should include

both regular foods and herbs. No one can obtain perfect health unless he has a complete diet program. Anyone who stops learning is older whether this happens at twenty or eighty. Anyone who keeps on learning not only remains young but becomes constantly more valuable, regardless of physical capacity.

WISDOM INCREASES LONGEVITY

The *Nei Ching* says:

The sages did not overexert their bodies at physical labor and they did not overexert their minds by strenuous meditation. They were not concerned about anything; they regarded inner happiness and peace as fundamental, and contentment as the highest achievement. Their bodies could never be harmed or their mental faculties dissipated. Thus, they could reach the age of one hundred years or more.

Those who rebel against the basic rules of the universe sever their own roots and ruin their true selves. Yin and yang, the two principles in nature, and the four seasons are the beginning and the end of everything and they are also the cause of life and death. Those who disobey the laws of the universe will give rise to calamities and visitations, while those who follow the laws of the universe remain free from dangerous illness, for they are the ones who have obtained the Tao, the Right Way.

Tao was practiced by the sages and admired by the ignorant people. Obedience to the laws of yin and yang means life; disobedience means death. The obedient ones will rule while the rebels will be in disorder and confusion. Anything contrary to harmony (with nature) is disobedience and means rebellion to nature.

Hence, the sages did not treat those who were already ill; they instructed those who were not yet ill. They did not want to rule those who were already rebellious; they guided those who were not yet rebellious. This is the meaning of the entire preceding discussion. To administer medicines to diseases that have already developed is comparable to the behavior of those persons who begin to dig a well after they have become thirsty, and of those who begin to cast weapons after they have already engaged in battle.

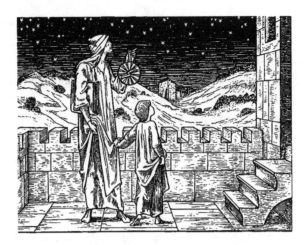

Fig. 6.4. "What the mind can conceive and believe, the mind can achieve" is inherent in the wisdom of the Tao.

No matter whether people are rebellious or obedient, there is method and regularity in the workings of the four seasons and yin and yang. Everything is subject to their invariable rules and regulations, which govern the relationship between external and internal influences.

Those who have the true wisdom remain strong while those who have no knowledge and wisdom grow old and feeble. Therefore the people should share this wisdom and their names will become famous. Those who are wise inquire and search together, while those who are ignorant and stupid inquire and search apart from each other. Those who are stupid and ignorant do not exert themselves enough in the search for the Right Way, while those who are wise search beyond the natural limits.

Those who search beyond the natural limits will retain good hearing and clear vision, their bodies will remain light and strong, although they grow old in years, they will remain able bodied and flourishing; and those who are able bodied can govern to great advantage. In their pleasures and joys they (sages) were dignified and tranquil. They followed their own desires and they never directed their will and ambition toward the protection of a purpose that was empty of meaning. Thus their allotted span of life was without limit, like Heaven and Earth.

Yang, the lucid element, ascends to Heaven. Yin, the turbid element, returns to Earth; hence the universe (Heaven and Earth) represents motion and rest, controlled by the wisdom of nature (the Tao). Nature grants the power to beget and to grow, to harvest and to store, to finish and to begin anew. Virtuous human beings matched Heaven when they cultivated their minds; they resembled Earth when they provided sufficient nourishment; and they were by the side of the people in the care of the five viscera.

The heavenly climate circulates within the lungs; the climate of the earth circulates within the throat; the wind circulates within the liver, thunder penetrates the heart; the air of a ravine penetrates the stomach; and the rain penetrates the kidneys. The six arteries generate streams; the bowels and the stomach generate the oceans; the nine orifices generate flowing water; and Heaven and Earth generate yin and yang (the two opposing principles).

The laws of nature are just, but terrible. There is no weak mercy in them. Cause and consequence are inseparable and inevitable. The elements have no forbearance. The fire burns, the water drowns, the air consumes, the earth buries. And perhaps it would be well for any people if the punishment of crimes against the laws of humans were as inevitable as the punishment of crimes against the laws of nature, were humankind as unerring in their judgments as nature.

PURE LIGHT

Ancient cultures worshipped the sun as a manifestation of the all-powerful Creator. They derived great benefit from its healing power. The Greeks and Romans built solariums where the sick came to fast and bask in the relaxing and healing ultraviolet rays. Ancient physicians were well versed in the knowledge of solar light therapy, in conjunction with fasting, herbs, natural foods, and physical exercise therapy. Pastries, sugar, white flour, and other junk foods were nonexistent; therefore, healing and rejuvenation through the use of heliotherapy (sun therapy), herbs, hydrotherapy (water therapy), and fasting was rapid and effective.

The bright solar orb (sun) is our most powerful source of energy and light. It sustains all vegetable food for human and animal life through the process of photosynthesis. It provides us directly with vitamin D, but it must shine on our bare skin for us to receive its benefits. We need the full spectrum of the sun, not artificial lights. Poor inside lighting is responsible for many physical and mental defects, from nervous conditions to cancer.

Fresh air and sunshine increase the quality and quantity of the blood by 25 percent within four hours time. Our blood has more hemoglobin in summer than winter. In the wintertime keep your rooms well ventilated to let in as much light and fresh air as possible. Sunlight directly affects the retina of the eye and the hypothalamus, which coordinates the nervous system and the pituitary gland, known as the master gland because of its influence on the endocrine system. Hormones from the glands directly influence metabolism, growth, sexual activity, and the overall health and vitality of the body.

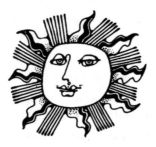

Fig. 6.5. Solar light

Sunlight makes better use of calcium and phosphorus for bone strength and development. Vitamin D from the sun helps the body's absorption of carbohydrates and the control of body weight. The powerful rays of the sun act as a disinfectant and help to overcome colds, flu, infections, TB, anemia, and so on. Sunlight helps more ailments than all the drugs in the world. The rays of the sun help us to utilize our vitamins, minerals, proteins, and fats. They distribute calcium in the body and tone up the muscles. They help to overcome insomnia.

The sun vitalizes the waters of the sea and the soil of the earth. Sun-dried fruits and vegetables are excellent sun-charged foods loaded with nourishment. Fruit trees take in the most sunlight of all food grown, because they are under the sun's rays throughout the year.

To stay in good health, we must enjoy the outdoors as much as possible. Sun and air baths help the body to eliminate its waste material daily. Fresh mountain or ocean air is the best tonic known for poor health. A few weeks in the mountains or on the ocean beach, with the sun shining

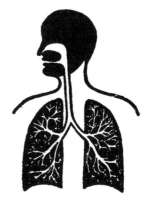

Fig. 6.6. Breathing and good blood circulation are inseparable. Physical exercises that enhance free blood and nerve circulation create superior health and freedom from disease and microbes.

on the bare skin, is the best-known physical and mental rejuvenator of all. Instead of lying in a head-shrinker's office, stretch out your nerve-wracked body on your favorite beach or mountain resort and let nature restore your health.

Solar Time Clock

It is well known that sunshine and solar energy are necessary for health and life on earth, but it is not generally recognized that there is quite a difference between morning and afternoon sunshine energy. At 4 p.m., on a clear day, we feel the heat of the sun more than at 8 a.m., although the sun is in the same position or height in the sky. The morning sun is tempered by the earth's atmosphere travelling in the opposite direction. Plants utilize morning sunshine better than that of the afternoon.

From dawn to noon the sun and earth forces are in opposition; the sun is radiating toward the west while the earth is revolving toward the east. All life depends on the opposition of these cosmic forces. In humans, from dawn until noon the eliminative powers are at their peak; toxins are neutralized or discarded, putrefaction and fermentation are inhibited, and infections are eliminated. During the predawn hours the cosmic energy is at its lowest; more people die at this time than at any other period of the day, especially sick people and hospital patients. In the afternoon the solar forces operate in the same direction as the rotating earth, east, and have a constructive and recharging influence; the food eaten at this time is thoroughly assimilated and absorbed into every cell of the body for constructive purposes.

The logical conclusion is that physical and mental activity should be at its height from morning until noon, and the afternoon and evening hours should be used for comparative rest and relaxation. To do otherwise is to work in opposition to the law of rhythm and universal yin/yang balance. Early daylight hours are yang—full of energy, activities, and heat—while early evening hours are yin—passive, restful, cool, and calm.

Vibratory Light Waves

One of the greatest scientific achievements of this century has been the discovery of the indispensable health benefits that are locked up in sunlight. Although sunlight seems to us to be merely brilliant white light, actually a single beam of sunlight runs the gamut of all colors. If a ray of light is divided by a prism into its different wave-lengths, the prism separates what the human eye recognizes as the seven colors of the scale of light (red, orange, yellow, green, blue, indigo, and violet).

When we speak of healing by sunlight, we mean, principally, the healing produced by the violet rays of the visible band of sunlight, together with the ultraviolet rays of invisible light. We are primarily healed by rays of light too short for the human eye to see. However, some of the therapeutic properties of sunlight are found in the infrared rays (invisible long rays of sunlight). In rheumatism or arthritis, bathing in sunshine has the effect of breaking up the harmful, tissue-stiffening uric acid crystals into disposable by-products. The uric acid is thrown off through the skin and kidneys, while some iron, curiously, is released from the crystals for constructive work in the bloodstream. This prop-

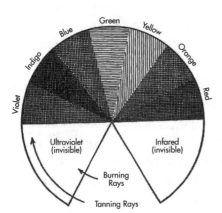

Fig. 6.7. Solar spectrum: the seven-color scale of life and birth. Rays just beyond the violet have the greatest effect in building vitality and health. Rays beyond red are very useful in reducing congested, inflamed tissues.

erty of the infrared rays in assisting the assimilation of iron by the system proves to be valuable in certain cases of anemia. The action of the infrared rays enables the iron (thus released into the bloodstream) to combine with oxygen in the formation of red blood corpuscles.

Sun Bathing

Wait at least two hours after eating your main meal before taking a sun bath. Sunglasses are harmful to the eyes, causing fatigue and tension. Use pinhole sunglasses to protect the eyes from glare, as they admit the entire spectrum of sunlight. Winter sun is just as good or even better than summer sun. Never sunbathe between the hours of 11 a.m. to 2 p.m., especially during the summer months. The best periods to expose the entire body to the sun are 9 a.m. to 11 a.m. and 2 p.m. to 5 p.m. Make every effort to get out into the sun, bathe in it, walk in it, work in it, learn to love it.

Overexposure to the sun where one becomes red or burned causes a negative reaction in the immune system. Gradual and slow tanning in five or ten minute increments benefits and enhances the body's immune system. The healing power of the sun's ultraviolet light is strongest at midday. One can burn very easy on cloudy days due to ultraviolet rays penetrating the clouds, so be cautious.

Scientific Solar Research

Millions of Americans eat diets heavy in refined and animal fats. These are the diets loaded with fried food, rich pastries, and fatty beef. These people should not be getting a lot of sunlight. Medical science has determined that one of the causative factors of skin, bowel, and breast cancer, as well as aging of the skin, is a high-fat diet. The National Cancer Institute has recommended that Americans cut down on total fat in their diets. Experiments have shown that animals fed a high-fat diet and exposed to intense sunlight suffer considerable cancer, whereas it is hard to induce cancer in animals getting the same amount of sunlight but eating a low-fat diet.

When there are a lot of fatty substances in the tissues, the sunlight acts as an accelerator of cancer but not as a cause. Wrinkling works the same way. It is the bad diet that has a lot to do with aging of the skin. (Excessive salt is the biggest culprit.) For extra protection, people should eat diets that are rich in vitamin C, E, and carotene, a form of vitamin A. These nutrients help prevent harmful chemical reactions in the skin.

In addition, a diet rich in natural complex carbohydrates, grains, legumes, fresh fruits and vegetables, germinated seeds, nuts, and sprouts, all eaten in season, will maintain the body in optimum health and superior protection from cosmic solar rays. When we learn how to live in harmony with the laws of nature, we are protected and nourished by all of her elements: fire, air, water, and earth.

Benefits of Sunlight Summary

1. Lowers high blood pressure and cholesterol levels.
2. Strengthens bones, teeth, hair, nails, and lessens cavities by increasing absorption of vitamin D and calcium.
3. Decreases susceptibility to bacteria, germs, and viruses.
4. Improves the immune system by increasing the amount and activity of antibodies and white blood cells; these cells manufacture interferon, an internal substance, which aids in healing diseased conditions internal and external.
5. Helps to overcome mental and emotional disturbances.
6. Helps to overcome hypoglycemia by lowering blood sugar.
7. Lessens frequency of colds, flu, and tuberculosis.
8. Aids in atherosclerosis, angina, cancer, and arthritis cases.
9. Decreases the need for insulin in some diabetics, in conjunction with proper exercise, herbs, and diets.
10. Improves overall health, well-being, and physical appearance.

FRESH OUTDOOR OXYGEN

We can live for weeks without food, a few days without water, but only a few minutes without air. Yet modern people stay cooped up in their homes or offices practically all day with the windows shut. They breathe in impure, stagnant air and wonder why they feel dopey and sluggish all day long. Have you ever noticed stale air in a room with closed windows after someone has slept in it overnight? The air is literally charged with auto-generated body poisons! If more people slept in rooms with good oxygen ventilation, many heart attacks could be prevented.

Breathing oxygen sustains our life on earth; when oxygen is withdrawn, existence ceases. The most mentally and physically active people are the ones who breathe deeply and use their lungs to the fullest capacity; they are full of energy, vitality, health, and youthfulness at any age! The joy of living glows on their faces: their cells, tissues, and blood are energized with life-giving oxygen. They enjoy life to the utmost, and people are attracted to their magnetic charm and vitality. Diseased, pale-faced, and anemic people are full of uneliminated toxins and poisons in every cell and organ; they do not obtain sufficient vital oxygen to burn up the wastes; they are weak breathers, with poor health force. Their thinking is poor due to oxygen starvation and poor circulation. On the other hand, the person who exercises and breathes power-charged vital oxygen functions on 220 volts with energy to spare. Fresh oxygen, sunshine, wholesome food, and exercise are key factors in building super health force.

When our body possesses a high health-force rating, four star and above, we are obtaining plenty of oxygen. There is a joy of living; we are happy to be alive; we bounce out of bed in the morning with a song in our heart. Depression, envy, hate, jealousy, worries, and anxieties flee like phantoms in the night. We enjoy our work and our creativity is enhanced; we are inspired to master life and accomplish great deeds without struggle. People who practice scientific breathing do not shun responsibility; they approach it head on with courage, fortitude, and determination; they create and invent, but do not follow fleeting fads. The weak, shallow breather, on the other hand, is an escapist, turning to drugs, alcohol, morbidness, perversion, fantasy, self-delusion, fads, and the make-believe tinsel world of material illusion.

Health Benefits of Deep Oxygen Breathing

1. Deep breathing builds a state of high-level health force.
2. Oxygen burns up and eliminates poisons in the lungs and bloodstream.
3. Deep breathing builds rich red blood cells.
4. Oxygen breathing helps to overcome the craving of artificial stimulants.

5. The body heals faster when sufficient oxygen is present.

6. It improves the memory and thinking ability and it cleans away the cobwebs from the gray matter.

7. It creates healthy circulation to all parts of the body.

8. It helps to overcome anemia and nervous diseases.

9. Deep oxygen breathing improves muscle tone, lung capacity, and the complexion; it flattens the abdomen and reduces wrinkles.

10. Diaphragm deep breathing aids digestion, assimilation, and utilization of food.

11. Fresh outdoor oxygen after meals helps us to digest our food efficiently.

12. Deep breathing improves the singing voice and makes the speaking voice beautiful and harmonious.

Oxygen: Blood, Flexibility, and Longevity

Why is deep oxygen breathing so necessary to health? Because our very life-blood depends upon it. Oxygen is a food for the body and it is absolutely vital in purifying the blood. All the blood in the body passes through the lungs every three-quarters of a minute and there it is purified and enriched by the oxygen we breathe.

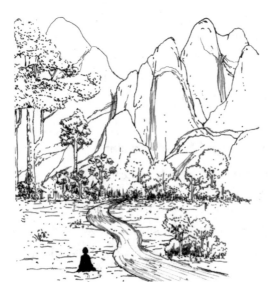

Fig. 6.8. Living and breathing the Tao

The native dancers of North Africa have amazing beauty, strength, and endurance. One of their tricks is their development of the breathing muscle, the diaphragm, for which they use special exercises. The diaphragm's action draws in large quantities of fresh air and throws out waste material. The blood-making spleen sends out that rich material that causes a person's cheeks to be red and ruddy; the other blood-making cells in the marrow of the bones voraciously grab the oxygen the diaphragm draws in. The whole secret of the exercises the dancers perform is to ensure correct breathing, so that all the internal organs are benefitted.

The same benefits do not come from the ordinary way of breathing. This is why so many men and women, who have lived thirty, forty, or more years, have stiffened intestines, cemented joints, hardening of the liver, inelastic arteries and veins, cold feet and hands, indigestion, and nervous dispositions. In fact, this is why so many individuals commence to deteriorate at a period in life when they should be in the best of physical and mental states.

We are oxygen creatures and cannot live without air. People with plenty of oxygen are the happiest, most influential people of all. We should be outdoors for several hours each day, even in cold weather (dress accordingly). A short walk should be taken in the open air after meals. Perfect digestion and assimilation requires lots of oxygen. During sleep there should be maximum ventilation, while making sure you are sufficiently warm. An abundance of fresh oxygen will make a great difference in the way you feel and think. Get your share! Large cities have a great deal of pollution, but outside air is still better than inside air. Go to the country, or near a lake or ocean, whenever possible, to obtain clean fresh oxygen.

Training Yourself to Get More Oxygen

There is a trick way of causing your lungs to change their position, to enlarge, and to assimilate more oxygen. This is done by the simple trick of flattening the small of the back, in conjunction with proper deep breathing techniques. After a few attempts you will see that more air is taken into your lungs and that you walk with the stride of youth.

1. Stand straight up with your back flat against a wall. Leave no room between any part of your back and the wall. It requires a little practice, but this brings all internal organs into their correct working position.
2. Learning to walk with the back flat is the trick. Stand, walk, and sit with the small of the back flat, and the head held erect, and then oxygen will take care of itself in the body. This carriage throws the hips forward and upward; practice gives grace and greater height to the figure.

WATER: LIQUID OF LIFE

Seventy-five percent of the human body is composed of water. Water flushes out internal wastes and purifies the cells, tissues, and organs. The finest of all water is that found in fresh fruit, vegetables, and juices; it is organic water of the highest quality. Pure rain water sent from the heavens is the cleanest liquid substance that nature has to offer, naturally distilled by the clouds and gently sent down in little organic droplets for

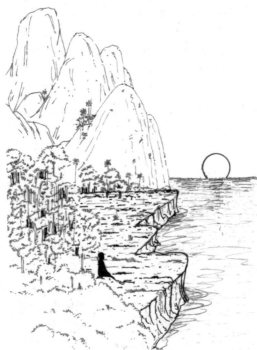

Fig. 6.9. Living in the Tao's liquid and light

the benefit of humankind. Cloud-distilled rain water is vitalized, energized, and aerated by the atmosphere on its journey to Earth; it is full of
life electricity and magnetism.

Rain water may be caught directly from the clouds and stored in a
clean, dry, and cool place. The easiest way to collect rain is during the
winter when nature pours her white snow flakes to earth in great quantities. The purest rain or snow is found in the country, or at the ocean or
mountains, where air pollution is at a minimum.

Pure rain or distilled (aerated) water acts as a solvent and dissolves
uric acid, mineral deposits, and toxic wastes within the body that make
one grow older years too soon. Pure vitalized water is a blood-builder
because it picks up the internal filth and cleanses the entire system.

Factory-distilled water is pure lifeless liquid and it lacks the electricity of vitalized rain water. The cosmic rays of the sun and atmosphere
are the life-giving principal ingredients that make rain water a superior
liquid. However, human-made distilled water may be vitalized and solar-
aerated by pouring it from one container to another outdoors in the
morning sunlight, thus imparting to it a degree of solar energized electricity. Still waters grow stagnant and lifeless; while moving and churn-
ing waters attract more sunlight, oxygen, and atmospheric life force. You
may also store the aerated water in colored glass containers and let it
stand in the direct sunlight, covered until ready to use.

The centenarians of high mountain regions utilize pure glacier
waters that have been energized by the unpolluted atmosphere; this water
is very fast-moving, causing it to remain in a constant aerated state for
daily use. Mountain or spring water does pick up some inorganic materials, but these have always been a part of our natural environment and are
not known to be harmful to the body. Inorganic mineral water does not
cause hardened arteries, as some people believe. Hardened arteries and
other civilized diseases are the result of a high intake of animal food and
junk food, stress conditions, and lack of pure wholesome natural foods.
Cholesterol deposits from wrong foods are the cause of hardened blood
vessels and other old age symptoms.

Do not be afraid of a few inorganic mineral substances or a couple of
harmless microbes; on the other hand, be intelligent enough not to use
contaminated sewers, stagnant lakes, or ponds, or chemically chlorinated
and fluoridated city tap waters. Water that flows in a living stream or that

comes to you fresh from the clouds, charged with solar energy and laden with cosmic electricity, is nature's sweet gift that you cannot improve on in any way.

Deep mineral waters as a rule are not as good as those that are clear, aerated, and fresh. It is a general rule, however, that young and growing persons need to drink water that contains lime, as it builds and hardens the bones and teeth; this is called hard water. It is likely that after a person reaches fifty years of age he or she will be benefited by drinking soft water, that is, distilled (aerated) or rain water, which prevents the rapid solidifying, hardening, and aging of the body.

Liquids should be taken only when thirst is present. Overconsumption of liquids causes polyuria (excessive passage of fluids or frequent urination). It also causes expanded kidneys and intestines, a yin condition. Overconsuming fluids causes the kidneys to excrete urine instead of cleansing the blood and ridding the body of uric acid and metabolic toxins.

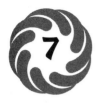

Rebalancing Your Health

It has long been understood that there is a link between the food that we eat and our health. The ancient Taoists developed a sophisticated understanding of health and wellness, including the use of herbs and food for rebalancing health.

These days we have a far more complex situation. This is due to several factors:

1. We have developed extremely sophisticated methods for the manufacture of food. There are huge numbers of highly processed and refined foods available to us that the ancient Taoists would never have dreamed of.
2. We travel more than our early ancestors. We expose ourselves to a wider variety of climates, seasons, and food types.
3. Our farming systems have developed a huge range of chemicals, factory farming, and modified food types that also affect our nutrition.
4. Our bodies are exposed to high levels of chemicals, pollutants, pharmaceuticals, and stress that our early ancestors would have had no experience of.

Thus we have to make adaptations in order to apply ancient principles to our modern situation. In the struggle to find the nutrition solution, the health world is overwhelmed with theories and suggested diets. One year we are told to eat only raw food; the next year the high-protein diet is in. How on earth do we know which one to follow to restore our health to balance? What we need to look for is flexible nutritional therapies that respond to each individual's needs.

Oriental nutritional theory emphasizes the importance of choosing the right treatment for the right person. To support this, a complex system of diagnostics was developed and is still used today by many practitioners of Chinese medicine. One of the gifts of modern medicine has been its sophisticated diagnostic procedures. We can use either system to enable us to choose the correct dietary therapy for each individual. Either way, we must choose a treatment based upon each unique person. To choose a diet without first diagnosing the person would be like taking a medicine without seeing what the illness was.

In either case, to improve our health, we need to start listening to our bodies, seeing where the imbalances lie, and finding the ways to restore balance to them. Rather than just applying the same dietary therapy to all people, we need to find ways of observing and measuring yin and yang imbalances and then use dietary therapy to restore health.

FOOD ENERGETICS

The ancient systems of nutritional healing regarded different foods as having different energetic qualities. They did not have access to reductionist science and thus did not know about micronutrients (minerals, vitamins, and so on). However, they did observe the different qualities of foods and the effects that they have on the people eating them.

Just as yin and yang can be observed in a person's energy, they can also be seen in a food. In food energetics, some foods are considered balancing: they do not have an extreme effect on energy but maintain the center. Other foods have an expanding quality: they expand our chi, making us feel lighter. Other foods have a contracting quality: they contract our chi, making us feel more grounded. We can understand these qualities better by considering a tree. A tree has a stable center, its trunk; it also has branches that reach upward to Heaven and expand their energy out. In addition there are roots that sink deep into Earth and contract the energy down.

We can apply this model to different foods to understand their energetic qualities. If we look at food groups we find that the most expansive are the simple carbohydrates, which release their sugars very quickly and thus rapidly lift our energy. Complex carbohydrates also give us energy, released more slowly. Thus they are expansive, but less so. Fats and proteins build our body cells and have a contractive and grounding effect. Physiologically these food groups slow down the release of sugars in the diet and thus help to regulate our blood-sugar levels. The denser the food, the more contractive it is. Thus meat is more contractive than beans and tofu.

Some foods are centering; those are the foods that are neither too sugary/refined nor too dense protein/fat. These usually form the center of most ancient time-tested diets. Most diets from around the world have both a protein and carbohydrate as the center. Commonly this will be a whole grain plus a bean.

Centering foods are often a mixture of carbohydrates and proteins, even within each food. For example, rice is thought of as a carbohydrate, but it does contain protein. Beans are often thought of as proteins, but they do contain carbohydrates. Such foods have a balancing and centering effect. These foods create the core of a healthy diet, and then other

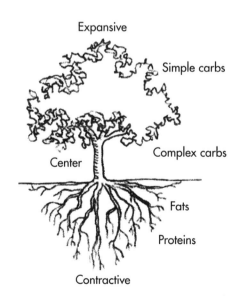

Fig. 7.1. Energetics of a tree. We can use the model of the tree and apply it to different foods to understand their energetic qualitites: simple carbs, complex carbs, fats, and proteins.

EXAMPLES OF TRADITIONAL DIETS

COUNTRY	PROTEIN		CARBOHYDRATE
India	Dahl	+	Rice
Mexico	Beans	+	Corn
Japan	Tofu	+	Rice
United Kingdom	Dairy	+	Potato
Europe	Cheese	+	Bread (wheat)
Middle East	Hummus	+	Bread

foods and flavors are used around these staples. Core foods help to maintain our sense of center. This is a very important principle in Taoism and Oriental therapy.

Center

Our center is about staying balanced. If we only have extremes in our life, then we become pushed and pulled about by circumstances. For example, if we eat only expansive foods we may feel high, but ungrounded. The opposite is if we eat an excess of contractive foods, then we may feel grounded but depressed and heavy.

If we choose one extreme, we will soon crave the other. Thus we become a victim to our own feelings and cravings. We are constantly swinging from one extreme to the other, the energetic equivalent of manic-depressive. This is reflected in the habits of yo-yo dieting and detox-retox in which people swing from a diet or detox program into their old bad habits as a response.

In Oriental therapy we seek to build a strong center. In Taoist Chi Kung (energy exercises) we focus our awareness on the tan tien area below the navel, where we store our chi. When we have more awareness in the center, then we are not so affected by outer circumstances. This gives us a gentle strength and stability. Building a strong center is an important aim. However, we also need to address any imbalances that occur, especially when we first start our practice.

In five-element therapy, the strength of the center can be seen by the power of our digestive ability. The ideal situation is one in which we can eat anything without a problem. This is called having a good digestive

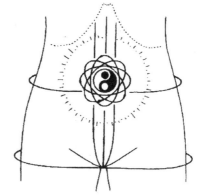

Fig. 7.2. Center force

fire; though even this does not want to be excessively strong. Digestive fire is a concept in many Asian nutritional systems; in ayurveda it is called *agni*. Five-element nutrition uses the model of a small fire burning in the belly, and the stomach is thought to be like a cooking pot; when we ingest food it enters the cooking pot and is broken down by the fire.

If our fire is not strong enough, we will struggle to digest the food that we eat. We may feel tired after eating, have constipation or loose stools, or even undigested matter in the stools. Feeling that we cannot absorb the food that we eat is frustrating to those who are trying hard to improve their health. There are several steps we can take to enhance our digestive ability, including:

1. Chew. This is the most simple and efficient way to boost digestive fire.
2. Eating root vegetables (such as sweet potatoes and carrots) can be very helpful to nourish the digestive fire.
3. Adding a few digestive spices, such as cinnamon, cloves, nutmeg, and garlic, can assist. Avoid these if there are signs of excessive heat.
4. Avoid foods that are cold, sweet, or mucus-forming, as these will diminish the fire! Ice cream is a prime example, but also iced drinks, refined sweets, and dairy.
5. Eat a good breakfast: this is the time that the earth element, which rules the digestion, is active. Therefore, a wholesome breakfast that is not too sweet can help our digestive ability.

6. Try not to get too scattered during the day, as this will scatter your chi and diminish your center. Avoid taking on too many tasks, seeing too many different people, being too long on the internet, or having different communication sources all going off at once. The more we can build a sense of center, the better our digestion will become.

ACID-ALKALINE BALANCE

As we have seen, the principle of yin and yang is the basis of the entire universe; it is the root and source of life and death. Similarly, the acid/alkaline balance affects every phase of life: from diet, to thought, to sleep, and physical activity. Everything we do in life either creates acidity or alkalinity. To attain good health it is necessary to thoroughly understand the causes of acidity and alkalinity and apply this knowledge to our life.

In order to grasp the significance of acid and alkaline, we must first understand the meaning of pH, which is a measure of hydrogen ion concentration in blood, urine, and liquids, and is used as a symbol to indicate acidity and alkalinity. A pH of 7 (0.0000001 gram atom of hydrogen ion per liter) is considered neutral, the measure of pure water. The acid end of the pH scale is from 1 to 7, and 7 to 14 is the alkaline end.

ACID/ALKALINE BODY FLUIDS

BODY FLUID	PH RANGE
Gastric juice	1.2–3.0
Vaginal fluid	3.5–4.5
Urine	4.6–8.0
Saliva	6.35–6.85
Blood	7.35–7.45
Semen	7.2–7.6
Cerebrospinal fluid	7.4
Pancreatic juice	7.1–8.2
Bile	7.6–8.6

Normal healthy skin can have a pH reading of 4.5 to 6, or acid. Blood pH is slightly alkaline, from 7.3 to 7.45 on the scale. Mouth saliva, in good health, should be 7.1 pH, slightly alkaline. The stomach must maintain between 4.0 to 5.0 acidity to digest and break down protein foods. If the stomach loses its acidity somewhat, and tends toward neutrality or alkalinity, protein and calcium digestion, assimilation, and absorption are lowered or decreased, resulting in indigestion and poor health. Urine measurements can fluctuate depending on the type of foods eaten beforehand. However, to ensure good health, the urine should be slightly acid or neutral, with an overall average range of 6.5 to 7.0.

Measured by urine analysis, above 7.50 pH is an alkaline condition, and below 6.5 is an overacid condition. Both of these conditions overtax the body, causing it to become tired and weak. The body organs are always working to maintain the blood in a slightly alkaline state, 7.22 to 7.35. Overacidity and overalkalinity both will eventually break down the organs (disease) because of the immense strain upon them to maintain the blood in proper balance.

Nitrazine pH paper can be purchased to check your urine and saliva readings occasionally. More important than checking these levels is heeding your inner voice or feelings as to what natural foods your body requires at any given time. Balance will be maintained by applying the universal yin/yang and acid/alkaline principles.

As the alkalinity scale in figure 7.3 shows, the normal condition of the blood must be maintained slightly alkaline. A slightly alkaline blood and lymph is a requirement for health and long life. Neutral blood would result in immediate death. An acid condition of the body and its organs

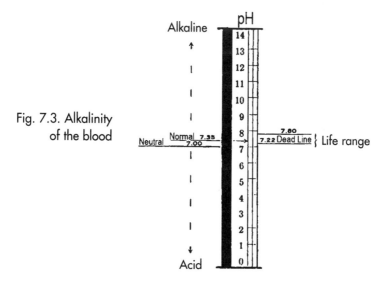

Fig. 7.3. Alkalinity of the blood

does not mean that the blood has become acid. Acidosis is not acid blood. If the blood were actually acid the body would immediately die from positive acidosis. Cells cannot live in an acid medium.

The body always maintains an alkaline reserve in order to neutralize acid elements. These alkaline reserves of sodium, potassium, calcium, and magnesium are called buffer salts. They maintain a balance between the alkalinity and acidity of the blood, which is normally 80 percent alkaline and 20 percent acid. An excess of either acid or alkaline in the body is quickly neutralized by the buffer salts. An exclusive acid-forming diet such as a high-protein or junk-food diet, combined with a lack of fresh fruit and vegetables, will cause a deficiency of these salts. This in turn will cause a drain on the alkaline reserves and irritation in the cells and tissues of the body, resulting in disease.

Overeating of alkaline foods will also cause a drain on the buffer salts in the cells as they try to neutralize the overalkalinity. The body expends much energy in overcoming or neutralizing either an overalkaline or overacid diet. The key is to consume both acid-forming and alkaline-forming foods in balance daily, adjusted to seasonal weather conditions. Solvent type foods such as watery fruits, juices, and non-starchy vegetables are alkaline. The heavier type foods are acid. The acid type foods are all proteins, starches, seeds, nuts, cheeses, and fats.

YIN/YANG AND ACID/ALKALINE FOODS

Yin and yang are generally believed to be the same as acid and alkaline, but in actual application they are not. From a broad universal perspective, yin is alkaline and yang is acid; from the food standpoint, acid-forming elements are made up of sulfur, phosphorus, and chlorine; alkaline-forming elements are made up of sodium, potassium, calcium, magnesium, and iron. The yin/yang scale is more variable than the acid/alkaline scale. For example, potassium and sodium are alkaline-forming elements, yet potassium is yin and sodium is yang. Another example is that meat, grains, nuts, and sugars are all considered acid-forming, yet meat and grains fall into the yang acid category, while nuts and sugar are classified as yin acid.

Yin foods such as nuts, dairy foods, and avocados are also high in fat. Yin/acid-forming foods, like milk, sugar, and nuts, are high in phosphorus and sulfur but low in sodium. Yang/acid-forming foods, such as rice, rye, eggs, and fish, are all high in phosphorus, sulfur, and sodium. Yin/alkaline-forming foods, such as oranges, pineapples, and tomatoes, are high in potassium, calcium, and iron but are low in phosphorus and sulfur. Yang/alkaline-forming foods, in the form of cherries, berries, garlic, burdock root, and ginseng, are high in sodium but low in phosphorus and sulfur.

Simply stated, yin and yang are on a deeper, more universal scale than acid and alkaline. Acid and alkaline pertain to chemistry and food. Yin and yang encompass all phenomena: physical (food, biochemistry), mental, emotional, and spiritual.

ACID-FORMING ELEMENTS	ALKALINE-FORMING ELEMENTS
Sulfur	Sodium
Phosphorus	Potassium
Chlorine	Calcium
Magnesium	Iron

There is a relative sliding scale between acid and alkaline. For example, meat is highly acid, but it contains some alkaline elements, while apples are mostly alkaline but contain a small amount of acid elements. Meat is on the yang end of the scale, and fruit is on the yin side. Pure sugar and fats are always yin. Pure starch and protein are always yang. Pure sugar, fat starch, and protein are always acid. Dairy fat is yin and acid. Watery fruits and vegetables are always yin and alkaline. Raw unsalted seeds and nuts are always yin and acid. Cooked grains, beans, eggs, meat, fish, and chicken are always yang and acid.

Yin foods cause expansion of the organs. Yang foods cause contraction of the organs. Consume only the proper quantity of protein, starches, fats, and natural sugars that the body requires daily, as excess or deficiency of these foods can cause disease. Consume mostly whole grains, seeds, and beans from the yang protein and starch category.

Meat eaters and exclusive grain and cooked food eaters have an acid/yang urine pH from 5.0 to 6.0, indicating that the internal organs are working hard to maintain slight alkalinity in the blood. To overcome low pH in the system, a little more raw food (fruits and vegetables in season) should be consumed. On the other hand, many fruitarians, vegetarians, and those who follow a strict raw food diet usually have a high (7.3 to 8.0) urine pH, which is considered alkaline and yin. High alkalinity in the stomach reduces its hydrochloric acid content, which can result in poor protein/calcium absorption and indigestion. Balance must be maintained with additional cooked grains, legumes, and vegetables.

Yin/Yang and Acid/Alkaline Food Classification

Extreme Yin Foods

High sugar and fat, white sugar and ice cream, fructose and glucose, margarine and lard, marijuana, chemicals, soda and cold drinks, grapes, cakes, pies, jams, coffee, alcohol, baking yeast and spices, chocolate, candy

Natural Yin/Acid Foods

Honey and maple syrup, carob and molasses, dried seeds and nuts, dried fruit, oils and butter, avocado, mushrooms, potatoes, nut butters, milk and cheese

Yin/Alkaline Foods

Tomatoes, eggplant, oranges, grapefruit, pineapple, fresh figs and dates, all juices, tropical fruits, melons, bananas

Yang/Alkaline Foods

Fruits: Apples, pears, plums, all berries, cherries, apricots, pomegranate, grapes

Vegetables: Cabbage, Romaine lettuce, green pepper, sprouts, alfalfa, squash, carrot, garlic, onion, celery, leeks, radishes, sea vegetables, broccoli, dandelion, kale, bib lettuce, artichokes, brussels sprouts, cauliflower, okra, Swiss chard, cucumber, endive, parsley, mustard greens, watercress, sorrel, beet tops, turnip root and greens, spinach, tomatoes

Yang/Acid Foods

Seeds/Nuts, soaked: Pumpkin, sunflower, sesame, almonds, walnuts, pecans, brazil

Grains: Rice, rye, wheat, corn, buckwheat, oats, millet, barley

Beans and Peas: Lima, pinto, kidney, adzuki, butter, black, and soy (tofu)

Dairy: Low-fat yogurt, buttermilk, skim and goat milk (sparingly)

Extreme Yang Foods (High Starch and Protein)

Yang/Acid: Meat, fish, fowl, eggs, white flour, burnt food, skim
milk cheese, high-salt cheese, and cigarettes

Yang/Alkaline: Salt, ginseng, burdock, miso, and tamari

Note: Consume yang/alkaline foods in cold weather and very sparingly in warm or hot climates.

Food Supplements

Yin/Alkaline: Chlorophyll liquid, alfalfa tablets, spirulina, garlic
pills

Yang/Alkaline: Kelp, dulse

Yin/Acid: Nutritional yeast

YIN/YANG AND ACID/ALKALINE CONDITIONS

The type of food we eat places us in a definite category. These different
categories are as follows: yin/alkaline, yang/acid, yin/acid, acid/alkaline
balance in a yin condition, yin/yang balance in an acid condition, and
lastly, acid/alkaline and yin/yang balance. Let us take a look at these different groups.

Yin/Alkaline Condition Above 7.5 pH

A yin/alkaline condition of mind and body is caused by eating an excess
of yin/alkaline foods, such as citrus fruits, tropical fruits, grapes, green
vegetables, sprouts, onions, tomatoes, and any other food that gives a
urine pH reading higher than 7.5. In the nonfood category, all drugs,
marijuana, alcohol, and soft drinks are yin (expansive). If one consumes
excessive amounts of alkaline/yin foods and not enough acid/yang foods,
the urine pH will rise above 7.5 to 8.0 or more.

Yin/alkaline diets are excessively high in potassium, which is an
expansive (yin) or centrifugal element. It expands cells, tissues, and
organs. If indulged in to excess, this diet can cause kidney expansion and
weakness, resulting in overurination. The kidneys are directly tied in
with the entire glandular and reproductive systems. Weak kidneys and
adrenals can diminish or stop the sex drive. In this condition the urine

turns light in color, like water, with a 7.5 to 8.0 pH reading. The kidneys lose their contractile or yang power and become loose, unable to synthesize protein and filter out waste products.

Excessive consumption of raw vegetables, especially lettuce, carrots, and carrot juice will cause liver congestion and yellow/orange or muddy colored skin (Caucasians only), which is so prevalent in many raw food dieters or vegetarians. The liver eliminates bile through the bile ducts, through the intestines, and out with the stools. If the liver is sluggish, due to improper foods or constipation, the bile will stagnate and flow into the blood, into the system, and out to the skin as a carrot complexion.

An overworked or diseased liver has long been associated with a mental condition called melancholia. *Melan* refers to the skin; dark bile reaches the skin from biliousness; it also causes mental depression and melancholy or a negative mental condition.

As a result of a yin/alkaline condition, a person tends to suffer with low blood pressure (expanded arteries and blood vessels), poor circulation, cold hands and feet, anemia, low blood sugar, diarrhea, asthma, impotence, yin arthritis, mental and physical laziness, nervousness, schizophrenia, poor memory, and loss of concentration.

Mentally, this condition causes fear, worry, anxiety, self-pity, irritability, criticalness, and self-righteousness. Yin/alkaline people are suspicious, with their nerves on edge, and are therefore easily intimidated and on the defensive, mentally and verbally. They attempt to make others perfect, instead of extending freedom to all. Usually unhappy themselves, they force their ideas or advice on others. Remember: these are extreme nutritionally affected psychological behavior patterns. There are variations of this type.

Yin/alkaline people lose the ability to center (contract-yang) their mind on a specific goal. With brain cells yin and expanded (confused thinking), they are unable to go within (one-pointedness) to find peace and contentment.

A yin/alkaline diet is deficient in protein, fats, sulfur, phosphorus, and chlorine. Many times these deficiencies lead to cravings and binging on yang/acid-forming junk food, such as pizza, flesh foods, and restaurant food. Or, due to lack of B vitamins and protein (which maintain normal blood sugar levels), an excess of cheese, ice cream, and other sugared foods are eaten. The diet is lacking in grains, beans, miso, cooked vegetables, and sea vegetables and consists of too much raw food in winter. The diet also lacks the pungent and salty taste according to the five elements.

Yang/Acid Condition Below 6.5 pH

A yang/acid condition of mind and body is caused by consuming an excess of yang/acid foods such as all meats, eggs, salt, fish, grains, nuts, fats, cheese, and all other foods that result in a urine pH reading of 6.5 or less.

Yang/acid diets are excessively high in sodium. Sodium is a contractive (yang) element. It contracts or restricts organs, tissues, and cells. Kidney contraction or restriction results in scanty urination and dark yellow or brownish and foamy urine. Healthy urine is straw colored or similar to a light beer. Dark urine indicates overworked kidneys. The kidneys eventually shut down operation and the end result is Bright's disease. Diseased kidneys are unable to synthesize protein and fail to filter out normal body wastes and environmental toxins. A yang toxic liver backs up bile into the blood, making it dark or black, causing biliousness, mental depression, and melancholia.

People in a yang/acid condition exhibit aggressive energy-force. They have high blood pressure, ulcers, heart disorders, kidney disease, gout, bone disease, and cancer. In physical diagnosis, their face and ears are reddish due to prominent veins in nose and cheeks, yellow eye whites, hot moist hands and feet, excessive sweating, and farsightedness. This is an extreme yang/acid condition.

If the urine pH drops to 5.5 and below, the kidneys, liver, bladder, lungs, skin, and other organs must operate under a heavy load to attempt to expel the excess acid toxins from the system and to preserve and maintain the blood in its normal 7.5 pH, a slightly alkaline condition. When the internal organs malfunction from overwork (overeating, toxins) disease is inevitable; if the blood pH falls to positive acidity, even slightly, death is certain.

The yang/acid person exhibits the following physical and mental traits: excessive sexual desire (irritated sex glands), menstrual disorders, hot temper, impatience, arrogance, possessiveness, dominance, grudge-holding, exclusiveness, demands immediate attention, and, in the extreme, being dictatorial.

Mentally, these people are self-centered, egotistical, and overbearing in manner and attitude. Unlike the yin spaced-out person, the yang person is more centered in his or her concentration and mental activity. Yang/acid people's brain cells are more contracted (yang and centered thinking) to a specific goal. Such people are not generally fearful or worrisome, like their yin counterparts.

This diet is deficient in alkaline minerals: potassium, calcium, magnesium, and iron. It also lacks raw foods, fruits, vegetables, seeds, grains, legumes, and sea vegetables. Yang/acid people crave many foods and substances, such as beer, wine, alcohol, coffee, marijuana, tropical foods, potatoes, juices, and all sugared foods. This diet lacks seasonal fruit and vegetables eaten daily in moderation; it includes too much meat, cooked foods, and fats, especially in summer. According to the five-element taste theory, this diet is too high in the salty, pungent, and sweet tastes and sometimes deficient in the bitter (almonds, raw vegetables) and sour (apples, plums, yogurt) tastes.

Yin/Acid Condition Below 6.5 pH

A yin/acid condition is caused by consuming chiefly yin (expansive) and acid-forming foods. Milk, cheese, and ice cream are yin because of their high fat (expansive) content and acid due to their acid-forming qualities, lowering body and urine pH below 6.5. All sugared foods, such as pies, cakes, donuts, soft drinks, and candy, are yin/acid due to their high sugar and white flour content. All sugar is yin (expansive), and all white flour products are acid-forming.

People falling in this category usually consume an excessive amount of devitalized junk food. Their urine pH is well below 6.5, and the blood and body are generally deficient in vitamins, minerals, trace elements, enzymes, and quality protein. Yin/acid individuals suffer from every known disease: arthritis, diabetes, hypoglycemia, gout, obesity, kidney and liver disorders, lung and blood diseases, skin and sexual diseases, fatigue, and all types of cancer.

Mentally, this condition produces weak-willed individuals, lacking in concentration and drive, with low self-esteem; they are usually followers, allowing others to use them; they do not think clearly for themselves, do not stand up for their personal rights, are duped by commercials and slick advertising, and believe without questioning what product to purchase or what alleged pain killers to use.

Acid/Alkaline in Yin Condition Neutral 7.0 pH

A yin condition along with an acid/alkaline balance results from consuming an excess of yin foods while at the same time eating the correct balance of acid and alkaline.

Such an individual typically consumes: 1) a large amount of tropical fruit and tomatoes, sprouts, cucumbers, raw greens, and fruit and vegetable juices, which are all yin and alkaline; 2) all high-fat cheeses, milk, avocados, seeds, nuts, oils high in fat, which are yin and acid-forming; 3) bananas, dates, figs, raisins, all dried fruit high in sugar, which are yin and acid-forming; and 4) potatoes, yams, eggplant, which are yin and acid-forming.

These people generally suffer with cold hands and feet, falling hair, skin disorders, colds, flu, fatigue, nervousness, low blood sugar (hypoglycemia), and sexual impotence or frigidity. Mentally, they tend to be docile, fearful, lacking in success drive, and they express little faith; they are usually peaceful but lazy. The diet of such persons is too high in potassium (yin) and deficient in sodium (yang). It also lacks sour, salty, and pungent tastes. To balance this diet, fruit should be consumed in season, more raw fruit and vegetables should be taken in summer and less in winter. More cooked grains, legumes, miso, sea vegetables, and soups should be eaten.

Yin/Yang in Acid Condition pH 6.5 or Below

An acid condition while in yin/yang balance is caused by eating an excess of acid foods, while eating the right balance of yin and yang foods. Such people generally eat a large amount of the following foods: all grains (rice, wheat, oats, and millet), beans, fish, cooked vegetables, soups, burdock, ginseng, and little or no raw food. These people generally suffer physically with lung problems, occasional fevers, yang liver congestion, anemia, and some skin disorders; they are usually underweight and sometimes emaciated. The body becomes too acid. Mentally, they are sometimes arrogant, generally desire leadership, and are too demanding.

This diet is usually deficient in alkaline elements, such as potassium, iron, and calcium. This deficiency sometimes leads to a craving for beer, coffee, and so on. If the diet is too strict, there may be occasional binging on extreme yin/alkaline fruits, ice cream, or other sweet foods or juices. This diet lacks seasonal fruit eaten daily in moderation and has insufficient raw food, especially in summer. According to the five-element theory, this dietary condition lacks two of the five tastes: sweet and sour.

Yin/Yang Acid/Alkaline Neutral Urine 7.0 pH

To acquire yin/yang and acid/alkaline balance, one should eat a sufficient amount of acid and alkaline foods, while balancing the yin and yang factors. In order to attain the correct balance, foods grown in the same climate should be eaten, ideally grown locally. In the south, some yin fruits and vegetables can be eaten daily in moderation, balanced equally with natural yang grains, legumes, sea vegetables, soups, land vegetables, and so on. In the north tropical food should not be used to any great extent. The diet should mainly consist of grains, soups, legumes, soaked or germinated seeds and nuts, apples, pears, berries, burdock, low-fat raw milk (sparingly), miso, sea vegetables, and so on. Those who constantly have a neutral 6.5 to 7.2 pH urine reading are in acid/alkaline balance. A yin/yang balance is achieved by adhering closely to a yin and yang balancing diet, which will automatically place one in the proper acid/alkaline balance.

An important aspect of achieving yin/yang balance is through regulation of potassium and sodium intake. Generally, the ratio should be 2.5 potassium to 1 sodium in the human organism. The formed elements of blood contain twenty times as much potassium as sodium. The main reason why strict grain eaters become underweight and lose muscle form and tone is because they lack sufficient potassium, which fills out the muscle tissue and imparts beauty. A 7 to 1 potassium to sodium ratio, as advocated by some, is much too low for health maintenance. A healthy person does not deny the body what it requires.

The healthiest and longest-lived people throughout the world do not consume extreme yin or yang diets: neither all raw foods nor all cooked foods. They eat a variety of natural foods, such as grains, legumes, vegetables, fruits, seeds, nuts, fermented and cultured dairy products, and meat (very sparingly or not at all), grown in their own climate and eaten in season.

EAT ACCORDING TO THE SEASONS

The influences of food, climate, and environment affect and intimately bind humankind to the inescapable natural laws of yin and yang. Cold weather creates an inner biologic need for warmth, fire, and yang foods. Hot or warm weather creates an inner biologic yin need for yin foods, which are cooling and refreshing, such as juicy fruits and vegetables, along with more water. An excessive consumption of cooked yang foods eaten in yang hot weather overheats the body, blood, and internal organs, resulting in extra heart beats, a rise in blood pressure, profuse sweating, and fatigue. An excessive consumption of raw fruits, juices, liquids, or raw vegetables eaten in yin cold climates will automatically lower blood pressure (due to expansion of vessels) and thin the blood, causing cold hands and feet and weakening the heart and circulatory system.

Changing weather conditions can affect us in a detrimental way if we do not learn how to acclimate ourselves to the changing environment. In arranging daily menus seasonal weather changes must be taken into account, especially for those who live in northern or seasonal climates. This is so important because cold weather is alkaline upon the body fluids. Consuming excessive alkaline foods in cold weather will cause overalkalinity within the body, resulting in cold hands and feet, low blood pressure, diarrhea, and so on. Therefore, the body requires more acid foods to balance itself correctly. Similarly, excessive acid foods in hot weather will cause overacidity.

To maintain internal balance during cold winter months, consume more protein, natural starches, and fats, and less alkaline foods. Use more raw food in summer and more cooked food in winter. Fall and spring generally require 50 percent alkaline foods and 50 percent acid foods. In tropical zones or during summer in the north, 65 percent alkaline foods can be consumed, while acid food requirements can be lowered to 35 percent.

If the temperature soars over 90°F, use more seasonal fruits and vegetables, and less grains, beans, and cooked food. By eating in this manner heat and cold will be more comfortable, mentally and physically. Hot weather has an acidifying effect upon the body fluids. Vacationers in Mexico and other tropical zones generally blame their diarrhea and stomach upsets on the water. In fact, eating rich, spicy acid foods, cold drinks, and ice cream creates extreme acidosis, digestive disorders, and loose bowels.

APPROPRIATE SEASONAL EATING PERCENTAGES

SEASON	ALKALINE FOODS	ACID FOODS
Summer	65%	35%
Fall	50%	50%
Winter	25%	75%
Spring	50%	50%
Very Hot	80%	20%
Very Cold	20%	80%

Note: These are only general percentages. Study and learn how to balance foods and learn to listen to your inner physiological needs; eventually you will know the right amount to eat of acid and alkaline foods.

EXTREMISM VERSUS BALANCE

In the modern world we have a habit of extremism. We are always trying to find the simple answer to solve all of our problems. The early Taoist models of thought show us that life does not operate in this way. Rather than trying to attain a single goal, life can be seen as a flow of energy. It is up to us to find harmony and balance within that flow.

For example, in modern thinking we may be tempted to try to reach a perfect goal: perfect weight, perfect health, ideal levels of energy. However, if we stop and observe nature we see that this is not reality. In reality, in the cycles of every day we flow between being tired to sleeping to wakefulness to high energy. We are in constant flux. The result of trying to force our bodies toward an unnatural goal is that we push ourselves farther away from balance and harmony. A lot of modern illnesses are a result of this disharmony.

Additionally, a lot of the current nutritional theories are based upon a movement in a single direction toward one extreme. For example:

Alkaline theory suggests that we all need to eat more alkaline-forming foods.

Raw food theory suggests that we all need to eat only raw uncooked foods.

High-protein diet suggests that we all need to eat a high-protein, low-carb diet.

Vegetarianism suggests that we all need to eliminate animal products from the diet.

Each of these diets works extremely well for some people, and various diet books are full of personal case histories to support the theory. The problem is that there is also a portion of the population for whom a given diet does not work at all, and may even cause further illness. For example, cold and thin people may become very weak on a diet of raw foods; others will put on weight from eating a high-protein diet.

According to ancient Chinese Taoist health teachings given in *The Yellow Emperor's Classic of Internal Medicine* as the five elements and transformation principle, there is no one perfect or ideal food to subsist on. Fruits and vegetables alone are too yin/alkaline; grains, beans, and meat alone are too yang/acid. Extreme diets, whether yin or yang, are unbalanced diets, creating imbalances in mind and body chemistry. If we choose an extreme diet we will always pull ourselves off-center, and building a strong center is so important for health and happiness.

One of the rules of yin/yang theory is that an extreme will always turn into its opposite. This rule applies also to dietary therapy. Thus overly yin people may benefit from the addition of a few extra proteins and quality fats. However, if they were to embrace a diet exclusively of these foods, they might in fact end up feeling too heavy and even more lethargic! This is an example of an extreme having the reverse effect. Similarly overly yang people will benefit from a few more carbs in the diet. A few salads and steamed veggies will cool and calm them immensely. However, if they were to go overboard on fruit juices and sweet foods, their blood sugar would rise up excessively, causing too extreme an energy rise.

The wiser course is to take our time and add a few foods into our diet for rebalancing. Once again the golden rule of the center appears: if we are eating some centering foods, plus the rebalancing items, then we will have a more successful result in the long term.

When necessary, a yin/alkaline diet can be used effectively as an eliminative or cleansing diet for a short period of time. All cleansing diets, fasting, juice diets, sprout/raw food diets can help tremendously to balance body chemistry and eliminate internal (yang/acid) toxins, and overcome yang constipation, yang liver disorders, and yang kidney trouble. However, they should be undertaken for this purpose only, not as a regular dietary program.

The same dietary principle holds true for counteracting a situation of becoming too yin and alkaline, as a result of excessive consumption of fruit, juices, sprouts, vegetables, liquids, and raw foods. A balance in the system can be created by discontinuing all raw foods for a few days or weeks and consuming only grain-based products, legumes, cooked vegetables, miso, soups, and sea vegetables. These are natural yang/acid foods, which will help to rebalance an extreme yin/alkaline system. After internal balance has been achieved, the exclusive yang/acid diet should be discontinued and a properly balanced diet maintained.

Beyond a certain point of cleansing, exclusive fruitarian, juicearian, or sproutarian diets generally fail to produce healthy results in balancing the body physically, chemically, and mentally. Blood, bone, and muscle are built by sixteen mineral elements, several vitamins, plus the proper amount of protein, natural complex carbohydrates, and fats. After a diet cleansing period, a true, lasting, and stable physical and mental healing must take place. A well-balanced diet is a definite requirement afterward in order to strengthen and build cellular structures, increase normal hormone production, impart muscle tone, and form and reconstruct blood and hemoglobin.

A balanced body chemistry is a prerequisite or necessary factor for internal healing and health maintenance. Each body cell is bi-polar: its nucleus is positive (yang); the cytoplasm is negative (yin). The cytoplasm is alkaline, which is surrounded by the nucleus, acid. For a proper balance the cells need an 80/20 ratio, that is, 80 percent alkaline and 20 percent acid. This is of vital importance and is essential for that spark of animation or electric potential between the nucleus and cytoplasm. If an excess of acid foods are eaten, the alkalinity of the cell is reduced. If an excess of alkaline foods are eaten, the acidity of the cell is reduced. An excess or deficiency of either acid or alkaline elements in the diet will result in a loss of that vital spark that is so necessary to maintain vibrant health.

Extreme yin or yang diets are much too rigid and create imbalances in body chemistry. Each causes its own kind of physical and mental disharmony. A person on a strict yin diet almost always binges on yang foods. A yang diet person binges on yin food. If people deny yin, they will crave yin; if people deny yang, they will crave yang. We are pulled toward what we need, if we deny it in our diet or elsewhere. Healthy and nutritionally balanced people have no need to fly from one extreme to another; they eat only according to their inner physiological needs and requirements and select foods from a wide variety of nature's bounty.

Although we can observe the techniques of others and imitate their diets, this is not enough. There are many people who, even after several years of following what they consider to be the ultimate diet, are still unable to make themselves healthy and happy. This is because they have not yet understood the principle behind the diet, without comprehension of which the technique is dangerous. For example, if a person living in a hot climate were to maintain a diet consisting of about 75 percent grains, 15 percent cooked vegetables, 5 percent beans, seaweeds, and pressed salad, that person would eventually become very sick (too yang). But such a diet would be a good approximation for the average person living in a cold climate (depending on such variables as age, activity, previous eating habits, and other factors). In short, the clearer your understanding of the unifying principle of yin and yang, the better you will be able to follow the correct diet successfully.

To achieve a proper yin/yang and acid/alkaline balance, it is best to consume food grown in your own local environment, which includes a daily quota of raw fruits and vegetables, cooked grains, and legumes. Then, listen to your inner physiological voice; our inner body intelligence knows what kind and how much food we require to maintain nutritional balance.

OVERWEIGHT PROBLEMS

Weight problems are one kind of imbalance that is an increasing concern in modern health care. In 2005, the World Health Organization (WHO) estimated that 400 million adults were obese. In 2010 the United States spent $168 billion on medical costs attributable to obesity. It appears that our modern consumer society has a cost.

In Oriental nutrition, not all overweight problems are seen as the same; thus they are treated differently. The yin/yang model can be used to gain a clearer insight into differences. The overly yang type of obesity is the result of a pattern of excess: excess food, excess alcohol, excess rich and fatty foods. An overweight pattern that is overly yang can be identified by characteristics such as: the body fat is solid and turgid and when pressed has little give and feels full; there may be signs of heat; the person may be loud and impatient or show other yang characteristics. Foods that can moisturize an overly yang and excessively dry situation include soups, sauces, salads, fruits, and water-rich vegetables. Those who are excessively dry may choose to consume a special moistening drink of psyllium husk or flaxseeds (linseeds) soaked in water overnight or a yogurt smoothie with seeds and fruit added.

On the other hand, the overly yin type of obesity is the result of a pattern of deficiency of quality foods and nutrients and exercise. An overly yin pattern may be accompanied by too much water in the body (water is yin), leading to fluid retention and dampness. It can be identified by certain characteristics, including: the body fat is soft, flaccid, and flabby; when pressed it gives way and feels empty; there may be signs of coldness; the person may be withdrawn and depressed or show other yin characteristics. If these symptoms exist, then it can be wise to pay attention to the water content or moistness of the food being eaten. We can tell a lot about the moistening effects of a food just by common sense and observation. If a food looks and tastes dry, then it usually is! If it appears moist, then it is. Foods that will dry up an overly yin and excessively moist situation include lightly cooked grains, foods without sauces, root vegetables, fish, and meat. Those with moistness and water retention may benefit from the addition of some diuretic herbal teas, such as roselle and nettle tea.

Treatment of Weight Problems

The overly yang weight problem requires a treatment protocol that reduces excess yang and adds a little yin.

Fasting works well with this type of pattern as it quickly removes excess yang.

The person can eat more cleansing and light foods: raw food, steamed vegetables, fruit, and juices.

Protein and fat should be avoided.

Toxins must be eliminated: caffeine, tobacco, alcohol, and drugs must be cut out, at least for the cleansing period.

Peace, quiet, and tranquility need to be sought: this person will benefit enormously from walking alone in nature and taking up meditation. It is difficult for such a person to lose weight without some level of relaxation.

Yang sports such as gym workouts could be reduced and replaced with yin exercise such as yoga and Chi Kung.

Treatment for an overly yin weight problem should be entirely different, as the whole situation is different. Excess yin needs to be reduced and a little yang needs to be added.

Sugars and fast-releasing carbohydrates should be eliminated, including fruit juices.

Fasting is unlikely to help with this kind of weight problem, though it may reduce toxins and water. This type has to be careful because if they go without food it increases the chance of a yo-yo dieting pattern, which will further weaken the body's metabolism.

Eating regularly is important, as it helps to balance blood sugar levels.

Increasing the levels of quality proteins (lean meats/fish) and healthy fats (cold-pressed oils such as olive and flaxseed oil) can also help this type to lose weight.

A little yang exercise, such as running, dancing, or jumping on a bouncer, should be added.

A little green tea can assist in stimulation of stagnant chi and assist with weight loss.

While these overweight problem types are not gender dependent, a larger proportion of men will suffer from the overly yang type of weight problem, whereas women are more prone to overly yin weight problems. If you are trying to deal with a weight problem, try to assess where you are imbalanced in your life (such as not enough exercise or too much alcohol consumption) and seek balance.

UNDERWEIGHT PROBLEMS

Being underweight is also an issue for some people. Even though our beauty magazines exalt extreme thinness, it is often a sign of weakness and deficiency, and an underweight situation may not support vibrant health. Once again, we can distinguish between overly yang and overly yin underweight problems.

An overly yang underweight problem is seen in people who are overly active, nervous, and jittery. They may be always moving or fidgeting and find it difficult to rest or be still. In order to gain weight, this type of person will need to eat more complex carbohydrates. Such people also have to rest and learn some form of relaxation. Deep breathing can be tremendously helpful. They need to avoid stimulants such as caffeine at all costs.

The overly yin underweight situation is one in which people are thin, quiet, and fragile. They are likely to get cold to the core and feel as if they have weak bones. They may find it very difficult to socialize and to express themselves. To begin to gain weight and restore health, this person may need to eat quality proteins and fats (such as olive oil and flaxseed oil). It is important for this type of person to eat very nourishing and high-quality foods, with an emphasis on warm and cooked foods. It always takes longer to restore a deficiency pattern. An overly yin underweight person is very deficient. Therefore, such people will need to take a lot of time and dedication to rebalance their health.

BALANCING THE LIFE CYCLE TRIANGLE

The two most fundamental ways to establish health, freedom, and happiness in our life are: 1) by improvement of our thinking ability toward the highest judgment, or awareness of absolute truth (yin), and 2) by dietary discipline in accord with the unifying principle (yang). Actually, these two ways are one, for without using our judgment, how can we eat correctly? And without eating correctly, how can we become aware of truth? A clear mind cannot exist in a disturbed body.

Everything in life affects the yin/yang and acid/alkaline balance. Activity, such as exercise, work, and study, creates acidity (yang), while rest and sleep create alkalinity (yin) within the body. Cold weather has a yin/alkaline effect upon the body, while hot weather has a yang/acid effect upon the body. Anger, hate, and jealousy create yang and acidity; peace, love, harmony in thoughts and actions, and enthusiasm create a natural body balance. Positive thoughts are yang; negative thoughts are yin.

Exercise creates acidity within the body. Vigorous exercise, where there is a breakdown of muscular tissue, as in weight training, distance running, and swimming, will cause much lactic acid to be generated in the system. In this case, the athlete will require more calories from complex carbohydrates (grains, legumes) to replace the broken-down tissues. However, yin/alkaline foods must also be consumed to balance the acidity of the exercise and to replace and renew electrolytes within the cells and tissues. This is not to encourage overeating; on the contrary, the demands made upon an athlete's body will automatically require eating enough to sustain endurance, stamina, strength, and health, while a nonexerciser cannot possibly utilize food as efficiently, due to slower blood circulation, poor stomach tone, and weak assimilation of food.

Only you can judge how much activity or rest you require and also how to balance your diet properly. You must listen to your inner voice to know when, what, and how much to eat, sleep, work, and exercise. Be moderate in all your activities. You can achieve superior health and harmony by understanding the universal law of rhythm. The life cycle triangle is the law of rhythm in dynamic action.

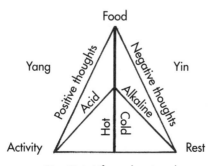

Fig. 7.4. Life cycle triangle

BALANCING YIN AND YANG

Yin and yang can also be viewed in terms of our feminine and masculine qualities. It is a common misconception that only women should have feminine qualities and only men should possess masculine qualities. Yin/yang theory is a theory of relatives, not absolutes. All of us are whole as we are, with our yin aspects and our yang aspects. These aspects include the following:

YIN AND YANG QUALITIES

FEMININE	MASCULINE
Intuition	Logic
Receptive	Creative
Passive	Active
Internal	External
Subconscious	Personality

We all possess all abilities and are complete. However, when we are with another person, we may be relatively feminine (yin) or masculine (yang) compared to them (regardless of gender). Often (but not always) a woman is relatively yin compared to a man, but she still possesses yang qualities within herself. These individual differences are what give us our individuality, and they do not need to be fixed or changed.

It is only when our inner harmony becomes unbalanced that we may need to take remedial action. For example, a person with a lot of feminine qualities may be always cooler than his or her more masculine partner who has a warmer body temperature. This does not need to be viewed as a problem; these are simply individual differences. However, if a person suddenly feels that he or she is much colder than previously, and begins to suffer discomfort from it, then there may have been a change in his or her own internal balance that needs to be addressed.

In terms of remedial action, we can see that proteins and fats enhance our masculine or yang qualities, whereas carbohydrates enhance our feminine or yin qualities. We often think of meat as being a masculine food, and we think of sweet foods as being a favorite of women. If the yin/yang imbalance starts to cause imbalances in health and well-being, then we may need to use the opposite food to bring ourselves back into balance. Five-element dietary therapy is a delicate art of listening to the body and responding accordingly.

Yin and Yang Dietary Guidelines

The balance between carbohydrates and proteins/fats is the broadest way to balance yin and yang. However, there are many different aspects of diet that can assist in this, including:

Cooking methods	Thermal properties of foods
Water content of foods	Flavors
Colors	Parts of plants eaten

In five-element dietary therapy these factors all have a subtle influence on the energetics of our food. Paying attention to them can enhance the effectiveness of our dietary therapy.

Cooking Methods

Raw foods and lightly cooked foods have a more cleansing and cooling effect on the body. Thus they can be used to treat an overly yang situation, especially where there is heat and toxicity. The longer a food is cooked, the more warming and nourishing it becomes. Therefore, these cooking methods can be used to treat an overly yin situation, especially where there is coldness and weakness.

YIN AND YANG OF COOKING METHODS

CLEANSING	NOURISHING
Raw	Grilled
Steamed	Baked
Stir-fried	Pressure cooked

Thermal Properties of Foods

The ancient Taoists discovered that each food has its own thermal property, regardless of its actual temperature. These can be chosen specifically to regulate internal temperature imbalances. Examples of warming foods include: ginger, oats, chestnuts, sesame seeds, sweet potatoes, garlic, kale, date, cinnamon. Examples of cooling foods include: lettuce, cucumber, celery, cabbage, tofu, wheat, yogurt, peppermint.

Water Content of Foods

One of the features of overly yin imbalance is to have an excess of water, such as fluid retention, dampness, and phlegm. A feature of the overly yang situation is to be too dry, such as dry skin, dry hair, dry nails, and dry lungs. Appropriate foods can be chosen from the charts given below to correct imbalances.

Flavors

In Oriental therapy, different flavors have different energetic effects on the body. The sweet flavor has the most uplifting and drying effect, whereas the salty flavor has a grounding effect. Bland foods have a more neutral effect. The body requires each of these flavors in a moderate amount daily. As shown in chapter 6, an excessive intake of one flavor will harm the associated organ and its corresponding organ. The key is to balance the five flavors according to seasonal changes and inner biological needs on a day-to-day basis. If you consume an excessive amount of salty foods, you will automatically desire or crave sweet foods to create a balance in the taste, which corresponds to an inner physiological (organ) need.

Someone who has an overly yin imbalance may want to reduce intake of sweet foods. Someone with an overly yang imbalance may want to reduce salty foods. The other flavors—bitter, sour, and pungent—have varying effects on the body and are used to make fine-tuned adjustments.

Colors

We are living in a universe of positive (yang) and negative (yin) magnetic energy fields, which continually vibrate at tremendous speeds and produce magnetic currents. These magnetic currents register on our brain in a color spectrum visible to the eye. The ultraviolet rays of the spectrum are yin and the infrared rays are yang. They go from yin to yang in this order: violet, indigo, blue, green, yellow, brown, orange, and red. Color is energy; different colors are different wavelengths of energies. Thus the colors of our foods have an energetic effect on our being when we consume them. Brighter and lighter colors have an uplifting energetic effect. Darker and duller colors have a grounding effect. Therefore, for example, someone with an overly yin imbalance may choose darker foods, such as meat, fish, and beans.

Parts of Plants

Yin and yang are relative terms, and thus they can be applied to any whole unit. Therefore, we can find yin and yang aspects within one vegetable. Some parts of the plant will have a more expansive effect, others more contractive, and some centering. Just as we saw with the tree example, the roots of a vegetable will have a more grounding and contracting effect. The shoots and stalks have a more neutral effect. Leaves and flowers have the most expansive and uplifting effect.

Eating all parts of a vegetable will have a balanced and whole effect, or we can choose specific parts for their specific qualities.

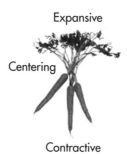

Expansive

Centering

Contractive

Fig. 7.5. Effects of plant parts

Summary of Yin/Yang Guidelines

We can attend to many different aspects of the food we eat when we are trying to regain balance. The relative amount of carbohydrates versus proteins and fats is the most powerful factor, but the others also can be used to rebalance on a more subtle level.

TO TREAT OVERLY YIN		TO TREAT OVERLY YANG	
QUALITY	**EFFECT**	**QUALITY**	**EFFECT**
Protein/Fats	Slow-release energy	Carbohydrates	Fast-release energy
Long cooking	Nourish	Light cooking	Cleanse
Warming	Warms	Cooling	Cools
Low water content	Dries	High water content	Moistens
Salty	Grounding	Wet	Uplifting
Dark color	Grounding	Light color	Uplifting
Roots	Grounding	Leaves	Uplifting

EATING HABITS VERSUS
MAKING CHANGES

Humans are the only animals that have taken the act of eating beyond the practical level. Eating is tremendously tied in with our emotional being; it does far more than meet our physiological requirements. Our eating behaviors are directly correlated with our psychological patterns. Therefore, to look only at the micronutrients in our food is to overlook a major aspect. Think about the emotional aspect of eating: we celebrate occasions with elaborate feasts; when we fall in love we exchange gifts of food (chocolates especially!) and we take our beloved out for dinner. As well as expressing joy with food, we can then use food to try to recreate that sense of happiness when we are no longer feeling it, hence the concept of comfort eating (one extreme being bulimia nervosa). Think of the woman who has just ended her relationship munching her way through a big box of cookies.

Other people are used to receiving attention through pain, so it is not uncommon for victims of abuse to develop eating behaviors through which they punish themselves with their eating habits. They may try to starve themselves (anorexia nervosa) or eat very plain foods or follow extremely strict diets. This is a way of reinforcing the belief that they are guilty and must be punished.

This emotional link with food operates at a subtle level, generating comfort or pain on a highly subconscious level. It is easy for us to develop eating patterns and habits that reinforce our psychological blocks, and this will create cravings for foods that do not serve us.

Intuition versus Addiction

We often talk about the body's wisdom and natural intuitive ability. We may assume that our body's desires are always for what will heal us or for what we need. But how do we know whether we are craving a food that we are addicted to, or our body is asking for what it needs? We can see how cravings arise when we look at the more addictive foods. If we have been drinking coffee for many years then our body adapts its energy system, as it expects a cup of coffee every morning. This leads to a craving for coffee, which will maintain our current equilibrium, though it

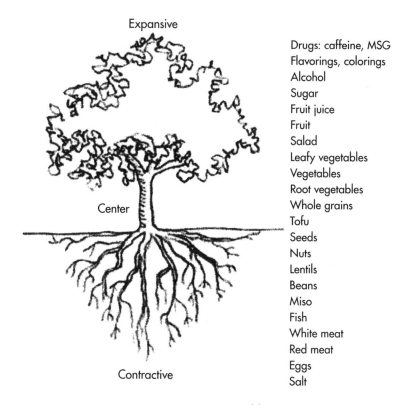

Expansive

Drugs: caffeine, MSG
Flavorings, colorings
Alcohol
Sugar
Fruit juice
Fruit
Salad
Leafy vegetables
Vegetables
Root vegetables
Center
Whole grains
Tofu
Seeds
Nuts
Lentils
Beans
Miso
Fish
White meat
Red meat
Eggs
Contractive
Salt

Fig. 7.6. Intuition versus addiction

will not bring us into vibrant health. This is a craving for what our body expects rather than a desire for what our body needs.

When we develop a habit of eating any food, then we may crave it as our body's way of maintaining routine. The further a food is from the center the more addictive it can become. Centering foods are the least addictive.

The more refined a food is, the more expansive and thus addictive it is. The most addictive foods are drug-foods, including MSG and caffeine, alcohol, and sugar. At the other end of the spectrum we have the most contractive foods, especially salt, but also an excess of meat and eggs. Dairy products may become addictive as they have the effect of protecting us from difficult emotions. More extreme foods are more addictive.

Balancing foods include vegetables, salads, whole grains, tofu, seeds, nuts, and lentils. It is unlikely that we will develop an addiction for these foods, unless they have been refined or have additives. Therefore we have to be on alert for what is a true instinctive desire and what is a habitual craving. It is important to learn to distinguish between the two so that we can choose healing. If we wish to restore our health we may have to address our habitual patterns and release the underlying emotions.

> ***How to spot a craving:*** the desire for a food tends to feel more urgent; our body may feel mildly panicky; sometimes there is a secretive aspect to the desire and we will consume the food where no one else can see us (we feel ashamed); or we may hang out with others who share our habit to justify ourselves; extreme contractive or expansive foods are the most addictive; it is a desire for the same substance over and over; we may want more, with an insatiable desire.
>
> ***How to know an intuition:*** the desire is deep, but not urgent; our body feels calm and relaxed; our desires change, as they are responses to the changing environment; once we have taken the food, we are satisfied and the desire is gone.

There is no right or wrong in this. We all have a choice at every moment. If you feel ok in your current situation, then do not try to make changes. If you are motivated to make a shift, then change your diet and make space for transformation. Do not change your diet for no reason. Rather, learn to listen to your body and act (or not) accordingly.

Replacing Bad Habits with Healthy Ones

Fasting and cleansing are great ways to clean the slate and start again. For example, just following a simple diet of organic centering foods, with no salt, sugar, caffeine, or additives, can help us to clear attachment to old patterns. Such procedures must be accompanied by consciousness: it is important to take time to look at what is going on in order to really make the shift at a deeper level. Often when we remove our comfort foods, emotions will arise that we have been suppressing. This needs to be met with awareness so that we can find ways to meet the underlying pain and thus heal it.

It can be a wise idea to go to a fasting center, where you will receive guidance throughout your cleanse and emotional support will be offered. Meditation is a great accompaniment to any cleanse or fast, as it helps to bring consciousness to our process.

In five-element dietary therapy, the focus is only to correct an imbalance if one exists. Once everything is back into balance, the person is encouraged to eat a wide variety of foods and a balanced diet. Obsession with food is considered an imbalance of the earth element and is a sign of a weak center. It can be the result of consuming too many extreme foods and of partaking of too many extreme activities.

If you have a strong mind, be wary not to let your mind overtake your healing process. You may feel great when you first make a dietary change, such as adding more protein to a protein-deficient diet. But then the mind may lead you to add protein to every meal; if you do not listen to your body, then you may not hear a signal that your diet has been rebalanced and it is time to move back to a more balanced diet. In this way, what starts as a healthy change soon becomes yet another mind-controlled habit.

We have become a very mind-dominated society in the modern world. This can lead to the situation in which we try to rule the body with the mind. However, a healthy relationship is one in which listening and acting are equal. If we listen to the body and then act, this will improve the relationship between mind and body. Controlling the body with the mind can result in the development of an eating disorder and take us a long way from feeling whole. Taoist practices always aim to harmonize the different aspects of the self. In this case the body is yin relative to the mind (yin = material; yang = immaterial), and so to harmonize the two is healing in itself.

MAINTAINING BALANCE

Often when people first become interested in nutrition, it is because a health problem has motivated them to make change. However, once that problem has been healed, we then need to switch our diet toward one that simply maintains our good health. There is a difference between using dietary therapy to correct an imbalance and eating to maintain health. Rebalancing diets involve going to the opposite extreme for a period until we come back to balance. Once balance is achieved, it is important to switch to a maintenance diet, or else we will swing the other way. For example, many people suffering from the results of an excessive lifestyle—too much fat, sugar, toxins, and stress—will benefit from a cleansing diet such as raw food. However, after a period, one should return to a more balanced diet or the body will eventually weaken.

Necessary Qualities of Maintenance Diets

1. They must be stable, and not extreme, so that they are easy to follow continuously.
2. There is evidence that they have been in use for long periods of time.
3. They promote well-being and health.
4. They promote longevity.

To find an ideal maintenance diet, it can be helpful to look into different cultures to find diets that have been in use for a long time and in which the members of that population enjoy good health and longevity. For example, the inhabitants of the island of Okinawa in Japan are known for their outstanding longevity. This population has been studied extensively to gain better understanding of their dietary habits. The average citizen of Okinawa consumes a diet made up of the following:

At least seven servings of vegetables daily, and an equal number of grains (in the form of noodles, bread, and rice, many of them whole grains).

Two to four servings of fruit.

Green tea (full of antioxidants).

Tofu and other forms of soy; various types of seaweed (soy and seaweed balance each other in terms of iodine).

Sweet potatoes, bean sprouts, onions, and green peppers are prominent in the diet.

Vegetables, grains, and fruits make up 72% of the diet by weight.

Soy and seaweed provide another 14%.

Meat, poultry, and eggs account for just 3% of the diet.

Fish rich in omega 3-fatty acids make up 11%; is taken about three times a week.

There is an emphasis on green vegetables rich in calcium.

Like diets of other Japanese, the Okinawan diet does not include much dairy (calcium comes from the dark leafy greens).

Okinawans do drink alcohol, but women usually stick to one drink a day, while men average twice that. Moderation is key.

In terms of vegetables, there is a special emphasis on sweet potatoes, which play a central role in the diet. This food has a very different effect on health than the normal potato. For example, a baked potato releases blood sugar very fast, whereas a sweet potato is slow-releasing. In five-element therapy, the sweet potato is known to improve digestive ability by enhancing the spleen-pancreas.

The diet of the Okinawans is in fact what five-element therapy would call a centering diet. It minimizes extreme foods and focuses on those that have a centering quality. Such a diet puts the least stress on the body (extremes cause most stress) and helps to maintain well-being.

Effects of Various Diets on Mind and Body

Grains, legumes, vegetables, fruits, sea greens, seeds, nuts (soaked); more raw food in hot weather and more cooked food in cold weather: More healthful; physically and mentally balanced temperament. Generally free from illness and disease. Intuition, creativity well balanced and more developed.

Grains, beans, cooked vegetables: Tendency to underweight or emaciation. This diet lacks raw food and sufficient potassium; may also lack protein and alkaline vitamins and minerals. Insufficient raw foods during hot weather may cause fevers, yang temperament, and contracted organs; anemia present; arrogance.

Exclusive raw fruit, vegetable, juice, and nut diet: Tendency toward possessiveness, nerve disorders, oversensitive, sentimental, and emotional, with a critical temperament. Disease symptoms: expanded (yin) kidneys, intestines, bladder, and colon; excessive urination, lung and respiratory weakness; weak digestion and sexual organs, glands, and hormones.

Alcohol, spices, stimulants, and drugs: Emotional instability and insecurity; heart and blood pressure weakness; expanded kidneys, skin diseases, falling hair on front and sides of head. Disorders in the sex glands and hormones, with excessive sexual desire; poor creativity and confusion in the mental realm.

Meat, fish, salt, and eggs: Tendency to be more aggressive, stubborn, and determined. More practical, mechanical, and materially minded. Fast and sharp thinking mind and senses. Disease symptoms: constricted (yang) heart, high blood pressure, circulatory problems, yang kidneys, pain in liver and gastrointestinal tract; constricted constipation, cancerous growths and tumors; farsightedness; loss of hair on top and back of head.

Sugar products, honey, dried fruits, all sweets: Mental instability and delusion, schizoid tendencies, and nervous disposition; expanded (yin) digestive systems and disorders, overweight; weak kidneys and bladder (hypoglycemia, diabetes); skin disorders; sexual weakness; liver and pancreatic disorders.

Dairy foods (cheese, milk, ice cream): More docile, mentally dull, and unresponsive; painful joints and lower back area. Disease symptoms: mucus conditions (colds, flu, lung disorders); skin diseases, cysts, tumors, heart and circulation problems; liver, gallbladder, and spleen congestion; sexual difficulties; prone to cancer and growths. Anemia and fatigue are generally present.

YOU ARE WHAT YOU EAT

As knowledge with regard to the effects of food upon humans increases, it is more than conceivable that those who avail themselves of the new values of nutrition may decrease the handicaps of disease, lengthen their lives, and so become the leaders of the future. Regimen is better than a physician. We ought to assist and not to force nature. We should each be our own physician by eating with moderation what agrees with our constitution. Nothing is good for the body other than what we can digest. What medicine can procure digestion? Exercise. What will recruit strength? Sleep. What will alleviate incurable evils? Patience.

"You are what you eat" is an old axiom as true today as it ever was. Food does make or break our mind, health, or character. If you are skeptical of this statement, you are urged to experiment on yourself by eating certain yin or yang foods exclusively for several weeks or months, and observe the change or reversal in your temperament, character, and overall health and well-being. Only then will you personally know that we are exactly what we eat, digest, assimilate, and absorb; nothing can change that fact. We can control our health and life by becoming masters of our habits. It is an extraordinary blindness to live without investigating what we are. A sound brain is not found in an unsound body, nor do we find a sound body nourished by an impure bloodstream.

Living and eating according to the universal principles of yin and yang, acid and alkaline, should be an enjoyable pleasure and experience for our creative imagination. It is a living, dynamic philosophy, a guide lighting our way to superior health and a well-balanced lifestyle. These life principles should never become a strict, inflexible, and austere ideology ruining all joy, happiness, and pleasure in life. Those who attain this proper balance, obtain sufficient exercise and sleep, and live in accordance with the natural laws of life will achieve super health physically, mentally, emotionally, and spiritually. These are the true compassionate teachers and leaders of the world; their judgment is always sound and useful.

Human beings have always longed for leaders/teachers to ease suffering. But what we really need is enlightenment from within. A healthy man or woman wants no followers and would never follow another person blindly. These are the true individualists, not carbon copies of another. The true teachers of the world inspire others to great heights and always extend others the freedom to live their own life without interference. Students learn to think for themselves under a true leader and teacher and are taught to be responsible for their own actions. They are positive, happy, magnetic, calm, patient, understanding, loving, kind, and full of pep and energy, with a clear, sharp mind.

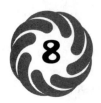

Avoiding Junk Foods and Food Poisons

In recent years, nationwide publicity on the subjects of natural living, health foods, and vegetarianism has made people more consciously aware of their health and well-being and helped them to take positive responsibility for their actions. The term "junk-food junkie" was coined during the surge of health awareness in the 1960s, and refers to those people who take little or no responsibility for their own health, who usually consume a great deal of processed, chemicalized, unhealthy junk food. This group generally refers to a health food conscious individual as a "health food nut."

However, many health food nuts who do not balance their diet carefully can be easily caught in the "junk-food syndrome." There is a difference between a junk-food junkie and one who is caught in a junk-food syndrome. The former consumes junk food at almost every meal; the latter eats healthy food most of the time but all too often gets caught in the vicious cycle of binging on junk food.

In addition, many people fast or attempt a raw food cleansing diet indiscriminately, when their body does not require one. Fasting has an extremely alkaline effect on the body cells and fluids, which is necessary to cleanse and purify a toxic and diseased organism. A very sick and diseased conventional eater will benefit greatly from a long fast or an extended juice diet. Their systems are acid, yang, and full of mucus, toxins, and wastes; fasting or raw juices will counteract, neutralize, and allow the body to eliminate these diseased conditions and to balance out their alkaline reserves and yin/yang polarities.

The people who mistakenly decide to fast or go on a raw food diet have usually been on a general health food diet for several years or have undergone several detoxification programs with some degree of success. They may believe that a fast or raw food diet of long duration will cleanse the body permanently. They have experienced the junk-food syndrome for many years and believe that fasting or eating only raw foods will cure their cravings for junk food. All too often, soon after a fast or raw food trip, such people will be found pigging out on their favorite type of junk food (pizza, ice cream).

Most fruits and some vegetables should be eaten raw. The body requires some raw fruits and vegetables daily; they furnish minerals, enzymes, and vitamins, especially vitamin C, which is lost in cooking. But there is no absolute necessity for anyone to consume all foods in the raw state. Grains can be sprouted, cooked, or made into bread and casseroles. Root vegetables, squashes, beans, and peas are more easily digested and assimilated when well cooked, steamed, or baked. In fact, there is no proof whatsoever of strict raw food dieters living any longer or being any healthier than a person on a well-balanced moderate diet. Many raw food dieters have digestive problems because of sensitive and expanded (yin) intestines and kidneys. Protein deficiencies are also common. A good natural food mixed diet, including raw and cooked foods, is better for most people.

In fact, most vegetarians and those who eat health foods do not need a raw food diet or a fast, as they are quite alkaline, yin, and flushed out from all the alkaline and yin foods they have been eating. What they need is proper and complete nutrition to put an end to the junk-food syndrome. An occasional short fast, or fruit or juice diet for a few days, should not cause any problems, provided a sound nutritional program is followed afterward. Eating too much fruit or juices, especially in cold weather (yin), will cause a swing in body polarity to excessive eating of heavier and more yang and acid-forming foods such as starches of all kinds and heavy protein foods.

The key to good health is to balance these two factors according to the weather, environment, and physical requirements on any given day or hour. You must listen to your inner voice and body intelligence about its daily food needs.

JUNK-FOOD SYNDROME: CAUSES AND CURES

The junk-food syndrome in people who are health-food conscious is brought on by poor dietary habits, bad digestion, poor assimilation and absorption, and malnourishment. Although health food fans consume much more natural, pure, and healthful foods than conventional eaters, more often than they would like to admit they also garbage-up or eat calamity junk foods such as Ding-Dongs, cakes, pies, soft drinks, cookies, moon pies, candy, pizzas, Twinkies, ice cream, fast food hamburgers, and on and on. The reader can easily add to this list.

How can we overcome insidious and incessant cravings for junk food? Are you beginning to wonder if it is possible for anyone to live on a natural food diet without experiencing those hidden hunger pangs and the junk-food syndrome? Is there something wrong with you, or does everyone experience these health food growing pains?

We have all experienced the junk-food syndrome in our own personal way. Each of you can relate a case history of your trials and experiments on various diets and junk-food trips. However, there is only one basic cause or reason for the junk-food syndrome, and it is this: the body is crying out for vital nourishment in every cell and tissue of its being. If your body could talk it would tell you that it needs an adequate supply of top quality protein, natural vitamins, minerals, trace elements, carbohydrates, fats, and enzymes, eaten in such a manner that it can easily assimilate, absorb, digest, and utilize the vital essences of those foods.

The diet and health suggestions as outlined in this book can help you overcome the junk-food syndrome and guide you to mastery of your eating habits. This syndrome can be overcome, and eventually you may look upon it as an experience or growing pain in your quest for super health. There are certain practices, misapplications, lack of thorough understanding of health principles, and poor living habits that cause abnormal food cravings and malnourishment, thus turning a person into a junk-food addict or health hypochondriac. An excessive daily consumption of raw foods, raw greens, dried (unsoaked) nuts and seeds, and dried fruits, combined with a lack of oxygen after meals, lack of exercise, too much fruit or juices, fasting when not required, lack of sufficient sleep, and lack of proper nourishing foods and food supplements, are some of the reasons why health food people turn into junk-food junkies.

Humans are an intimate part of nature's finer forces; it is the natural law or urge within humans that strives for eternal balance within the body. An extreme raw food diet will create a binging syndrome, which pulls one to consume large quantities of junk food or yang or acid foods, such as grains, bread, potatoes, nuts, cakes, and pies. These yang/acid foods are beneficial in moderation, to create balance. Raw food fans believe that these natural yang/acid foods are poisons or mucus-forming in the body and therefore should be avoided like the plague. However, they are constantly pulled toward these heavier yang foods like a magnet to a bar of steel. Their conscious lower mind or will tells them to eat more and more yin foods, while the subconscious mind constantly seeks equilibrium and creates an insatiable craving to overeat yang/acid foods.

This same principle of binging can be applied to any strict dieting program: for example, a strict grain and bean diet, which is too yang and acid, will create an internal, subconscious, and physical craving (physiological need) or binging syndrome of consuming large quantities of yin foods such as fruit, juices, vegetables, or yin junk food, such as beer, coffee, ice cream, or sweets. Cravings for unwholesome foods and poisons are always a sign of malnutrition, poor eating habits, and bad digestion and assimilation, which are the effects of lack of knowledge and misapplication of universal and natural health laws.

Overcoming Junk-Food Syndrome

The foods and the health suggestions listed here will nourish and vitalize your body. They will halt all cravings for junk food.

1. Consume a well-balanced diet consisting of whole grains, beans, peas, sea vegetables, seeds, nuts, fruits, vegetables, miso, and tofu.

2. All seeds and nuts should be soaked and germinated overnight for proper assimilation and protein absorption. These can be

blended into a seed or nut shake the next day. Eat germinated seeds and nuts more in hot weather and sparingly in winter. Seeds/nuts can be roasted in winter.

3. Use whole food supplements daily: nutritional yeast, alfalfa seeds (powder or tablets), carrot calcium, kelp, dulse, nori, raw vegetable juice (more in summer), fresh raw wheat germ, miso, and soybean powder.

4. Drink cereal grain coffee, dandelion tea, bancha twig tea, Mu tea, jasmine tea, alfalfa tea.

5. Consume highly nourishing vegetable stock soups.

6. Eat more cooked grains, beans, vegetables, and soups in winter, according to inner bodily requirements, and more seasonal raw food in summer. Use the various methods of cooking: sautéing, boiling, steaming, and baking.

7. Consume some raw food daily, more in summer, less in winter. Best fruits: apples, peaches, all berries, cherries, pomegranates, apricots. Best raw vegetables: celery, green peppers, sprouts, cucumbers.

8. Avoid tropical foods as much as possible, unless you are in the tropics, including tomatoes, oranges, avocado, eggplant, potatoes, yams, pineapple, and so on.

9. Avoid all animal fats, high-fat dairy, fried foods in grease, meat, soft drinks, sugars, white flour, white vinegar, hot spices, MSG, saccharine, coffee, commercial tea, and foods that are canned, packaged, or served in restaurants. Sweeteners such as honey, maple syrup, barley malt, and rice bran syrup can be used sparingly.

10. Use the following natural low-fat dairy products occasionally: yogurt, buttermilk, cottage cheese (raw milk). Tofu can be used to supplement dairy products. Yang people should not use eggs and all others should use them sparingly.

11. Go outside after meals for proper digestion and assimilation. Oxygen is necessary for proper metabolism and absorption.

12. Get daily exercise such as yoga, running, swimming, cycling, bodybuilding, breathing/stretching exercises, and Chi Kung.

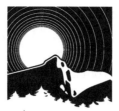

Fig. 8.1. If you smile, the world smiles with you in return.
If you frown, you will be frowned at.
If you sing, you will be invited in joyous company.
If you love the world, you will be surrounded by loving friends,
and nature will pour out the treasures of the Tao.

Flowing with the Tao and Yin/Yang Forces

As we give up our junk-food habits, such as coffee, alcohol, sugar, ice cream, milk, meat, and pastries, we begin to crave and desire these products as they are being eliminated from our system. An outright denial of these cravings can be disastrous to both mind and body. The reason we desire these foods is because they cause an addiction; when they are eliminated too fast we experience withdrawal symptoms, the same as a drug addict. However, this is only temporary, until elimination of internal toxins is complete and the body becomes balanced.

When we totally deny our addictions to junk food, with the attitude or affirmation of never eating them again for the rest of our lives, we become obsessed with denying that which our body craves. If the mind denies junk food strongly enough, it will run to what it dwells upon, and cause us to eat large quantities of junk. A better method to overcome junk-food addiction is to say to yourself, "I will avoid junk food for as long as I can, then, when I desire some junk food, I will eat it in small quantities only." This will satisfy the addiction or withdrawal symptoms, and your mind and body will be more at peace. As your body continues to cleanse and slowly eliminate poisons, over a period of weeks or months the junk food that once tempted you will no longer do so. Your cravings will vanish like magic, and you will become the master instead of the slave of your dietary habits.

The reason this method works is because we are not negating or feeling guilty about eating a small amount of junk food occasionally. When we affirm to our mind that we may eat anything at any time, the struggle between our mind and body ceases. This method removes the tension and stress that accompany the attempt to live up to our perfect dietetic expectations or ideals. Tell yourself that you cannot have something, and you will want it even more. An extreme yang action will change into an extreme yin reaction.

When the mind/will/ego are used (in a yang way) to overcome, control, or deny physical or physiological cravings and addictions (yin), which are still present in the system, extreme junk-food binging is generally the result. If the yang mind strongly denies an inner craving, the craving usually wins out. If yang will not bend, it will break. Yin and yang must be balanced within the body for optimum health. This is the unifying principle of physical life. Deny something, and you will be pulled toward it. Place a "Wet Paint" sign next to a freshly painted fence, and people will touch it to see for themselves if it is wet or dry. Vow to become a celibate, and your sexual cravings will overwhelm you, unless your whole being has overcome the desire without struggle. Tell a child a fire will burn and hurt him, and, in spite of the warning, he will play with fire and get burned. Deny him the real experience and he will be attracted to it unconsciously. Denying or struggling against something takes us away from the flow of life and from harmony with the Tao.

Eat too yang, and you will crave extreme yin, and vice versa. The mind and body operate in unison; an unbalanced body creates an unbalanced mind, and an unbalanced mind further unbalances the body. A sound mind in a sound body is what we should strive to attain. May you eat in peace. We are creatures of habit. We succeed or we fail as we acquire good habits or bad ones, and we acquire good habits as easily as bad ones. Most people do not believe this. Only those who find out succeed in life.

In this physical, three-dimensional world, all is duality and change. Nothing here remains forever the same. All phenomena are constantly spiraling onward and upward, evolving into higher and greater things. Change *is* the illusion of the physical world; the spiritual worlds never change; they are absolute and nondual; it is where the dual physical world is born. The One (Wu Chi) becomes the two (yin and yang), the two become the three (trinity), and the three become ten thousand things.

FLEXIBILITY IS THE KEY TO YIN AND YANG BALANCE

Second-generation teachers of macrobiotics like Michio Kushi, Michael Abehsera, and Herman Aihara modified the practices of early macrobiotic proponent George Ohsawa. They recommended a somewhat wider application of grains and vegetables. Michio Kushi's standard diet of 50 percent cereal grains, 25 percent cooked vegetables, and 25 percent supplementary foods such as miso soup, beans, seaweeds, fruit, is an example. While this diet is generally sound for the temperate zones, it can still create complications if its practitioners do not understand how to apply the unifying principle of yin and yang. This is a good example of the saying that "a principle without a practice is useless; a practice without a principle is dangerous." On such a diet many people become too yang, that is, contracted, rigid in their thinking, and subject to a variety of symptoms associated with overstimulation of the parasympathetic nervous system. Aside from the discomfort of being too yang, such people suffer from an inability to discharge old, poor-quality, stored yin, such as cholesterol, crystals, stones, and cysts.

The simple fact of the matter is that the heart must expand as well as contract, we must breathe in as well as out, and so on. Yin is necessary to life. In fact, as a general rule we need at least seven or eight times as much yin as yang in our diet, and the ratio can go much higher if, for example, we are very active (yang) in hot weather (yang). If we become too yang the body will necessarily retain its stored animal fats and yin toxins, particularly if we consume too much salt and other minerals such as those contained in seaweed. The farther we move toward yang and away from balance, the more desperately will the body hold on to yin.

The frequent practice of macrobiotic dieters is to deny cravings until they build up to a point of irresistibility, at which time many people binge wildly, eating pints of ice cream, sugar-rich foods, meat, or even on occasion turning to drugs such as marijuana, LSD, or cocaine. The law of front and back is undeniable. Balance will be made sooner or later.

We must learn to change and be flexible in our diet and health program. What worked for us in the past may not work for us now. We become a different person every second, every minute, every hour, every month, and every year. Without constant change, growth, and flexibility, we would die of stagnation. Accepting change and flexibility in this physical yin and yang world spirals us onward in our quest for perfection, toward the universal force.

EXTREME YIN AND YANG FOODS AND POISONS

Did you know that the average American diet is costing this nation over 30 billion dollars annually in doctor bills? Per person annually, Americans are consuming 102 lbs. of refined white sugar, 53 lbs. of processed oils and fats, 100 lbs. of white flour, 7 lbs. of white rice, many gallons of alcohol, and thousands of cigarettes.

Disease is on the rise. Hospitals are filled to capacity. Jails and mental institutions are overcrowded. One of the main causes of these confusing problems can be attributed to very poor living and eating habits over decades, such as the consumption of processed and demineralized foods and poisonous substances (drugs, marijuana, coffee, sugar, alcohol).

It is crucially important for us to avoid consuming the substances that are poisonous to our bodies, and to limit our consumption of foods that are extreme yin or yang. They include:

1. Meat, fish, and fowl
2. Pasteurized milk and its products
3. White flour and its products
4. White sugar and its derivatives
5. Vegetable oils, animal fat, and derivatives
6. Tobacco, alcohol, vinegar, tea, coffee, sodas, and cocoa
7. Processed peanut butter, other nut butters, ungerminated seeds and nuts, and dried fruit
8. Salt and condiments
9. Marijuana
10. Commercial eggs

Meat, Fish, and Fowl (Extreme Yang Food)

The flesh of an animal is not food; it is the result of food plant life. All animal and human life is dependent upon the plant kingdom for its sustenance. Meat-eating animals are not the strongest and longest-lived animals in nature; the elephant, rhinoceros, and gorilla (all vegetarians) are the true kings of the jungle.

Flesh foods affect the body. Meat contains urea (uric acid or the urine of the animal), creatinine, creatine, and phenolic acids. It may contain synthetic female sex growth hormones and other chemicals, such as PCBs and DDT, antibiotics, drugs, nitrates, and red dye coloring used to preserve and make the otherwise grey cadaver flesh more pleasing to the eye at the butcher's counter. These are all cancer-causing agents. Meat is loaded with trichina worms, parasites, and putrefactive bacteria. Pork contains 31,080,000,000 putrefactive bacteria per ounce; steak and beef, 24,500,000,000; hamburger, 21,000,000,000; sausage, 20,000,000,000.

Excessive flesh eating produces toxic metabolic wastes in the system, causing toxemia, malnutrition, high acidity, purine bodies, and intestinal putrefaction. It contributes to diseases such as cancer, kidney and liver disorders, arthritis, hardened arteries, mental disorders, bone and blood diseases, and many others. Meat eaters generally age faster, have less endurance, develop more diseases, and have a lower life expectancy than vegetarians.

Growth drugs have been used for over fifty years as a cattle feed additive or injection to increase growth quickly, without using extra feed. There is a close link between these growth drugs and human cancer and other diseases. In the mid-1970s the government placed a ban on feeding DES to cattle to stimulate weight and growth. However, the FDA has currently approved six growth hormone promotants (HGPs), three naturally occurring hormones and three synthetically prepared hormones. Profit is clearly more important than health or honesty. This is just one very good example and reason for you to consider alternative sources of nutriment, relatively free of hormones and poisonous substances, such as found in plant food.

Pasteurized Milk and Products (Extreme Yin or Yang/Acid Food)

Drinking milk may be hazardous to your health. Some milk supplies have been found contaminated with penicillin and chloramphenicol, two antibiotics that are supposed to be forbidden by law, plus insecticides, lethal drugs, and radioactive material. Among the ailments attributed to milk are: pesticide poisoning, adverse drug reactions, drug resistance, salmonella, staphylococcus poisoning, anemia, hypocalcaemia (excess calcium in the blood), diarrhea, asthma, and liver damage. If you are eating pasteurized cheeses, ice cream, sour cream, powdered milk, cottage cheese, cream cheese, or anything else made from the pasteurized milk, you are getting a dose of the above poisons. Think about that the next time you go shopping in your local market.

Cow's milk contains hormones that are secreted by the cow for the purpose of stimulating growth in a calf, to move its weight from about 80 pounds at birth to 1,000 pounds two years later. You probably weighed about 7 pounds at birth and it took you a full twenty-one years to reach your present weight. Dr. F. Pottenger Jr. of Monrovia, California, conducted an experiment on cats in which he fed them pasteurized milk. In three generations they displayed homosexual tendencies and were unable to produce offspring. They developed brittle bones and lung diseases.

Pasteurized milk and its products lack the enzymes, vitamins, and minerals so necessary to maintain health. Pasteurization is for the purpose of keeping bad milk in a saleable condition and for no other purpose. Pasteurized cow milk products are primary factors in causing body cramps, allergies, arthritis, fatigue, indigestion, gas, and diarrhea, due to fat and lactose intolerance. Lower back pains can also be attributed to milk consumption. After the weaning period most humans do not produce enough of the enzyme lactase that digests the milk sugar, lactose, which causes trouble. Cheeses and cow milk are extremely high in lactose and fat, both extreme yin elements and contributing factors in heart disease, high cholesterol, diabetes, colds, skin diseases, and cancer. Cheese is so concentrated that it takes 5 quarts of milk to make 1 pound of cheese. Regular cheese has more fat than most meats.

Scientists have discovered that pasteurized cow milk products remain unmetabolized in many adults because they lower hydrochloric acid in the stomach, which is required for protein and mineral assimilation. The body cannot utilize 42 percent of the protein contained in pasteurized milk according to Dr. S. C. Deal, in his book *New Life Through Nutrition* (1974). Milk causes the intestines to generate excessive amounts of the lubricating substance called mucus, to help keep foods moving through the system. This material has the ability to harden and forms a coating on the inner lining of the intestines that makes it almost impossible for nutrients to pass through into the bloodstream, which of course means poor absorption. Poor absorption leads to chronic fatigue. Milk drinkers are always full of mucus, coughs, headaches, colds, and flu. An excessive build-up of mucus travels up to the lungs, bronchial tubes, nasal cavity, and head, causing colds, flu, headaches, pneumonia, and asthma.

Milk is an excellent source of calcium but many people just don't seem to be able to metabolize it properly. It may be because the pasteurization of milk destroys enzymes in milk or because the heat of pasteurization distorts the calcium. No one really knows, but laboratory animals raised on pasteurized milk have exhibited all the symptoms of arthritis. Low calcium intake can cause muscle cramps. But anyone who depends upon milk for calcium is making a mistake. Nondairy sources of good quality calcium include sesame seeds, cabbage, okra, parsley, watercress, wheat, kale, cauliflower, lemons, strawberries, and collard greens.

High-fat dairy foods (butter, processed cheeses, sour cream, cream cheese, and regular raw and pasteurized cheeses, such as cheddar, muenster, edam) are all extremely yin and should be eaten very sparingly. Low-fat yogurt, buttermilk, and skim milk are more yin and yang balanced and can be consumed in moderation. Low-fat skim milk cheese, Swiss cheese, low-fat cottage cheese, and highly salted cheeses are extremely yang due to their fat-free concentrated protein and high salt content and should be eaten very sparingly. Goat milk, goat cheese, and feta cheese are yang.

White Flour and Its Products (Yang/Acid Poison)

White flour and its derivatives affect the body. White flour products, such as white bread, noodles, and pizza, are considered yang and are the main cause of constrictive constipation. The stools are dry, small and hard, and bowel elimination is difficult. White flour contains calcium sulfate, a chemical name for plaster of Paris; if continually indulged in, it will plaster, clog, and close up the eliminative channels of the body. Intestinal statis or constipation causes anemia and pasty complexion, which can be attributed to white flour products. Such products are also totally lacking in the entire vitamin B complex family. They also deplete these vitamins from the body if eaten exclusively. They contain zero roughage, which is necessary for healthy digestion and proper intestinal and bowel action. They add empty calories and unhealthy weight to the body.

White flour products maintain long shelf life, due to their lack of whole food value, while whole grain flour products cannot keep long because of their freshness and high nutrition. Bugs and insects will not eat white flour due to its lack of nutritional qualities. Ironically, farmers feed wheat bran and wheat germ to livestock for health and prize-winning reasons, while poisoning themselves unwittingly by avoiding them. The show animals are thus healthier than most humans.

All soft, fluffy supermarket bread is puffed with air in big vats, to blow it up for shelf life. If bread can be squeezed like an accordion, it is not fit for human consumption. To make white flour, bread millers remove all of the vitamins, minerals, protein, and bulk elements from the wheat and enrich it with a tiny amount of synthetic vitamins and minerals, which cannot be absorbed by the body. Twenty-six natural elements are removed from the flour, and a fraction of a penny's worth of inorganic vitamin/mineral elements are added back. This goes for all white flour supermarket products, such as macaroni, gravy, and spaghetti. Supermarket cereals are made from white flour, with added salt, sugar, BHA, BHT, artificial additives, pyridoxine hydrochloride, colorings, cottonseed oil, hydrogenated oils, and preservatives. Cheap cereals contain as much as 70 to 85 percent refined sugar and white flour starch. Cheap hydrogenated oils and salt come next as chief ingredients in cereals; artificial colorings are also high on the list. Cereal was named after the Roman goddess of grains, Ceres. The real cereals are whole grains: rye, rice, wheat, corn, barley, buckwheat, oats, and millet.

White flour is devoid of nourishing elements and fiber bulk; as a result, eating white flour will make you fat. Whole grains are not fattening. Whole fiber foods cause you to eat less; they also move the stomach and bowel contents along, thus aiding weight loss. White flour products do not fill you up, therefore you can keep on eating them, while chalking up the calories and fat. You can make your own whole grain flour products and avoid obesity, disease, and a thin wallet. Avoid all products containing white flour, sugar, and additives. Use only 100 percent whole grain products. In the long run, whole foods natural cooking can save you loads of money, prevent disease, increase your health force, and, most importantly, save your life.

To make white rice, the bran, which contains the valuable B complex vitamins, has similarly been removed. As a result, white rice is constipating and does not promote health. It contains some or all of the following inorganic chemicals and unwholesome substances: plaster of Paris, polysorbate 60, calcium bromate, azodicarbonamide, sodium stearoyl-2-lactylate, amomonium phosphate, carrageenin, propylene glycol, diacetyl tartaric acid, monoglycerides and diglycerides, and synthetic vitamins. Propylene glycol is used in antifreeze; carrageenan is a possible cancer-causing agent; be suspicious of the other chemicals also.

White Sugar and Derivatives (Yin/Acid Poison)

Sugar, its derivatives, and other unnatural sweeteners and food additives affect the body. Sugar is an extreme yin substance, which is psychologically and physically addicting. It contains zero minerals, vitamins, enzymes, protein, natural fiber, trace minerals, or other food value. It contains empty calories and can make you obese and lethargic. It uses up insulin and causes diabetes, obesity, heart disease, poor eyesight, skin diseases, bad memory, cancer, and kidney and liver disorders. It places a drain on the alkaline buffer salts and causes calcium to be depleted from bones, teeth, hair, nails, and eyes, causing tooth decay, soft nails, blindness, bone disease, and hair loss. It robs the body of iron, the major blood-building mineral.

Sugar is a main ingredient in most processed foods: ice cream, 30–50%; white bread, 10%; commercial cereals, 40–50%; peanut butter, mayonnaise, salad dressing, ketchup, 20–30%; nondairy coffee creamer, 30–40%; imitation fruit juice, 98%; gelatin desserts, 85%; cigarettes, 50%; cigars, 20%; pipe tobacco, 40%; canned fruits, 20%–35%; candy, 85–95%; baby food and infant formulas, 20–30%; spaghetti sauce, 10–20%; colas and soft drink sodas, 40–60%; hot dogs, 10%; cookies, cakes, pies, donuts, and so on, 30–50%.

Sugar in any form is harmful. Any of the following is just another name for sugar: sucrose, fructose, glucose, maltose, lactose, galactose, cane syrup, corn syrup, corn sugar, invert sugar, dextrose, saccharin (coal tar product), and cyclamates. Most fast foods contain high percentages of both sugar (yin) and salt (yang). Sugar is sold to the tune of 32 billion pounds and $6.4 billion per year. Dental bills cost Americans $6 billion a year, while isolated societies and rural cultures, which do not consume sugar and its derivatives, are free from tooth decay. Excess sugar in the blood can result in brain damage, schizophrenic tendencies, depression, and extreme mood changes. Sugar consumption is now up to approximately 200 pounds per person per year.

As sugar intake increases, degenerative diseases also increase. Refined sugar, fats, and empty calorie carbohydrates exhaust the pancreas, which results in diabetes. The death rate from diabetes has increased 52 percent in seventy years. Diabetes, hypoglycemia, and skin diseases are all unknown in societies that do not consume sugar and refined foods. Diabetes and hypoglycemia can be controlled and prevented on a sugar-free and junk-food-free diet. The diet must contain whole grains, legumes, vegetables, fruits, seeds, nuts, and low-fat dairy.

Brown sugar is white sugar colored with molasses, and it reacts exactly the same in the body. Honey, rice bran syrup, molasses, barley malt syrup, dried powdered dates, carob powder, and malt powder are natural sweeteners and substitutes for all forms of white sugar and its derivatives. However, these substitutes should be used very sparingly and in small quantities in cooking or flavoring food. All sweet foods and substances are extremely yin (expansive to mind and body) and can cause disease if used indiscriminately. Intestinal mucus is usually simply an extension of mucus of the stomach, and it is always aggravated and instigated by the use of white sugar and other similar irritants. Chronic diarrhea is often the result of the free use of sugar in its various forms, causing intestinal (yin) expansion and loose stools. Dilation or distention of the stomach with enormous quantities of gas and fermentation can be attributed to sweets and sugar. Gastric ulcers can be caused and greatly aggravated by sugar products.

The stomach requires a good calcium supply to function properly; sugar causes rapid calcium loss. Gout, chronic rheumatism, nervous headache, neurasthenia, eczema, apoplexy, leukemia, MS, TB, MD, and other chronic diseases require entire abstinence from white sugar and its derivatives, if there is any chance or hope of a healthy recovery. White sugar is not digested in the mouth or stomach but only in the small intestine, where it comes in contact with the intestinal juice. Several hours pass after eating a meal before the intestinal fluid is able to digest white sugar and prepare it for absorption. This is not true, however, of fruit or other natural sugars.

It is evident that cane sugar is a crude vegetable product not well adapted to human nutrition. In many cases stomach acidity, catarrh, indigestion, gas, ulcers, and hyperacidity are due to this cause. The extensive use of candies, preserves, sodas, and sweets of various kinds, as well as the free use of white sugar and corn syrup with cereals and pancakes, in coffee, tea, and in other ways, may be directly held responsible as the cause of the indigestion and chronic disease that prevails throughout the civilized world. Millions of men, women, and children are suffering from disordered conditions of the body due to the excessive use of white sugar without being aware of the real cause of their distresses. Not a few intelligent, observing people have discovered that sugar is productive of sour stomach and various other gastric disturbances.

It is evident, then, that white sugar and its derivatives are totally devoid of properties that are found in wholesome natural foods. No healthy human being can suffer physical ills from consuming whole grains, legumes, fruit, seeds, yogurt, or vegetables, because these foods are natural to the human digestive process.

Vegetable Oils, Animal Fats, and Their Derivatives (Extreme Yin/Acid)

Vegetable oils, animal fats, and their derivatives affect the body. Fats are used as fuel in the body. The amount of fat required daily is quite small. The body's preference is to store up fat for use in an emergency. It is deposited under the skin between the layers of muscles and serves as a padding around the internal vital organs; it is used to nourish the nerves also. Fats are converted into soap in the intestines by the action of the digestive fluids. Soap is soluble in water and in this form the fat is absorbed after the soap is decomposed and the original fat is reconstructed. Kidney stones and gallstones are nothing more than hard round soap balls, developed in the system from an excessive consumption of fatty foods and oils. The less oils and fats in your diet, the healthier you will be; there is no secret about this.

Bottled oils, even vegetable oils, will cause liver and bladder trouble if eaten to excess. Why is this so? Because all oils, from either vegetable or animal sources, are super concentrated food derivatives, which the human body was never designed to handle. For example, several pounds of nuts are required to manufacture one small bottle of nut oil; it is the same with all other oils. The whole food factor has been removed from the original product (fractionated), and we are left with a highly concentrated food substance, which burdens the human chemistry system and internal organs beyond their capacity. The result is malnutrition, indigestion, chronic fatigue, liver and bladder disease, anemia, falling hair, malabsorption of food, poor eyesight, and ultimately cancer.

The body was designed to handle foods in their whole form, with oils intact, such as found in all seeds, nuts, legumes, beans, grains, olives, and cultured dairy products. By consuming whole foods we can be assured of obtaining the whole food factor in the right combination and proper proportion. We should consume no more than 1 to 2 tablespoons of free oils or other fats daily. One famous health writer and researcher has discovered that any consumption of fractionated fats, as found in vegetable oils or other animal fats that have been placed in bottles, is deleterious to health. So heed the warning: the less fractionated oils in your diet, the healthier and longer you will live. Animals in nature do not consume such things; it is common sense that we should follow that line of logic also. Cold pressed vegetable oils should be used mostly in cold weather (winter) and very sparingly in summer.

The body requires a very small percentage of fats in the daily diet; these can be acquired mostly from whole natural foods, without injuring our health. Most Americans consume from 50 to 60 percent fat daily, which is why we have the highest death rate from heart disease in the world. With the excessive consumption of animal protein, sugar, salt, and fat, it is easy to see why the United States is one of the most chronically diseased countries on earth. Most people consume more than 2,000 calories in fat per day. The human body is an amazing work of art, and it can do many things on its own if we feed and take care of it properly. However, overconsumption of fatty foods and oils robs the body of the opportunity to manufacture its own fat. Left to its own, the body will form its required fat from natural complex carbohydrate foods such as whole grains, legumes, seeds, nuts, fruits, and vegetables.

The fat formed in this way is different from other fats because it contains the special characteristics of human fat, specifically designed by nature for the human body.

One ounce of fat contains 240 calories, more calories than the same amount of carbohydrates or protein. Excessive oils and fats take several hours to digest, create chronic digestive disorders, and lead to a multitude of illnesses. Expensive margarines are an extremely yin and inferior product. Margarines made from soybean or other oils are all hydrogenated and artificially flavored and colored. For example, soybean oil is heated to high temperatures, and hydrogen gas is bubbled through it, which causes the liquid oil/fat to become solid and made into bars of commercial brightly packed margarine. This hydrogenation process does two things to the unsaturated oil: 1) it makes it hard; 2) it changes polyunsaturated fats into saturated fats, which are more cholesterol-forming than butter or eggs. Avoid all margarines, including corn, safflower, soybean, and any others made from cheap oils. Use yogurt, tofu, natural cooking herbs, and miso to make your own fresh toppings and salad dressings. They are all fast, easy to make, inexpensive, and will save you doctor bills.

Metallic nickel is also used in the process of turning unsaturated liquid vegetable oils into a hard stick of phony imitation butter. Free nickel in the system can cause ill health. Imitation margarines will raise your cholesterol, not lower it; they will clog up your organs and arteries, not clear them out. Lard and other animal fats are all highly saturated: 100 percent fat. Cottonseed oil is another highly processed, non-nutritive product used in many commercial foods, including potato chips, candy, pastries, and ice cream. This harmful oil has been reported to lower the sperm count in the testicles of male animals. In simple terms: cottonseed oil will lower your sex drive and reproductive powers. Read labels, even the ones in health food stores, and avoid these disease-producing poisons.

If you must use polyunsaturated vegetable oils, the best are: cold-pressed virgin safflower oil, dark sesame oil, and olive oil. Safflower oil contains the highest amount of linoleic acid (75 percent), which is the most polyunsaturated oil of all. The lower the linoleic acid content, the more saturated a fat or oil is. Foods deep fried in oils, especially rancid, cheap commercial oils, can cause severe organic health disorders.

Sautéing vegetables in a small amount of pure dark sesame oil or saf-flower oil is permissible during the cold winter months. Use less oil in summer.

Tobacco (Yin/Acid Poison)

The nausea and sickness that follow a person's first attempt to use tobacco are definite evidence of the poisonous character of this drug. Vertigo, pallor, high pulse rate, pounding heart beat, breathing diffi-culty, vomiting, and in extreme cases unconsciousness are produced by a very small quantity of tobacco smoke in persons not accustomed to its use. Almost no one dies of nicotine poisoning when they first begin to smoke because the human system possesses great powers of accommo-dation to circumstances. In this way the worst poisons may by degrees be tolerated until enormous doses can be taken without immediate fatal results. However, the system is still slowly poisoned and remains in a lowered state of health, until the smoker suffers and dies ten to twenty years or more before his or her natural life span.

There are nineteen poisons in cigarettes, including nicotine, arsenic, and methene. Smokers are known to take on Buerger's disease, which lowers skin temperature and causes gangrene. Smoking pregnant women can easily pass on the habit to their offspring. In many cases, the chil-dren of smoking mothers are sick from birth. Smoking is a contributing factor in heart disease and circulatory disorders. It lowers the red blood count and causes anemia. Heavy smokers do not generally have a taste for natural foods, so everything they eat is heavily sugared, salted, or spiced, which further imbalances the system. Stomach ulcers are greater in smokers than nonsmokers.

Smokers generally appear ten to fifteen years older than their actual age. The heavy tar substances in cigars or cigarettes adhere to the lung walls, coating them thick and black, and obstructing the oxygen and blood exchange within the lungs. They cripple the brain cells, causing them to harden, thicken, and finally lose their finer nerve tissue. Brain cells do not regenerate or grow back when destroyed through smoking or other nerve poisons. Tobacco dulls the finer senses and severely weakens the pineal and pituitary glands, the very receptors of higher values and intuition.

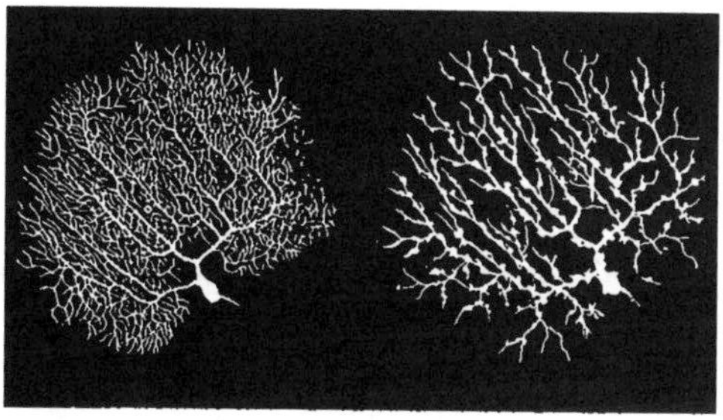

Normal brain cell | Tobacco-crippled brain cell

Fig. 8.2. Tobacco affects the brain.

A single cigar or several cigarettes will, in thirty minutes, produce a rise of blood pressure amounting to twenty points. One pound of tobacco contains 350 grains of nicotine. One drop kills a dog. One-thirtieth of a grain causes toxic symptoms in humans. Nine-tenths of a grain will kill a person. One pound of tobacco, then, contains more than enough poison to kill three hundred people. When smoking is stopped, it takes about a month to get the nicotine out of the body. It takes several months to a few years to completely clean out the lungs and internal systems, provided a wholesome dietary and exercise program is adopted.

Alcohol/Vinegar (Yin/Acid Poisons)

Alcohol and vinegar are protoplasmic poisons. Vinegar is extremely acid and harmful to the stomach, kidneys, and liver. Both destroy red blood cells and lessen the functioning power of the brain. Alcohol over-stimulates the brain and body, leaving the drinker fatigued and washed out after its effects have worn off. It eats away the stomach lining, leading to ulcers and cancer, and hinders the formation and action of the gastric ferments, in as little as 0.5 percent in water. It expands the liver and kidneys, causing chronic disease symptoms. Alcohol is a narcotic, which impairs intelligence and weakens the memory, judgment, and the reasoning faculty. Alcohol always diminishes, never increases, the energy of the heart and is therefore detrimental rather than beneficial in cases of shock, collapse, and fainting.

The craving for alcohol, in many cases, can be traced to poor nutritional habits and deficiencies, lack of exercise and fresh air, and stress. Any extreme always creates a craving for its opposite. Alcohol is extremely yin, and heavy drinkers generally crave meat (yang). A healthy, well functioning liver will feel the effect of even one drink. Heavy drinkers do not feel the effects after a few drinks because their liver has become diseased and unable to react to any further poisoning. Alcohol produces a profuse flow of mucus in the stomach, the purpose of which is to protect the mucous membrane from the irritating effects of the alcohol. It increases the liability to infectious disease and prevents the development of immunity by hindering the formation and accumulation of glycogen in the liver and diminishing the alkalinity of the blood. Also, healthy blood corpuscles help to prevent disease, and a pint of alcohol puts 20 percent of our blood cells out of commission. Alcohol diminishes muscular vigor, nerve sensibility, and vital endurance. It causes depression and mental degeneracy.

Tea, Coffee, Sodas, and Cocoa (Yin/Acid Poisons)

Coffee and commercial tea are artificial mild narcotic stimulants, and they are definitely addicting and habit-forming when continually used. They are extremely yin and acid-forming in the body, containing poisonous substances that narcotize the brain, nerves, and blood. They excite the nervous system temporarily, followed by physical and mental let-down, fatigue, and depression. Strong cravings for these substances are definite indications that they contain mild narcotic poison-stimulants, which create a dependency-addiction syndrome, with withdrawal symptoms when they are abruptly taken away from the user. They cause transitory stimulation, followed by marked increase of fatigue. Commercial tea contains tannic acid; it interferes with gastric juice in the stomach. All of these yin poisons expand and weaken the kidneys, bladder, liver, and intestines, causing their acids to flow into the blood, poisoning the system. Many tea and coffee drinkers develop discoloration of their teeth and skin. Coffee contains pyrimidine, a smoke poison produced by the roasting process.

Caffeine's effects on the nerves cause wakefulness, nervousness, excitability, insomnia, and muscle twitching. It also causes raised blood pressure. Eight ounces of coffee contains 85 to 90 mg of caffeine; colas about 75 mg. Colas and soft drinks also contain 7 to 8 teaspoons of white sugar per bottle (about an ounce). Orange or lemon flavored imitation drinks contain brominated vegetable oil, corn and cottonseed oil, and the poisonous chemical bromine. All colas and soft drinks eat away at the vital organs, including the reproductive glands. Cocoa contains a mild narcotic called theobromin, equal chemically and pharmacologically to caffeine in tea and coffee; its effects on the body are the same.

In light of these facts it should not be difficult for any intelligent person to reach the conclusion that these poisonous stimulants do not build health or instill vitality within the body; they only waste vital energy, exhaust the body's reserve force, and lower immunity and resistance to disease. Rest and sleep are the only natural and healthful remedies for fatigue. Addiction to these deleterious substances confuses and dulls the body's natural signals for rest and sleep, thereby resulting in nerve exhaustion, nervous disorders, and mental confusion. If you value your personal well-being and are interested in building your vital health force, avoid these artificial stimulant/poisons like you would arsenic capsules.

Processed Nut Butter and Ungerminated Seeds/Nuts (Extreme Yin/Acid Food)

Nut butters and dried seeds and nuts affect the body. Commercial peanut butter contains salt, sugar, cheap hydrogenated oils, about 80 percent fat, and nickel, which can cause lung infections. All nut butters and nuts are extreme yin due to their high fat content. These products should be used sparingly. Excessive fats expand the liver and decrease normal bile functioning. A diseased liver causes poor eyesight, jaundiced eyes, dandruff and falling hair, skin diseases, and other maladies.

Dried seeds and nuts can cause severe digestive disorders. Unsoaked or ungerminated seeds and nuts are only about 10 to 20 percent digestible and assimilable, due to the fact that their life force is lying dormant. The life force becomes active only when moisture (liquid) is added to them. They then become active and start growing or germinating; only then will they become almost 100 percent digestible and assimilable in the human system. Seed and nut germination has been a regular practice of the ancient yogis, Chinese Taoists, and other long-lived people throughout the world for centuries. Make it your practice too, and experience the vibrant health force that you are capable of attaining.

The following seeds and nuts can be soaked overnight in water: sunflower seeds, pumpkin seeds, sesame seeds, almonds, walnuts, and pecans.

After soaking, they can be placed in a blender with some added apple or pineapple juice and you can enjoy a zesty seed or nut milk. Soaked cashews also make a delicious cashew milk, creamy and good tasting. Soaking and blending seeds and nuts makes their protein value more easily digestible. You can use 2 to 3 ounces of a single seed or nut, or using them in any combination will add variety to the milk. You may also soak a couple dried figs or apricots with the seeds and blend them together; add ½ teaspoon of licorice powder to the moving blender for a pleasant taste. Use this blended seed/nut mixture more during hot weather, two or three times per week. The value of seed and nut germination (and the soaking of dried fruit; see below) is one of the most important health secrets that we have investigated and researched in the health field.

Dried Fruit

Dried fruits include apricots, raisins, apples, pineapples, figs, and peaches. The maximum benefit is received from dried fruits if they are soaked first, as unsoaked dried fruits almost always cause gas before the digestive juices can get to them. The normal digestive process for dried fruits lasts about ten hours, and before the unsoaked dried fruits are adequately soaked up by the digestive juices, the body is ready to expel them. Thus, we do not get the good out of them unless they have been presoaked.

There is an art to soaking the dried fruits properly. Wash, add cold water to cover, and bring slowly to a boil. Remove from heat and allow them to stand all night. The boiled water kills all insects and parasites that might otherwise cause trouble. Remember to start with cold water, so that the increasing heat will penetrate into the inside of the fruit. They also may be soaked overnight and liquefied with juice in a blender. Soaked dried fruit can also be used in bread and other baked dishes.

The natural fruit liquid has been removed from dried fruits, which turns them into a very concentrated sugar. All dried fruit is extremely yin and acid, and it is the cause of much distress and ill-health among dieters today, who use it excessively. It almost always causes skin eruptions when eaten dried, or even when soaked, if eaten excessively. Dried fruit should not be used as a staple in the diet but rather as a supplement, mostly in cold weather when fresh fruit is not available. It should be taken sparingly: no more than one or two apricots or figs, a few dates, or a teaspoon of raisins per day maximum. When on a vegetarian or health diet, do not become a health nut and attempt to live on dried nuts and fruit, as some have attempted to do with disastrous results in poor health.

Salt and Condiments
(Yang/Alkaline, Poison in Extreme)

Today, our lands are demineralized and chemically fertilized, and the topsoil is very poor due to bad agriculture methods. The more soluble sodium salts have washed away from the soil, leaving it high in potassium. This sodium loss has led to the use of a deadly substitute, sodium chloride or common table salt, which is composed of the caustic alkali, sodium, and a poisonous gas, chlorine. It is an inorganic compound that cannot be assimilated by the body. It has no nutritional value because it cannot be dissolved and utilized by the cells and tissues. For optimum health we need about 200 milligrams per day from sea salt or kelp.

Salt eating is a habit, just like tobacco, alcohol, coffee, or drugs. The average person who eats processed commercial food consumes more than 2,000 milligrams of cheap salt, which contains the following chemicals: silicon dioxide (common sand), aluminum calcium silicate, tricalcium silicate, sodium calcium aluminosilicate, sodium aluminosilicate, calcium silicate, magnesium silicate, yellow prussiate of soda, and sodium ferrocyanide.

Excessive consumption of salt causes high blood pressure, hypertension, kidney disease (yang), hardened arteries, eye disorders, and unbalanced chemistry. It also depletes calcium from bones and teeth and irritates the mucus lining of the stomach and intestinal tract; it affects the nervous system, causing nerve disorders and irritability. Poor capillary circulation, hot or cold hands and feet, anemia, dizziness, headaches, nose bleeds, and sexual hyperesthesia are all symptoms of excessive salt in the system. Biologists have shown that ½ ounce of salt absorbs and holds 4 pounds of water in the body, thus leading to edema and obesity. It draws the vital fluids from cells, tissues, glands, and organs, causing them to atrophy or dry up. It degenerates the lymphatic and endocrine systems. The thymus is known to be very sensitive to salt; rapid aging accompanies the deterioration of the thymus gland. In China, salt in a saturated solution has been used as a means of suicide. Do you agree that commercial salt should be labeled with skull and crossbones?

The use of salt and salted foods, plus the use of other table condiments such as monosodium glutamate (MSG) and black pepper, is largely responsible for the desire to overeat, especially devitalized foods. Salt deadens the sensitive taste buds on the tongue. Regular salt eaters generally have no desire to eat fresh raw foods because they have lost the finer sensitive nerves of taste on the tongue. The more salt we eat, the more we will crave junk food and the less we will desire fresh, wholesome, poison-free food.

The only salts that the body can actually use are the organic salts formed in plant life from air, water, soil, and solar energy. From the plant, we can digest, assimilate, and fully utilize the organic salts. We require more than just one mineral salt. We need all of them in the right combinations: potassium, silicon, calcium, iron, lime, and chlorine. Inorganic table salt destroys the electrochemical balance between the natural combination of organic salts in the body and the sixteen mineral elements.

Common salt causes an imbalance of the sodium/potassium elements that make up cell life. Salt smothers or crowds potassium out of the cell, where it rightly belongs, and the inorganic table salt overloads the cell, causing local irritation, yang inflammations, and hypertension. It hinders the digestion of albumen by interfering with the secretion of gastric juice. Gout is aggravated by the use of salt, and attacks of gouty pain subside when salt is stopped. Eczema, skin diseases, and dropsy, along with swelling, are directly attributed to salt eating.

Salt removes water from blood and lymph, which is needed for its excretion by the kidneys. This causes abnormal thirst, only satisfied by copious drinking of water, alcohol, and sodas. Heavy salt eaters are generally also heavy meat eaters and drinkers. Salt is also used in meat products to preserve and mask the taste and appearance of the dead, decaying, and decomposing flesh. Ancient civilizations used salt to preserve and embalm the mummified bodies of their dead royalty. It is ironic, and rather sad, that today we are preserving and mummifying living bodies in early preparation for burial.

Here is a list of foods that are commonly eaten by millions of people, which contain large quantities of salt and other unmentionables: all cheeses, except the low-sodium variety; commercial bread; processed boxed cereals; ketchup, sauces, and spreads; frozen dinners; salad dressings; cottage cheese; margarine and butter, except unsalted butter; cakes, cookies, pies, candy; dried soups in envelopes; canned soups, vegetables, and beans. The list goes on and on.

We strongly urge and recommend that young and old alike drastically reduce their salt intake. For your improved health, use the following salt substitutes: powdered kelp, Dr. Bronner's Balanced-Mineral Salt, vegetable (dried powder) seasonings, miso (from soybean), soy sauce (from health store), and sea salt. Awareness is the key; be aware of what you buy from food stores. Read labels. Ask questions. Think. Think. Think. It requires little effort to cease the consumption of junk food when a sound nutritional program is adopted.

Marijuana (Extreme Yin Poison)

Marijuana is twenty times more yin than sugar. We can only shake our heads in wonder every time an educated person says marijuana is harmless or repeats the comment that there is no scientific evidence that marijuana is dangerous. In the thirteenth century, religious leader Ali al-Hariri reported the dangers of marijuana smoking. Warnings kept cropping up over the next six hundred years, and in 1893 the Indian Hemp Drugs Commission urged great caution. In 1924, the League of Nations unanimously classed marijuana as a dangerous drug. It remained a dangerous drug until the early 1960s when "due to a lack of solid evidence" researchers decided that marijuana was harmless. The evidence was there; it was just being ignored. A few researchers tried to get their antimarijuana views before the public and were hooted down. Others conducted research and published the results in obscure medical journals rather than face the public ridicule that an antimarijuana stance brought.

Finally, in 1974, the Senate Judiciary Committee conducted hearings on the marijuana epidemic and antimarijuana research was made public. The collective testimony of twenty of the world's leading medical researchers unquestionably revealed that

1. THC (intoxicating chemical in marijuana) tends to accumulate in the brain, glands, and fatty tissues.

2. Marijuana causes massive damage to the entire cellular process.

3. Smoking marijuana causes irreversible brain damage.

4. There is danger of genetic damage from marijuana use.

5. Chronic marijuana smoking (three joints or pipes per week) for six months produces lung damage equal to twenty years of heavy smoking of normal cigarettes.

6. Marijuana and tobacco smoke in combination are far more damaging to lung tissue than either by itself.

7. Prolonged use of marijuana results in emotional problems.

These opinions were not the result of a single, isolated study as the nation's media reported and implied. Instead they were compiled after the study of many, many research projects. Nor were the studies conducted by unknowns trying to make a name for themselves. Dr. Julius Axelrod, who won the Nobel prize for his study of drugs and the brain, said that marijuana causes irreversible damage to the brain. Dr. Phillip Ze, senior research psychiatrist at New York State Psychiatric Institute, said that chronic marijuana smoking causes bronchitis, diminished lung capacity, and changes in lung tissue. He went on to say that it was very much more dangerous than had been expected.

Dr. Harvey Powelson, a research psychiatrist at the University of California, Berkeley, was highly praised for his promarijuana stand in 1964. Then he was attacked in the press and in person when he changed his views. Dr. Powelson's views changed as his psychiatric study deepened. He found that marijuana disrupts the thinking process and that memory and time awareness become distorted. Dr. Powelson said that three years of chronic smoking left the smoker with permanent brain damage equal to ten years of heavy drinking.

In those hearings, opposition to the decriminalization of marijuana laws was unanimous. The committee was opposed and the witnesses were opposed. Facts supported their decision and logic refuted every promarijuana argument. The medical evidence filled four hundred pages in the record of the hearings. Here we are summarizing only a tiny bit. The main reason for the opposition was the conclusion that marijuana can cause death. This view may be shocking but scientific evidence proves that the dangers of death are great because marijuana: 1) increases the heart beat and blood pressure, enhancing the danger of a stroke; increases the possibility of fainting, without advance warning, which could come while working or driving a car; 3) increases the potency of barbiturates and thus the chance that a nonlethal dose could be turned into a lethal dose without the knowledge of the barbiturate user.

These are the hard facts. The effect of cannabis (marijuana) is subtle and insidious, but harmful reactions in the heart and circulatory system are suspected. Medical evidence also revealed the dangers of chromosome damage, sexual impotence, and emotional changes, all of which the marijuana user may not be aware of until it is too late. Marijuana decreases the sperm count and volume in males aged eighteen to twenty-eight, and reduces blood plasma to 50 percent below normal. According to Dr. Henry Brill, regional director of the New York State Department of Mental Hygiene, there are indications of adverse reactions in the body's anti-infection chemistry. While no one suggested that all marijuana users will move on to heroin, the results of the studies stated that marijuana is the universal threshold drug through which young people make their entry into the drug culture: the more use of pot, the more the use of other drugs. This remained unchallenged by the promarijuana groups.

But the biggest reason for opposing marijuana, both its use and sale, was brought out by Dr. Hardin B. Jones, perhaps the world's most respected authority on drugs and drug abuse. Dr. Jones is professor of medical physics, a professor of physiology, and assistant director of the Donner Laboratory at the University of California at Berkeley. He has taught drug abuse courses and interviewed over 1,600 drug users. Jones's findings, after many years of research, show that marijuana use kills cells in the area of the brain necessary for the awareness of pleasure, the very part of the brain that allows the full awareness of the joys of being alive. There is perhaps no greater hell, said Dr. Jones, than not to be able to feel alive, even if pain accompanies that awareness. And that is the hell that is projected for those who use cannabis.

Commercial Eggs

Eggs may be used by those on transition diets away from the use of flesh foods, or by extremely rundown and protein-deficient individuals. One egg contains 6 grams of protein, of which about 94 percent is utilized by the body. Egg yolks are rich in all the elements necessary for complete nutrition, including iron, minerals, vitamin B complex, and fats. Powdered eggshells are very high in calcium. Eggs are one of the few foods high in vitamins D and A.

Although eggs contain complete proteins of high biological value, egg whites, when taken to excess, are capable of producing intestinal putrefaction to a great degree. Many people are very sensitive to egg albumen and suffer symptoms of toxic poisoning, causing nausea, vomiting, and diarrhea. The free use of eggs, especially egg whites, is found to be injurious in many cases of Bright's disease. Nonfertile, unhygienic commercial eggs increase stomach putrefaction to an even greater degree. The best eggs from the health standpoint are the ones bought locally from a farmer who allows a rooster to roam freely in the chicken coop, which produces fertile eggs. The chickens should also be allowed the freedom to soak up the outdoor fresh air and sunshine and be fed pure whole grains and food substances.

Eggs encourage the growth in the colon of germs of putrefaction, which have been proved to be the cause of membranous colitis and appendicitis. The regular and excessive intake of eggs overworks the liver, causes gas, constipation, and an oversupply of albuminous matter in the body.

It can be seen, then, that eggs, as a class of food, cannot be recommended without qualification. Infants, young children, and invalids should eat them very sparingly, or not at all. Such persons can better utilize raw goat milk products, which contain high-quality proteins with less danger of toxic residues. Cooked eggs are harder to digest than raw ones. Raw eggs are practically liquid. All foods must be turned to liquid before the body can digest them. The longer an egg is cooked, the more difficult it will be to assimilate. Cook eggs as little as possible, never allowing the white to set. Coddled, soft boiled, or poached eggs are the easiest to digest.

Eggs, being an extreme yang food, should not be eaten in warm weather; they can be digested and utilized easier in cold (yin) weather. People with yang livers, kidneys, heart, colon, and intestines should avoid the yang effect of eggs. Meat, fish, and eggs are not absolutely necessary to reach and maintain the highest level of optimum health, nutrition, and longevity. If at first you succeed, try to hide your astonishment.

THE DANGER OF FOOD FADS

Webster defines a fad as a trend, craze, or short-lived fashion. There are literally dozens of dietary fads in vogue today. It is the thing to do. Each fad has its own set of prejudices, rules, and regulations. Ignorance, prejudice, fashion, gullibility due to fear tactics or false hope, and a relaxing sense of security that comes from allowing someone else to think for them are all forces that make people susceptible to dietary fads.

People who are bored with life have nothing constructive to accomplish. They lack exercise and physical fitness and seek excitement and stimulation in artificial things. They are the ones who zoom like bees to a hive, to the first dietary fad that sounds plausible to them. If results are not forthcoming, they look to other dietary cults for further guidance or relief from their health phobias. We are living in an age of the food crank. Many theories are expounded concerning the natural food of humans and how to prepare food. Here are just a few now in vogue:

Cooking is evil and against nature, only raw foods should be eaten.

Eat lots of meat; humans are carnivores.

Eat only cooked grains and vegetables; raw food is for apes.

Eat only raw fruits and nuts; humans are like apes.

Drink only fruit juices, humans are fruitarians and were not originally meant to eat solid food.

Eat only sprouts and fruit, the body requires no protein.

The high-protein diet is necessary for health and strength.

Live on air alone; human are breatharians and should fast as much as possible, drinking only water.

The fact that a cult or organization has a large following, or that its followers experience certain benefits, is not conclusive proof for or against the philosophy it teaches. People can be helped temporarily by almost any change in diet away from the conventional "meat and potato, coffee and donut" mode of existence. Dietary and reducing fads are more fashionable than sensible. People are commercially exploited by fast and slick salesmen who prey on the credulous and fearful. Propaganda is the tool used to rake in enormous financial profits. Many people often experiment on themselves, changing from one dietary program to another, without learning sound and scientific nutritional and health principles. In most cases, the fad diet does not meet their own individual and physiological requirements. Confusion reigns supreme and many people give up in disgust and return to the realm of junk food.

Some food fads are harmless, while others can be very dangerous to the body. An occasional exclusive fruit or eliminative cleansing diet when the physiological need arises is definitely beneficial and health building, but carried to extremes it can lead to malnourishment and ill-health. The same is true for an all-grain diet; it is very cleansing and healthful for a specific period of days, but carried on exclusively or permanently, it can be damaging. An exclusive fruit diet, vegetable diet, or grain diet is referred to as a mono-diet. A mono-diet can improve physical and physiological health. Each such diet is based on simplicity, which makes digestion much easier, to allow for healing, cleansing, rebalancing the internal organs, and rejuvenating the blood and lymph system.

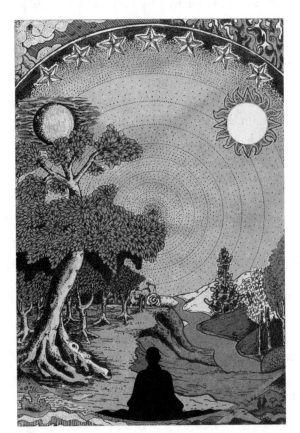

Fig. 8.3. Whatever you do, or dream you can do, begin it. Boldness has genius, power, and magic in it. We can live in the Tao by just deciding to do it.

Many strict dieters limit themselves unnecessarily in their choice of foods, in the false belief that these foods are fattening, mucus-forming, or acid-producing. Some people cannot tolerate fruit due to gas; others shun grains and beans; some are strict food combiners; and some cannot tolerate nuts or dairy products. These notions are generally not based on a solid foundation of facts. Such people make themselves miserable by attempting to live by a set strict standard of rules and regulations, of do nots and cannots. So, for the bewildered dieter, what is left to eat?

All is not lost; there is bright hope for survival in this nutritional/ dietary jungle; a healthy, vibrant life can be achieved by thinking, studying, contemplating, and applying the secrets of the ancients as set forth in this book.

The longest-lived and healthiest people throughout the world do not follow any dietary fads; they are usually much too busy working. They achieve good health by living close to Mother Earth, making work their exercise, and remaining physically fit well over the century mark; sunshine, fresh air, and outdoor activity are part of their daily living habits.

Generally if a person's diet is well balanced in all food elements and if he or she exudes energy, glowing health, and vitality constantly, that person is cultivating good eating and living habits, such as getting complete rest and pursuing mental poise, exercise, and pleasant and healthful environmental. This person is not a food faddist. He or she is balanced mentally, physically, spiritually, and emotionally.

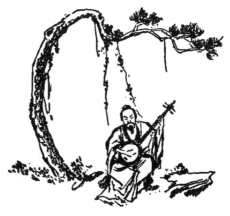

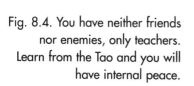

Fig. 8.4. You have neither friends nor enemies, only teachers. Learn from the Tao and you will have internal peace.

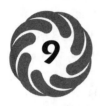

The Great
Physician Within

We cannot possibly attain health without cleansing the body. That is how important it is. Never eat when ill; instead, rest in bed, drink distilled water when thirsty, have proper ventilation and warmth, and in a few days to a few weeks, you will feel like a million. Fasting and eliminative diets are the greatest means of cleansing the body, as they strengthen the nerves, aid digestion, and help to build a powerful organism. When your body requires a thorough internal house cleaning, make up your mind to call on nature's maids in the form of the water fast, raw juice cleansing, or eliminative diet. Do not make a thousand excuses why you cannot begin on a sound health program. Only failures quit. The successful people in life are the ones who follow a truly logical and correct plan of living in harmony with nature's laws. You will be amazed at how much better you will look and feel after a fast or an eliminative diet, maybe even years younger.

FASTING IS NATURAL

The phenomenon of fasting is probably the least understood and the most abused health measure that has ever been used in human history. Understood and used with the proper knowledge of its processes, fasting is life-saving and health-promoting. Misunderstood and abused, without thorough knowledge of its principles, it can be disease-producing and death-dealing.

To set the record straight, fasting or abstinence from food is an intimate part or process of every breathing life form, either plant or animal (including human), that has ever existed since the beginning of creation. It can be said that we all fast during sleep and we customarily break-the-fast with the morning breakfast. Just as we must all rest, mentally and physically, from our daily activities and give our body a chance to recharge its batteries through sleep, so must we allow our digestive and eliminative organs a rest (fast) from all food for the purpose of cleansing, purifying, and revitalizing worn out cells, tissues, blood, and all physiological functions.

There is nothing mysterious or occult about fasting. Although fasting has been used in various religious cults throughout history, it has not been generally recognized for its true value in the scientific care of the sick, the maintenance of health and the extension of life. The word *occult* means "secret." Fasting is an occult mystery only to those who have not taken the time to study it. And it will continue to be a mystery to all those who condemn it without first giving it a thorough investigation and fair trial.

A great sage once said: "Condemnation before investigation is the greatest bar to all knowledge." Let us not condemn the natural process of fasting, for it has been proven through scientific research and testing

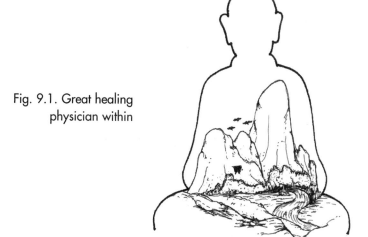

Fig. 9.1. Great healing
physician within

to be of true value in all states of health and disease. Abstinence is one of the best of all remedies and alone cures without danger. Instead of using medicines, fast a day. Fasting is the royal road to internal purity.

Fasting Defined

Fasting is defined as a complete and total abstinence from all food, including juices, for a shorter or longer period of time and for any number of purposes, such as illness or weight loss. We all fast in rest or sleep whether we know it or not. Continual eating without periods of fasting would cause internal toxemia or food poisoning. However, nature dearly cares for us by taking away our hunger after a certain amount of food is consumed. It is a built-in safety valve; otherwise we would all die from gluttony.

Any food eaten in excess of bodily needs and natural hunger will cause a toxic overload in the system of undigested waste products (toxemia) within the cells and tissues. This in turn overworks the body's eliminative organs. We can now detect the first state of the disease process: overworked organs of elimination, followed by toxemia or poisoned blood, and ending with pathology, disease, and an early grave. The cure of disease lies in preventing the cause of disease.

Fasting allows the eliminative organs to catch up on their work. The body is always striving to maintain a balance, and when it is given a physiologic rest (fast), it will carry out its prime objective without the aid of drugs, medicines, or any other unnatural cures. The most sensible health policy we can follow is to eat only when truly hungry, which is indicated when the mouth waters, and there is a zest and relish for natural unstimulating food. If food is not relished at regular mealtimes, skip the meal and fast until true hunger returns.

Fear of Fasting or Starving

Fasting has been feared by many people, due to misinformation and fear tactics by the press, radio, and TV, including the unwillingness or ignorance of medical authorities to investigate and reveal the truth of the matter. At the same time, the press has run articles telling of plane crash victims and survivors of other natural disasters, who survived for many days or weeks without food and medical help. Subsisting almost entirely on water, survivors often come out of it with improved health and freedom from previous disease conditions. These cases definitely substantiate the claim that the human body is inherently capable of surviving under adverse situations with no ill or adverse effects.

Those who are supposed to know about our health and welfare are completely ignorant about the distinction between fasting and starving, which are two completely different conditions. The first is beneficial and rejuvenating; the latter is destructive and death-dealing. Starvation begins where fasting leaves off.

Fasting is a process whereby the body exists on its stored reserves of fat, protein, and minerals, until they are used up or exhausted. Then it is time to break the fast. To go beyond the stored reserves is starvation. Fasting does not use up the vital tissues or organs. Starvation is a pathological skeletal condition that ends in death. Proper fasting eliminates bodily poisons and adipose tissue and breaks down destructive cells. Countless people have fasted with or without supervision for a variety of reasons from a few days to many weeks. The results of these fasts have been proven to be of utmost value in achieving superior health. If carried out properly and scientifically, the fast is a means of acquiring complete rejuvenation and vigorous, robust health.

Experimental and Scientific Fasting

It is unfortunate for the American people that the medical profession refuses to acknowledge, recognize, or teach the value of fasting as a natural form of correct care in sickness. In European countries, fasting, juice diets, and other natural therapeutic measures are used by the best doctors in clinics and sanitariums. One such well-known clinic is the Buchinger Sanitarium in Bad Pyrmont, Germany, where more than seventy thousand fasts or juice fasts have been conducted. In Australia, Dr. Alec Burton has conducted thousands of fasts at his Natural Hygiene Resort for many years. In Sweden, in the year 1954 and again in 1964, Dr. Lennart Edren led a 300-mile walkathon of fasting participants. A total of thirty people started and finished the walk with no ill effects. All medical tests on the fast-walkers proved to be positive, with no adverse side effects. This experiment clearly proves that we are able to fast even under strenuous physical exertion.

In this country, Dr. H. M. Shelton has personally supervised more than thirty thousand fasts in his fifty years of practice in Texas. He writes about some interesting cases of feats of strength while fasting. In volume 3 of *The Hygienic System*, chapter 16, he states that Bernarr Macfadden, the "father of physical culture," held a fasting and strength contest in Madison Square Garden in 1903. After a seven-day fast, J. H. Waltering captured first place by running a mile in six minutes, considered quite fast at that time. Even more fantastic was Mr. Gilman Low, a weight-lifter from Boston. He lifted 500 pounds twenty times in fifteen seconds and 900 pounds twice in twenty seconds. On the seventh day of his fast (completely without food), he lifted a ton twenty-two times in nineteen seconds. All of this was closely observed by medical doctors.

Does this indicate a state of starvation, weakness, or death? No. It simply means that the human body has a tremendous storehouse of reserve food material by which it sustains itself during periods of fasting or food shortage.

Dick Gregory, the famous comedian, writer, and author of many books, one being on natural health and vegetarian nutrition, has undergone many fasts while engaged in long distance running (15 miles).

We have personally gone on extended water fasts up to two to four weeks, and on watery fruit diets for up to forty-eight days, thus regaining our health and well-being. However, we do not recommend a fast or fruit diet for this length of time unless you have proper supervision or are well versed in the procedure.

Animals and Fasting

We all can learn a lesson about fasting by observing the habits of wild and domestic animals. Animals will not eat when sick or wounded, but they will retreat to a quiet location and rest, drinking only water until well. It has also been observed that some animals will consume a small amount of grass when sick. There is something in the grass and plant life that the animal craves when sick. The green chlorophyll supplies the missing elements or cleansing properties that are needed in sickness. The household animal will recover of its own accord when left alone. It will let you know when it is ready to eat.

It has been noted by research scientists that scores of insects and animals abstain from food for a few days up to many months during the winter season. The breeding season of numerous lower animals is a period of fasting and resting. The silver salmon fasts for weeks while swimming hundreds of miles upstream to its spawning ground. The queen ant eats nothing until her eggs are hatched, and then the hatched workers finally bring her food. An incredible period of many weeks passes before she is again ready for food. The common earthworm has been kept alive for well over fifteen generations in laboratory experiments because of periodic fasting.

It would be well for human beings to follow the same course of action as do all animals; that is, when sick, diseased, or emotionally upset, take a physiological rest: abstain from all food (fast), rest in bed, keep warm and quiet, and drink only pure water as thirst demands until recovered. We are the only creatures that eat at all hours of the night and day and that continue to do so when sick, diseased, and emotionally upset. Humans are the only living beings that refuse to resort to fasting when sick, instead foolishly partaking of food and imbibing poisonous medications in a futile attempt to restore sick bodies to health. Nothing adds to the fires of disease like drug treatment and forced feeding. This procedure has caused much suffering and agony, sending millions of unwary souls to an early grave.

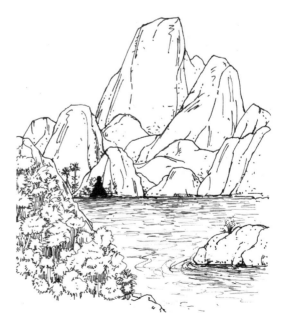

Fig. 9.2. Fasting is internal resting.

All living organisms, from the one-celled amoeba to the human, the highest form of intelligent life on Earth, are subject to the same universal natural laws of life and existence, namely, the inherent qualities of self-healing, self-regeneration, and self-rejuvenation. It behooves every medical scientist and nutritional researcher to investigate the truths nature has to offer, and to use her natural principles for the benefit of all humankind.

Historical Fasting

Let us again remind our medical brethren that the father of medicine, Hippocrates, recommended fasting in the care of the sick. He said that if a sick person is fed, the disease is also being fed. On the other hand, if food is withheld from the sufferer, the disease is fasted out. All nations of antiquity followed the natural principles and methods of fasting and frugal eating as advocated by their great philosophers and sages: Socrates, Plato, Pliny, Seneca, Pythagoras, Moses, Jesus, Buddha, Mohammed, Galen, Benjamin Franklin, Thomas Edison, and many, many more.

Jesus reportedly fasted forty days in the mountains and thereafter could not be tempted by the devil. Likewise, Gandhi subjected himself to fasting and prayer frequently. Moses fasted and prayed, and he descended from the mountains a wiser man. In early Rome, certain drug doctors were not allowed to dispense their concoctions. Paracelsus once said that fasting is the greatest remedy, the physician within that heals us. Confucius, Buddha, Lao-tzu, Christ, Moses, and others fasted for internal purity and illumination.

By following the advice and example of these great men, you too can become disease-free. The old adage "there is nothing to fear but fear itself" can be applied to the fear of fasting. Fear not, for you will be guided by the spirit of the great ones who have also tread the straight and narrow way.

What to Expect While Fasting

The length of a fast cannot be determined beforehand. Each case is unique and every person has different quantities of toxic poisons within his or her body and various degrees of organic constitutional weaknesses.

Nature will always indicate how long one should fast. Take it day by day.

The first two or three days of a fast are the most difficult, especially for sick people. This is because the faster has, perhaps for the first time, missed the accustomed stimulating meal. Like a drug addict, the food addict will go through two or three days of withdrawal symptoms. At this point of the fast, the tongue may become coated white and the breath may smell bad. There may be a foul taste in the mouth and nausea, accompanied by dizziness upon arising, topped off by an empty feeling in the stomach. After three days these symptoms will usually disappear as the body's reserve forces draw on themselves for nourishment.

These symptoms may also reappear as the fast progresses, as the elimination process continues. It must be understood that the elimination of toxic material thrown out into the bloodstream for expulsion is a necessary cleansing process. Near the end of the fast these unpleasant effects will subside and a feeling of well-being will take their place.

Addictions to stimulating foods will cause withdrawal symptoms during a fast. Stomach rumblings, headaches, nausea, weakness, fatigue, irritability, and a coated tongue are definite signs that a fast is needed, along with a change to a more wholesome, natural, nonstimulating diet afterward. If a crisis overtakes you during a fast, do not panic. Here are

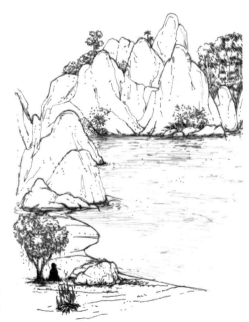

Fig. 9.3. Short and long
fasts in nature

some of the temporary eliminative symptoms you may experience before reaching normal physiological balance and high-level health: feverishness or chills due to toxic material being thrown into the bloodstream for elimination, cramps, retention of urine, diarrhea, headaches, and insomnia.

To facilitate internal healing, fasters require plenty of rest, sleep, fresh air, sunshine, and freedom from all stress; this especially holds true for those weakened by a debilitating disease. Many people prefer to drink warm water during a fast and to place a ginger compress or hot water bottle on the stomach, intestines, or bowels to attract blood to the area for healing.

It is amazing how hunger will vanish after the fifth day of fasting. In fact, then the mere mention of food will sometimes cause nausea. As the reserve food supply within the body takes over the job of sustaining the body, other inner functions work to maintain balance, such as the pulse rate slows down, blood pressure decreases, and stomach secretions are reduced. The eyes become brighter and hearing becomes more acute. The blood cells increase in number.

You will know that your fast is nearing completion when the symptoms of elimination disappear. Your breath will smell sweet, and foul tastes and nausea will be gone. Your pulse rate, blood pressure, and temperature will return to normal. The stomach secretions and hunger that were lacking will return in full force. Your mouth will water and you will desire the simplest of food. You will have a feeling of well-being and a new zest for living.

Long Fasts

One fast will never completely cleanse the body. It requires from one to three years of periodic fasting and correct eating to obtain a thorough cleansing of the system and a return to vibrant health. A single long fast may produce a clean, pink tongue, but this does not necessarily indicate a totally pure and cleansed body. When the tongue has become pink, it either indicates that the body is pure or that its reserve fuel supplies and vital force have been used up for cleansing during that particular fast.

Many times a person who is fasting will run out of energy and vitality well before the tongue clears up and becomes pink. In this case, it is imperative to break the fast. Nothing is ever gained by trying to break records while fasting, at the expense of the recovery ability of the body. Fasting too much and too often can make a nervous wreck out of the strongest-willed person, not to mention a sickly one.

Most people can withstand a seven- to ten-day fast without supervision, provided some studying has been done on the subject. Longer fasts must be taken only under the proper supervision of one who knows the procedure thoroughly. The sicker the body, the more crisis reaction it will have; that is why it is so important to be supervised by a competent health doctor. Between each fast, maintain a well-balanced diet, obtain sufficient exercise, sunshine, fresh air, rest, sleep, and emotional poise.

Precautions in Fasting

Fasting is most beneficial in acute diseases but not in degenerative conditions. An acute disease is a violent or quick release of toxins in the system; it is a sign that the body has enough reserve vital power to discharge and eliminate the internal poisons and heal the organism. A chronic disease is a condition of long standing (degeneration) leaving an individual with weak healing power.

Degenerative diseases, such as cancer, diabetes, rheumatoid arthritis, Parkinson's disease, tuberculosis, heart disease, and extreme malnutrition (anorexia nervosa), do not readily respond to long fasts. Other natural health and biological therapies are recommended to regain health and balance body and blood chemistry. Some of these therapies include: herbs, acupuncture, vitamin/mineral food supplements, balanced individual dietary measures, color and music therapy, hydrotherapy, corrective exercise movements, shiatsu massage, sunshine, sufficient rest and sleep, harmonious environment, and positive physical and mental conditions.

Dr. John Tilden, an early 1900s fasting physician, advocated only short fasts from three to ten days for certain chronic diseases, and thereafter fed his patients only one meal per day until they recovered. He never advocated long exhausting fasts, as he believed they were too depleting to the nervous system.

A note to the seriously ill: If you have either an acute or chronic condition, before undertaking a fast or an eliminative diet, please consult a natural health practitioner or a competent doctor who thoroughly understands the process of fasting, natural healing, nutritional therapy, and the yin and yang principle. A professional of this caliber can determine more accurately what can be accomplished in your individual case. Disease is nature's effort to get you well. Regain your health by living away disease.

Breaking a Fast

Extreme care should be taken in breaking a five- to ten-day fast. The first day after the fast, drink a mixture of 4 ounces of apple or orange juice and 4 ounces of water, one glass every two hours. The second day eat fresh fruit according to your hunger. The third day eat a well-balanced diet. It is best to consume fruit and vegetables grown in the region and climate where you live, that is, apples, berries, peaches, cherries, and winter vegetables in the northern region and oranges, grapefruits, and melons in the southern region.

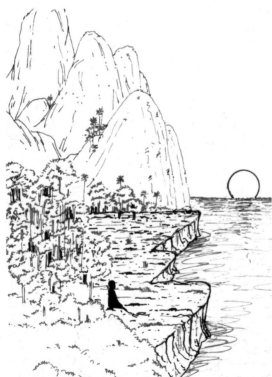

Fig. 9.4. Breaking a fast

Reasons for Fasting

1. For body and blood cleansing
2. For colds or flu
3. When mentally and physically fatigued
4. For spiritual development
5. For rejuvenating internal glands and hormones
6. For losing weight
7. To prevent acute and chronic disease
8. To feel and look better
9. To eat less and save money
10. To lower cholesterol levels and blood pressure
11. To overcome drugs, smoking, and alcohol
12. To overcome stress and sleep better
13. To improve digestion and bowel movements
14. To increase mental and physical discipline

Fasting Recommendations

We do not recommend that raw food dieters or strict fruitarians fast for any length of time; what is needed in these cases is a well-balanced natural diet. These extreme alkaline diets are already naturally cleansing to the system, but they are deficient in many nutrients that are necessary for tissue repair, healing, and body-weight maintenance. Any further fasting in these cases will lead to disease and compound the problem.

The ancients teach that it is more beneficial to fast when ill or not hungry; all animals in nature follow this procedure. This is in conformity with the natural flow of life. Many people attempt to set a scheduled day for fasting, but when their prearranged day arrives, they may find themselves hungry or in no mood to fast. Instead of heeding their inner psychological voice, they fast anyway. This is not a healthful practice, because the body is not in need or ready for a cleansing at that time; what is needed is wholesome food.

Many health enthusiasts believe the erroneous concept that fasting is a cure-all; it is not. Fasting too long and too often, when one is not physiologically ready, can lead to junk-food binging, and, more seriously, to nervous exhaustion and anorexia, conditions that can be fatal.

The best advice is to fast only when necessary, especially when hunger is not present or when physically or emotionally exhausted. Missing a meal or two occasionally improves digestion and elimination, clears the mind, and increases health and longevity. Fasting in its proper time enables us to cleanse, heal, and balance the body chemistry in a normal cycle. The beneficial results of any fast will be enhanced provided the person adopts a natural food diet and healthy lifestyle afterward, as suggested in this book.

Fasting Summarized

To clarify mistaken beliefs and sum up the benefits of fasting in a condensed version, we quote the mid-twentieth century advocate of fasting in America, Dr. H. M. Shelton.

Fasting does not:
1. Cause the stomach to shrink up.
2. Cause the walls of the stomach to grow together.
3. Cause the digestive fluids of the stomach to turn upon it and digest the stomach.
4. Paralyze the bowels.
5. Impoverish the blood or produce anemia.
6. Produce acidosis.
7. Cause the heart to weaken or collapse.
8. Produce malnutritional edema.
9. Produce tuberculosis nor predispose to its development.
10. Reduce resistance to disease.
11. Injure the teeth.
12. Injure the nervous system.
13. Injure any of the vital organs.
14. Injure the body's glands.
15. Cause psychosis.

On the positive side, fasting does:
1. Give the vital organs a complete rest.
2. Stop the intake of food, which may decompose in the intestines and poison the body.
3. Empty the digestive tract and dispose of putrefactive bacteria.

4. Give the organs of elimination an opportunity to catch up with their work, and promote elimination.
5. Reestablish normal physiological chemistry and normal secretions.
6. Promote the breaking down and absorption of exudates, deposits, diseased tissues, and abnormal growths.
7. Restore a youthful condition to the cells and tissues, and rejuvenate the body.
8. Permit the conservation and recanalization of energy.
9. Increase the powers of digestion and assimilation.
10. Clear and strengthen the mind.
11. Improve function throughout the body.

REJUVENATING PROGRAMS

If you are an extremely busy person and do not have the time or inclination to go on a total fast for a few weeks at a health spa, then the eliminative diet and the raw juice cleansing rejuvenation program are for you. The program consists of consuming only raw fruits and vegetables and their juices, to be eaten at mealtimes or at any other time during the day that you feel hungry.

Raw Juice Power

Natural science has rediscovered the regenerating and rejuvenating properties of raw foods and fasting as passed down throughout the ages from ancient teachings. In the days gone by, humans were known to have lived to great ages in perfect health and vitality. Today, European health clinics are utilizing the principles of this secret youth formula in the form of therapeutic juice fasting, including the use of fresh raw fruit and vegetable juices, vegetable broths, youth-giving herb teas, and mineral waters.

In unhealthy, diseased, and acid/yang conditions, raw juice cleansing therapy is a beneficial alternative to the conventional water fast method. Both methods are useful and will rejuvenate and cleanse the body, but program of juices, vegetable broths, and herbs will provide a demineralized and depleted body with the necessary elements such as live raw enzymes, trace mineral elements, vitamins, and minerals, which are extremely necessary factors in supplying life-giving elements for the glands, organs, tissues, and blood to increase the recovery ability and healing of the entire body. The blood-sugar level remains close to normal during a raw juice fast, while alkaline reserves are built up to neutralize the excessive acids in the tissues and blood. The morality of clean blood ought to be one of the first lessons taught us by our pastors and teachers. The physical is the substratum of the spiritual; this fact ought to give to the food we eat and the air we breathe a transcendent significance.

Raw fresh fruits and vegetables contain highly nutritive solar-energy electricity and enzymes that operate to preserve and prolong the life of the living cells. Juices and liquids do not impair or tax the digestive process and are very effortlessly absorbed quickly into the bloodstream, cells, and tissues. A person fasting on juices thus does not experience much weakness or low energy lags during or after the fast, as often occurs on a strict water fast. Similarly, it is often the case that the recovery after a juice fast is quicker and more stable than after a water fast.

Eliminative Diet

The eliminative diet is a superb method of cleansing the body of internal impurities. It consists of consuming only raw fruits, vegetables, and juices, excluding proteins, fats, and starches, as well as the heavier acid-forming fruits and vegetables such as bananas, dates, dried fruits, potatoes, nuts, and avocados. Raw fruits, vegetables, and juices are easy to digest and assimilate, thus enabling the remaining body energy to expend itself on self-healing and cleansing. If a person consumes starch, fat, or protein foods during a cleansing diet, the healing process will be delayed. Heavier yang/acid foods are more difficult to digest and take longer to be absorbed into the bloodstream; they should therefore be avoided during a cleansing period.

A few days to a week on juicy fruits and vegetables, with sufficient rest, will allow the body to eliminate accumulated waste products, fatty deposits, and excess weight. The best time for this type of yin-eliminative diet is during hot summer months. You can expect to lose from 7 to 10 pounds of body weight and fat per week on this diet; it will also normalize blood cholesterol levels and lower high blood pressure.

During an eliminative diet you may experience varying degrees of aches, pains, headaches, diarrhea, dizziness, and nausea. These temporary symptoms indicate that the organism is working to eliminate years of accumulated internal waste products. A crisis resulting from an eliminative diet or fast is a physiologically preventative measure much less painful than the possibility of degenerative or chronic disease years later. Note, however, that an eliminative diet or fast is not recommended for those with diabetes, hypoglycemia, or other degenerative diseases.

Acute and chronic diseases can be attributed to the overconsumption of protein, fat, and high-calorie processed starch foods. You do not need to be too concerned about eating high-protein or other acid-forming foods; the main concern here is internal cleanliness and a return to a wholesome nutritional program that includes grains, legumes, vegetables, fruits, germinated seeds and nuts, sprouts, and a moderate amount of low-fat yogurt, buttermilk, and cottage cheese (all raw).

Cleansing Foods

The following raw foods are excellent blood cleansers and purifiers.

Apples	Cucumbers	Nectarines	Pineapples
Apricots (fresh)	Grapefruit	Oranges	Plums
Blackberries	Grapes	Papaya	Raspberries
Blueberries	Honeydew	Peaches	Strawberries
Cantaloupe	Huckleberries	Pears	Tomatoes
Cherries	Mulberries	Persimmons	Watermelon

The following foods may be used as disinfectors and mucus dissolvers in a salad consisting of tomatoes, cucumbers, green peppers, and tender celery:

Cayenne pepper	Leeks	Onions
Garlic	Lemon juice	Radishes

The following vegetables are utilized more efficiently to cleanse the cells and tissues, build the blood, and purify the internal organs. They must be freshly squeezed in a juice extractor and sipped slowly. Use

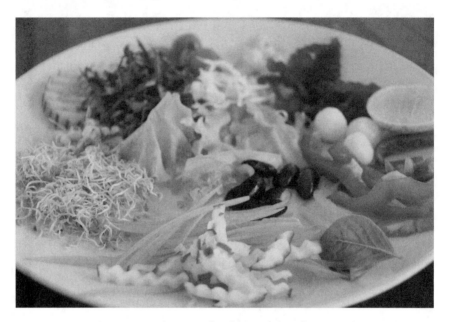

Fig. 9.5. Cleansing foods (see color plate 14)

carrot juice as a base, about 5 ounces, and add 3 ounces of any of the vegetables listed here.

Alfalfa	Endive	Spinach
Asparagus	Green pepper	Squash
Beet	Kale	String bean
Brussels sprouts	Kelp	Swiss chard
Cabbage	Lettuce	Tomato
Carrot	Parsley	Turnip
Celery	Parsnip	Watercress
Cucumber	Potato	Zucchini
Dandelion	Sorrel	

Daily Ration of Juice

Juice is best taken on an empty stomach, or one half hour before a meal. The daily ration of vegetable juice should be from 4 to 6 ounces, unless you are on a juice cleansing program for a specified period of days, in which case you can drink a quart or more per day. Any more than 4 to 6 ounces of vegetable juice on a daily basis may overwork the liver, causing yellow/orange skin, or what is known as carotene anemia. This is a result of the liver's inability to utilize vitamin A in large amounts. The darker races should observe the whites of the eyes for yellowness.

Likewise, no more than 4 to 6 ounces of fruit juice should be taken daily. An excessive consumption of fruit juice overworks the kidneys and pancreas because of the concentrated sugar content. A healthy body produces only a small amount of insulin daily. An excessive intake of sweet juice will make the body produce excessive insulin and lead to hypoglycemia (low blood sugar). An excessive consumption of fruits and juices creates high alkalinity (yin condition) in the system and overworks the adrenal glands in their effort to maintain the pH of the urine between 6.5 and 7.0. This yin condition also decreases the hydrochloric acid in the stomach, thus lowering protein and calcium absorption.

As mentioned earlier, balancing the potassium/sodium (yin/yang) content of foods and juices basically involves using the food grown in the climate where you live. If you live in the north, you will obtain much better results if you consume the fruit and vegetable juices that are grown in that region: apple, pear, plum, berries, cherries, grapes, peaches, melons, carrots, beans (green), squash, celery, green pepper, cucumber, parsley, and so on. These foods are grown in cold (yin) climates and they are classified as more yang than tropical foods because of their higher sodium content. Northern (sodium/yang) foods are more sustaining and warming in cold weather.

Yin (potassium) foods are grown in hot southern (yang) climates. Southerners can best utilize the foods grown in their region, such as all citrus fruits, tomato, papaya, persimmons, mangoes, melons, peaches, berries, and all vegetables grown in the south. These plant foods are high in potassium (yin) and very cooling to the system.

Consume fruit in season only, and not to excess. More fruit can be eaten in the summer for yin and yang balance. Use good judgment in the choice and amount of raw foods at all times.

CONSTIPATION

Constipation is a worldwide problem. However, it seems to be more concentrated in the so-called civilized Western nations. Constipation is virtually unknown in undeveloped and agricultural-based countries. Wild men and wild animals do not suffer from this malady, which is perhaps responsible for more human misery and mental and moral disaster than any other single cause.

Constipation was known back in the time of Hippocrates, when certain days of the month were set aside for taking purgatives, enemas, and emetics. Hippocrates claimed that chronic disease came from autointoxication, that is, self-poisoning due to constipation. He said that the deposits of accumulated waste in the colon release toxins, which inflame the nerves, producing rheumatism, neuralgia, melancholia, hysteria, eczema, acne, headaches, and many other health problems. Since his time, constipation has grown to epidemic proportions, especially in stress-filled modern society where unnatural living habits are more prevalent, and tons of refined, processed, and artificial junk foods and drugs are consumed daily. Constipation precedes most disease conditions.

Constipation can be defined as the inability to evacuate the bowels; impacted colon; lack of intestinal strength and peristalsis activity; lack of complete bowel movement; improper stools and infrequent movements. There can also be constipation of the liver, kidneys, and bladder because of a clogged condition from overeating. See the comparison below of a normal, healthy colon and an abnormal, diseased colon, and resolve to eat healthfully and perform internal exercises daily to maintain a normal colon and good health.

Atonic constipation is a yin condition of expanded colon and intestines. The symptoms of this disease are lack of muscular tone in the

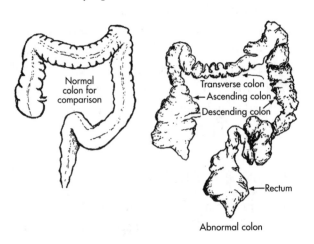

Normal colon for comparison

Transverse colon
Ascending colon
Descending colon

Rectum

Abnormal colon

Fig. 9.6. Normal colon and abnormal colon

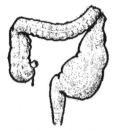 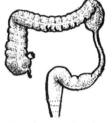

Fig. 9.7. Colon in atonic
and spastic constipation

Atonic constipation   Spastic constipation

colon and abdominal cavity and fallen and pushed out intestines with gas pockets and clogged with fecal matter. It is caused by overeating; eating fruits, fats, liquids, sugars, and other yin foods to excess; excessive use of cathartics; and improper and overuse of enemas.

Spastic constipation is a yang condition in which the colon is constricted or tense and the fecal matter is evacuated in small lumps and stringy. It is caused by excessive intake of meat, fish, fowl, eggs, white flour products, and salt.

The Most Common Causes of Constipation

1. Constant overeating and improper diet
2. Too many food combinations at meals
3. Improper mastication
4. Drinking with meals (excessively)
5. Eating when not truly hungry
6. Ignoring nature's call
7. Eating when emotionally upset, angry, or tired
8. Eating too many constipating foods
9. Not eating enough fresh, raw foods
10. Lack of abdominal tone and physical fitness
11. Excessive fruits, liquids, and sugars
12. Excessive meat, eggs, white flour products, and salt

Causes of Constipation

1. Constant overeating and improper diet: overeating bloats and overtaxes the digestive system and organs. An overloaded

stomach cannot digest food properly and the resulting mass of fermenting food coats up the walls of the intestines and colon, making it very difficult to evacuate waste matter. Internal secretions also fail to handle the excessive amount of food eaten. Improper foods make the condition even worse.

2. Too many food combinations at one meal can easily upset the body and blood chemistry, causing indigestion and toxemia. A mono-diet of just one food such as grapes or apples per meal can do wonders in overcoming constipation.

3. Improper mastication overburdens the stomach and digestive organs. Food must be chewed into a semi-liquid state before the digestive system can handle it without trouble. Swallowing foods half chewed places all the work on the stomach and intestines, causing blockages in the colon.

4. Excessive drinking with meals dilutes the digestive juices, causing indigestion and constipation; it also hampers proper salivation of foods, which impedes digestion. If liquid is taken at a meal, simply sip slowly and mix with the saliva. Chinese herbalists recommend a small cup of herb tea after meals to help cut any fat (vegetable or animal) eaten during the meal and to aid digestion.

5. Eating when true hunger is not present is a burden to the stomach, internal secretions, and intestines. True hunger is present when the mouth waters for wholesome, unprocessed foods. Stomach pangs, pain, or rumblings are all signs of indigestion and false appetite cravings. It is best to eat at regular hours, but if not hungry, skip that meal and wait until true hunger returns, or eat a light meal of fruit or vegetable broth.

6. Ignoring nature's call to evacuate causes an accumulation of fecal matter in the lower bowel, making it insensitive to further movements. This directly leads to colitis, piles, prolapsed colon, autointoxication, and constipation. No matter what you're doing at the time, always heed the call of nature.

7. Eating when emotionally upset, angry, or tired. Food is very poorly digested and assimilated when eaten in a state of emotional turmoil; the mouth becomes dry, saliva does not flow freely; stomach secretions stop or slow down. There is no real

appetite and therefore no nerve power to digest and utilize food properly, resulting in constipation. It is the same with fatigue; rest when tired. If you cannot sing or laugh before a meal, skip it until you can.

8. Eating too many constipating foods—such as meats, cheeses, nuts, white flour, white sugar, pastries, nut butters, oils, fatty foods, fried foods, and popcorn—and the excessive use of lettuce or raw spinach lead to disease, if not counterbalanced by high-fiber or anticonstipating foods, such as whole grains, fruits, sprouts, vegetables, juices, beans, and yogurt.

9. Not eating a sufficient amount of fresh raw foods can cause constricted kidneys and liver and also hardening of fecal matter in the colon and bowels, which is a yang condition. Lack of raw food deprives one of vitamins, minerals, and enzymes necessary to the proper functioning of the digestive and eliminative system.

10. Lack of abdominal tone and physical fitness can cause prolapse of the internal organs. The diaphragm muscles must be strengthened to build up tone and health in this area. Those who exercise daily (especially the abdominal region) rarely experience constipation. An overall exercise program also stimulates internal secretions, hormones, and organs.

11. Overeating of fruits, liquids, and sugars causes atonic or yin constipation.

12. An excessive intake of meat, eggs, white flour, and salt causes spastic or yang constipation.

Detecting Constipation

Health and disease can be detected by observing the form and color of the feces. The stools should be firm and shaped like a banana or cigar, without odor; odor is a sign of internal stasis or constipation. When eating wholesome foods, thoroughly chewed and digested, the feces will be medium brown, firm, and will float. If feces are dark or black, excessive animal products have been consumed or there may be internal bleeding. Reddish feces are usually an indication of bleeding hemorrhoids. Greenish stools mean an overconsumption of yin fruits and sweets.

Light-colored feces are caused by an excess of raw fruits and vegetables. A baby's feces are yellow and soft. If the feces do not float, excessive yin foods, fruits, sugars, and liquid have been eaten or eating has happened without thorough mastication and bad food combinations.

Excessive salt consumption causes intestinal water absorption, which results in small and dry feces. Excessive use of dairy products, fruits, sugar, and fats (all yin) results in shapeless feces or diarrhea. The bowels should move after each meal. If you eat three meals per day and have only one movement, you are constipated. In this case your body wastes are usually retained for two days or more. If you have small or scanty bowel movements three times per day, you are still constipated.

Foul smelling stools are an unnatural and unhealthy condition, common to meat eaters only. Meat eaters invariably have coated tongues and foul breath, along with bad-smelling stools. In the case of the dog, tiger, lion, and the human meat-eater, fragments of decaying flesh are always to be found in the colon, while in the colons of vegetarian animals like sheep, cow, deer, and nursing infants and flesh-abstainers among humans, there is no decay or foul odors. Vegetarian gorillas and apes, who are physiologically built like humans, have odorless stools, which are large and mushy. Their intestines and skin are free from parasites. Pinworms and parasites are a sign of intestinal toxemia and constipation. More than 80 percent of all people have pinworms and many other types of worms. A diet of processed junk foods, meats, fried foods, and sugar will surely attract worms in your system.

Overcoming Constipation

Constipation is not overcome in a day or two; it takes time for the body to eliminate years of toxic wastes and to rebuild and strengthen itself. Relax and get plenty of rest, exercise, fresh air, sunshine, and natural foods. Be persistent in performing the Intestinal Cleanse (see below) each morning. Within a couple days or weeks on this program you will experience normal and complete morning bowel movements. The key point to remember is to strengthen the entire abdominal cavity, that is, the diaphragm, stomach muscles, and internal organs. When these vital body parts are strengthened, you will vibrate with healthy personal attractiveness.

Oriental belly dancers have excellent control of their abdominal muscles and diaphragm. Through their action of drawing in large quantities of fresh air and exercising, these girls have marvelous complexions, skin tone, sparkling bright eyes, and the grace of a fawn. Include some abdominal exercises, hula, or belly dancing movements in your morning routine; be imaginative.

Intestinal Cleanse for Internal Health

Practice this intestinal program every morning.

1. Upon awakening in the morning perform from 10 to 15 sit-ups. Increase the number up to 20 as you become stronger.
2. Next, drink a glass of herb tea.
3. Now do some more abdominal exercises, such as toe touching, side bends, pulling the stomach in and out. Try to pull the contents of the abdomen upward, then force it downward. Wiggle your insides, tossing them from side to side. Strive to control these vital muscles and make them work at will.
4. Continue the exercises until you feel the need for a bowel movement; usually 5 or 10 minutes will be enough.

Abdominal Lift

Practice this Abdominal Lift on an empty stomach throughout the day, or preferably with the morning Intestinal Cleanse. This super exercise is great for the wasp-like waist appearance. It will provide your internal organs and intestinal canal freedom from unnecessary wastes, and it will keep the muscles and skin firm and youthful.

1. Stand with feet apart, knees slightly bent, and lean a little forward from the hips with the back straight.
2. Inhale deeply and then exhale as much air as possible from the lungs.
3. Next, pull in the abdominal muscles with a firm upward movement until a hollow appears under the rib cage. Hold this position for a few seconds without inhaling, and then relax.

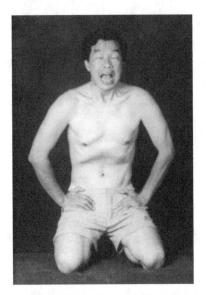 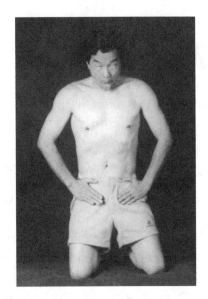

Fig. 9.8. Abdominal Lift, rolling the abdominal ball

If these instructions are carried out regularly, you will receive the marvelous results of superior physical health and well-being. Drugs, laxatives, stomach and bowel remedies, along with their injurious side-effects, can be thrown out with the rest of the garbage!

Stomach, Intestines, and Chest Strengthener

This exercise also tones and trims the waist, hips, legs, arms, shoulders, and back.

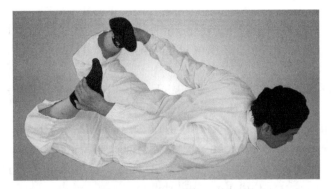

Fig. 9.9. Rock the body to and fro on the abdomen as shown for 30 to 60 seconds.

Raised Legs Sway

This exercise tones and strengthens the abdominal muscles, stomach, and lower intestines and reduces the hips.

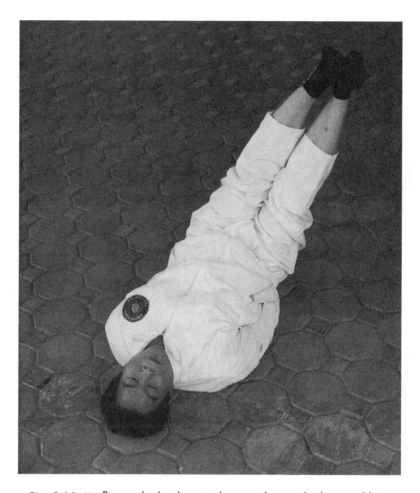

Fig. 9.10. Lie flat on the back, raise legs, and sway the legs and hips
from side to side. Repeat every day.

Stretch and Swing

This exercise massages the stomach, intestines, and internal organs, trims the waist, and strengthens the chest and back.

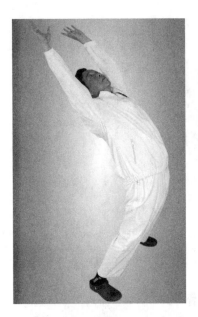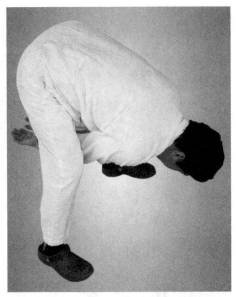

Fig. 9.11. Spread feet 3 or 4 feet apart, knees bent. Inhale while stretching backward with arms overhead; while swinging forward and downward, exhale completely and vigorously. Repeat movement 6 to 8 times per day, especially mornings.

 Internal Bath to Overcome Constipation

A high enema will soften the deposits of the large intestine or colon and should be taken at least three days in succession to eliminate hardened waste matter.

1. Fill a 2-quart enema bag with 1½ pints of hot water (100°F). Hang the bag 3 feet above the floor so that the pressure remains steady, allowing the water to penetrate the deep crevices.

2. Lie on your back; draw knees up and relax the abdomen. Insert the regular 6-inch nozzle at the end of the tube, well-lubricated with Vaseline, into the anal opening. Do not hurry the water into the

colon; pinch the hose if necessary to avoid stomach cramps; discomfort will pass if the water flows in slowly. Massage the stomach area with your hands for 1 or 2 minutes. Get into a squatting position and expel the water and fecal matter.

3. Repeat the above process again with warm water. This time hold the water in for 10 or 15 minutes and pump the stomach in and out several times.

4. Repeat a third time with cold water. This tones the entire bowel area.

If your system is extremely toxic, continue with three enemas per day for a three day period. You can never get all the waste out in one enema or in one day. Afterward, use an enema when you have the flu, colds, sickness, fatigue, or toxemia. It will work wonders for your health and well-being. You may also add lemon juice to your enema bag, or garlic and cayenne, to help cleanse the bowels.

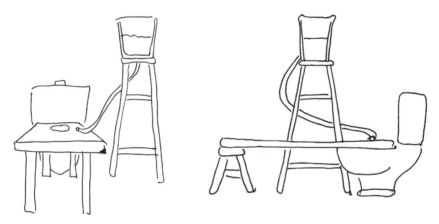

Fig. 9.12. Colonic cleansing equipment for internal bath

Flaxseed Cure for Colon Cleansing

Cook or soak a handful of figs and prunes and blend them thoroughly; make enough to last a few days. Also add enough water to blender to allow for a liquid consistency. To 2 ounces of the fruit, add about 2 or 3 tablespoons of cleansed flaxseed, mixing it thoroughly. Eat this mixture after breakfast and before retiring at night. Flaxseed taken in this manner is tasteless and slides down easily. If the constipation is really stubborn, increase the flaxseed to 6 tablespoons per meal. This is necessary to cleanse the walls of the colon.

Flaxseed is not only lubricating but healing and nourishing as well, as much of the oil is taken by the tissues. To be effective the flaxseed treatment requires drinking enough water so that the seeds can absorb the fluids in the intestines. They swell up and produce a slimy mass that not only cleanses the colon but will in time restore the elasticity of the intestines with the resultant effect of a complete evacuation or bowel movement after each meal. Try this wonderful treatment and watch your health improve.

Use this treatment only to overcome constipation; never remain on it after the condition is corrected. Maintaining a wholesome diet, plus sufficient and proper internal exercises, will give you healthy and regular bowel movements indefinitely.

Banana Diet for Intestinal Disorders

Bananas are one of the best cures for most intestinal diseases. In terms of our personal health, the gastrointestinal tract is the most vital area in the body. Experts in autopsy state they have found that 60 to 80 percent of the colons examined have foreign matter, such as worms, accumulations of old feces-stones, and decaying undigested food residues. The average so-called healthy person of today is continually carrying several pounds of never-eliminated feces. Poor intestinal health can easily lead to serious metabolic and organic complications.

However, do not lose hope; the mighty banana can rescue you from this internal disorder and restore intestinal fortitude. Bananas are an excellent laxative food; they aid the tiny intestinal villi to expel old waste matter; they increase the absorbing surfaces of the entire gastrointestinal tract. In all intestinal disorders the body loses the ability to extract any nutriment from all types of carbohydrate foods, but the mashed pulp of fully ripened (brown speckled) bananas contains powerful digestive enzymes that tremendously alter the internal chemistry of the digestive tract, restoring its ability to digest, absorb, and totally assimilate complex carbohydrates and other food elements.

When feeling bloated, lacking appetite, constipated, fatigued, and cranky, try an exclusive banana eliminative diet for a day or two, or up to a week. Mashed ripe bananas are easier to absorb than a whole banana; they also taste like pudding. Mash them into a creamy pulp with a fork. Eat a bowl of this delicious banana pudding at your regular meal times, or when feeling hungry. Mash three to five bananas per meal, and eat as often as hungry.

For best results, eat no other food during the banana diet, except for pure water. We recommend this for occasional use only as an internal house cleansing. The whipped banana pulp diet feeds and helps to increase billions of friendly intestinal bacteria, or intestinal flora.

Other Laxative and Digestive Aid Foods

Apples: Contain natural bulk, fruit fiber, iron, malic acid, all acting to produce a healthy digestive tract.

Prunes: Rich in iron and potassium; highly laxative and cleansing.

Pineapples: Contain bromelin, an excellent aid in protein digestion and enzyme action; helps to relieve yang constipation.

Pears: Abundant in malic acid and kidney flushing action; beneficial in overcoming congested kidneys and impacted yang colon.

Figs: Highly laxative due to its natural fiber, tiny seeds, and fruit sugars feeding colon germs; high in iron, minerals, and vitamins.

Whole Grains: High in B complex vitamins, bulk (cellulose), and natural laxative qualities; use grains in diet for superior health.

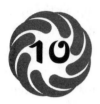

Tao Garden's Healing Meals

Tao Garden Resort and Training Center in northern Thailand is the home of Master Chia and the worldwide headquarters for Universal Healing Tao activities. This integrated wellness, holistic health, and training center is situated on eighty acres surrounded by the beautiful Himalayan foothills near the historic walled city of Chiang Mai. Year-round classes as well as retreats are offered in this serene setting, which includes a health and fitness spa and flower and herb gardens. At Tao Garden the food is grown and prepared in accordance with the suggestions given in this book but also with awareness that we are all at different stages in our journey toward healthful eating. (For instance, limited amounts of meat and sugar are occasionally used.) Before sharing some of Tao Garden's menus and recipes, we will review some of the principles and factors that underlie them.

GENERAL DIETARY PRINCIPLES

The key to good health is to balance our eating habits with our daily work, exercise, and living habits, and thus maintain the body in a constant youthful condition. We learn a thing by constantly doing it. If you constantly cultivate healthy habits, you will reap or create healthy bodies and freedom from disease. The ultimate choice is yours; you can be master of your destiny if you truly understand that your health can be no better than what you eat, assimilate, absorb, and digest, and the effort,

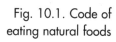

Fig. 10.1. Code of eating natural foods

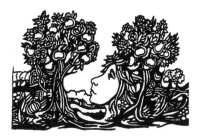

discipline, and value you place on internal and external physical fitness. By daily cultivating the dietary and health principles given in this book for the rest of your life, you can attain excellent health and long life. You will not need to worry about vitamin or mineral deficiencies, malnourishment, calories, or ill-health.

Eating Habit Tips

We all eat too fast: slowly enjoy your meal. Eat normally: not too much, just enough. Eat to fill your stomach halfway and double your life. When you overeat it takes too much energy to digest the food. If your waistband gets tighter with every holiday party, give yourself a ticket for speed eating. It is tempting to blame your aunt's triple chocolate rum balls and that box of sugar cookies in the office coffee room, but a compelling new study suggests that how fast you eat may be as important as what you put on your plate. Researchers already know that speedeaters are twice as likely to be overweight as those who munch in a leisurely fashion. Scarfing down food reduces the release of appetite-regulating hormones into your bloodstream. These chemicals normally tell your brain to get your hand off of those sugar cookies.

In an Athens University study, volunteers who wolfed down two and a half scoops of ice cream in five minutes were compared with another group whose members made the treat last for thirty minutes. The researchers measured blood levels of two types of appetite-lowering hormones, PYY and GLP-1, before and after; they discovered that when people savored their ice cream slowly, the levels of appetite-regulating hormones were 25 to 30 percent higher. PYY and GLP-1 are two of more than a dozen hormones responsible for making us feeling full and satisfied. Other mechanisms, such as stretch receptors in the lining of the stomach, play important roles too.

Fortunately, we know more than ever about how these checks and balances work and how modern food choices and eating habits can short circuit them. There is no better time to help your body's natural appetite-control systems. Begin with a crunch. Filling your stomach with raw veggies will activate stretch receptors that signal your brain that you are full. Studies have found that people who start meals with a large, low-calorie salad eat 12 percent fewer calories during the meal than those who do not.

Dine in the slow lane. Take small bites, chew thoroughly, and put utensils down between bites. Fill your senses by noticing the colors, aromas, flavors, textures, and temperatures of foods before and while you eat them. When you eat till you burst, your stomach feels fuller and fuller for nearly an hour afterward. That is a delayed reaction. Fill your tank only to 80 percent. Wait twenty minutes and you will feel fully satisfied. In Japan, they call this trick *ham hachi bu* and consider it a key to longevity.

Your emotional state is important: eat with joy and happiness in a good environment. Allow four hours between each meal, keeping in mind the following digestion times: fruits, two hours; grains, two to four hours; animal products, four to eight hours. Your first meal should be easy to digest and it should be hot food, as the body is slow to start and it needs to warm up with grain soup or cereal. Keep in mind the following guidelines:

> **Breakfast:** eat like a king (9:00 a.m.–10:00 a.m.)
> **Lunch:** eat like a prince (1:00 p.m.–2:00 p.m.)
> **Dinner:** eat like a pauper (5:00 p.m.–6:00 p.m.)

Do not take liquids with food with the exception of thick soups. Warmth is needed to digest your food, so drink no iced or cold drinks; drink only herbal tea or hot water. Rice (only) soup stops diarrhea. Chinese tea draws oils, fats, and mucus out of the body, but it can hurt the heart. Oranges activate lungs.

Prayer: Chi Charging Your Food

By connecting to Heaven and Earth you will maximize the holistic healing potential for your physical and subtle bodies. To aid your digestion, we recommend that you spend a few minutes placing your hands over your food and sending chi into it. Connect your center to the infinite source of the universe, the Tao. If there is no energy in your tan tien, then there will be no energy to work with. When you are aware of your chi, you can direct heavenly light straight into your food and energize your body. Always perform this sacred chi food practice before each meal and give thanks after.

Cooking

To cook or not to cook, that is the question that has been hotly debated by health food fans for many years. It is true that some articles of food can be eaten without preparation or cooking with full benefits of health and nourishment, that is, most fruits and some vegetables, such as cucumbers, all germinated seeds and nuts, green peppers, celery, and other tender juicy greens. Fruits eaten raw in season can be absorbed and digested easily, but they cannot sustain the body in superior health exclusively. Since cold weather is extremely yin upon the body, properly cooked natural foods are a physiological necessity to keep the body warm and in yin and yang balance. This is the law of nature. We need more cooked yang food in winter and much less in summer. If we try to deny our physiological requirements by consuming either raw or cooked food exclusively, the body will not function efficiently and in good health.

Heat energizes food. It has been argued that all wild animals take their food raw. This is true. However, they have digestive systems adapted to digest tough raw vegetables. The human system cannot possibly assimilate and digest raw legumes, grains, and root vegetables. Raw starch is indigestible; the starch molecule must be broken down by the use of fire so that we can absorb the food value. Fire is one of the five elements of nature. Fire is what separates human from beast. Without fire, we would still be like the animals in a wild or primitive state: no advancement, no civilization, no evolution, no great intelligence, no art, no culture, no mental and spiritual upward movement. Humankind was given the knowledge of the use of fire to advance and to populate the globe, including the cold northern regions. To accomplish this task, fire was a necessity to keep warm, survive, and grow.

It is true that cooking has been abused in modern times, but this does not mean that proper cooking is bad; it is good. Because water drowns people is no reason to stop drinking it; because fire can burn and destroy life and property is no reason to not use it to heat the house or cook food. In general, foods that are palatable raw should be eaten in that form. Other foods not suitable to the human stomach in a raw state are better cooked and thus more readily acted upon by the digestive juices of the stomach.

Cooking Tips

1. Cook with a loving heart.
2. Plan meals not only for nutritional content but also aesthetic interest. Blend and harmonize colors, textures, and flavors.
3. How vegetables are cut determines how they are cooked: for steaming, chop food in bigger pieces; for stir fry, chop in thinner pieces.
4. Combining certain foods while cooking brings out food flavors.
5. Use pure vegetable oil (corn, safflower, or soy) in cooking or salads; no more than 3 teaspoons/day. Olive oil is too heavy for cooking but is good for salads.
6. Cooking heat sources: charcoal results in juicy food; gas results in neutral food; electric results in dry food.
7. Use your sense of smell to determine correct timing for adding foods and completion.

ULTIMATE SUPER DIET

The kind of food you eat is even more important to your existence than the kind of air you breathe. More good health or ill health can be traced directly to food than to any other of the outside factors surrounding your existence. The consensus of worldwide research and observation indicates that the ideal diet for humankind should consist of foods that are high in natural carbohydrates and low in animal protein, especially meat.

This diet consists of the following foods and nutritional elements: seeds, nuts, and grains, which contain fat-lowering and energy-building elements, high-quality B complex vitamin factors, vitamin E, natural fatty acids, lecithin, phosphorus, iron, magnesium, zinc, proteins; fresh fruits and vegetables, especially berries, sub-acid and sweet fruit fresh squeezed vegetable and fruit juices. These foods contain a super abundance of essential organic vitalizing vitamins, minerals, trace minerals, enzymes, alkaline cleansing, purifying, and blood enriching elements.

Golden Nuggets of Nutrition

SEEDS	NUTS	GRAINS	LEGUMES
Sunflower	Almonds	Buckwheat	Peanuts
Sesame	Walnuts	Rice, corn	Soybeans, peas
Pumpkin	Pecans	Millet, oats	Adzuki, garbanzo
Alfalfa	Filberts	Wheat	Black beans
Chia	Cashews	Barley	Lima beans
Flaxseed	Pine nuts	Rye	Pinto beans

This ultimate super diet may be supplemented with moderate use of the natural protective foods: yogurt, buttermilk, whey, nutritional yeast, kefir, sea kelp, alfalfa liquid, brown rice polishings, and soybean powder with enzymes.

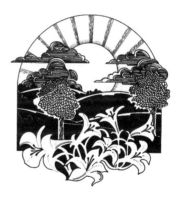

Fig. 10.2. It is better to light one candle (light of the sun) than to curse the darkness. There is not enough darkness in the world to put out the light of one candle; nor is there enough ignorance or wrongdoing on earth to submerge what is corrected (The Way of the Tao).

Grains Are Nourishing and Strengthening

Natural whole grains are excellent sources of B vitamins and contain six of eight essential amino acids. The other two amino acids can be supplied by adding seeds, nuts, vegetables, or legumes to grain meals; together they form nutritionally complete proteins. Grains are high in sodium, a yang element, and phosphorus, an important mineral for proper brain functioning. Grains are heat producers and impart sustaining energy.

For example, two slices of whole grain bread, well chewed, will impart more energy and working power to the body than 2 pounds of steak.

European centenarians are known to work all day in the fields on a bowl of vegetable soup, raw fruit, and a few slices of dark whole grain bread. The hard working, enduring Chinese consume whole rice and seaweeds as their energy- and strength-sustaining foods. The Turkish people are extremely hardy and robust and eat grains, sesame seeds, dates, and raw camel or goat milk. The strong Russians use buckwheat and millet. The Mexicans use corn and beans. The lactovegetarian Bulgarian diet includes whole grains (mainly barley), sunflower seeds, honey, sauerkraut, fresh fruits, and vegetables.

Grains are high in natural carbohydrates and should be used mostly during the cold winter months for heat and body energy. They should be used in smaller quantities in warm weather. Warm weather is yang, and the body needs more fresh fruits and vegetables to maintain its fluids in proper yin/yang balance. In addition to being cooked, grains can be sprouted or used in making bread.

Rice

Brown rice is an easily digestible starch, good for weak constitutions and for building overall good health. Rice, and all other grains, should be chewed very well, from 30 to 50 times each mouthful; this will ensure perfect digestion and assimilation. Rice can correct conditions of diarrhea and constipation, due to its balanced qualities. A regular diet of rice can lower blood pressure and help arteriosclerosis. Due to its high amount of B complex, rice calms the nerves and brain. Brown rice contains phytic acid, which eliminates toxins and poisons from the body; rice also helps to overcome allergies. There are two types of brown rice: long grain and short grain. Long grain rice is a summer food; short grain rice is more yang and imparts more heat energy for the cold weather.

Oats

Oats, flaked or rolled, are good in cereals, soups, breads, and cookies. They are high in fat and are valuable in cases of underactive thyroid and overweight conditions. They have been used with success to combat sterility and sexual impotence. Oats are high in silicon, a mineral element that fosters a healthy complexion, shiny hair, strong nails, and sparkling eyes. Diabetics can become stronger and healthier with the regular use of oats in the diet. Oats help to eliminate stored protein and toxic wastes from the body. Lungs and large intestines are most benefited by oats and rice. Oatmeal or steel cut oats are best eaten in the winter and late fall.

Millet

Millet is rich in phosphorus, magnesium, iron, silicon, fluorine, manganese, vitamin A, and B complex, making it excellent for all nervous conditions and mental fatigue. It is a good source of protein. Millet has been used to help prevent miscarriages and correct deficiencies in pregnant women. Millet's nut-like flavor makes a delicious and nutritious meal. It is the most alkaline of all grains, therefore it aids conditions of toxemia and acidosis. The spleen is the organ most benefited by millet, as is the stomach. Yellow millet aids digestive problems and can help repair the gastrointestinal system. It should be used mostly in the fall or Indian summer. Red millet is more yin and is a summer grain.

Rye

Rye helps improve the circulation and clean the blood vessels, therefore helping arteriosclerosis. Rye helps strengthen and tones muscles and imparts high energy and endurance. It is very low in gluten. Rye strengthens and purifies the liver and gallbladder. Rye is a hearty grain used by many European cultures. Rye is used to make bread or as a cooked cereal. Rye is a spring food.

Buckwheat

Buckwheat is rich in minerals and vitamins, especially C and E. It is the most yang grain, high in protein. In fact, buckwheat has the highest amount of protein of all grains: 12 to 16 percent. The amino acid lysine is very high in buckwheat, giving it the same high biological value and nutritive quality as the protein found in animal food. The darker the buckwheat, the more protein it contains. Its magnesium helps to calm, relax, cleanse, and balance the nutrients in the blood. Buckwheat also contains a large amount of manganese, a mineral generally deficient in many people, which is necessary for muscle control, growth, metabolism, and the reproductive system. Manganese strengthens the nerves and muscles and helps build good posture and courage to carry on the responsibilities of life. Buckwheat is rich in rutin, one of the bioflavonoids, which is vital in reducing capillary fragility and maintaining sound blood vessels. Buckwheat helps to overcome environmental radiation poisoning and fallout.

Buckwheat should be used mostly in winter, as it imparts high energy and heat. The kidneys and bladder are most benefited by buckwheat. It can be used in noodles, cereals, casseroles, loafs, and takes the place of meat products. Buckwheat is also a good blood builder and helps to overcome anemia.

Corn

Corn builds the blood and imparts high energy; it is high in natural complex carbohydrates. Corn is very rich in calcium and vitamins B, C, A, and F. Corn oil contains vitamins F and E. Corn builds strong bones, teeth, and muscles. Corn aids conditions of underweight and overactive thyroid; it slows down the metabolism. It is beneficial for the heart and small intestines. Our ancestors thrived and survived on corn. The early Native Americans and Mayans cultivated corn for centuries. They built great civilizations, and their people were robust and long-lived. Corn can be eaten on the cob or made into corn bread and soups. It imparts good vitality, aids digestion, and builds rich red blood. Corn is the sweetest of all grains, and it is converted into sugar within the system very quickly, giving quick energy and endurance. It is the most yin grain and should be used mostly in summer.

Barley

Barley is used by many cultures around the world. It imparts much heat and energy and gives strength and endurance. It contains vitamins B_1 and B_2. Barley is beneficial for the lungs and large intestines. Barley is very easy to digest and is good for those with weak digestive systems, making it valuable in conditions of underweight, stomach ulcers, and diarrhea. It can be mixed with vegetables, used for bread making, and is excellent for soups; it is also used in making barley miso, which is not as yang as soybean miso. It is also used as a poultice for skin diseases and burns. Barley is a fall food.

Wheat

Wheat contains the highest vitamin and mineral content of all grains. Wheat is high in protein and gluten. The bran in wheat imparts good digestion and elimination. The germ in wheat contains a rich source of vitamin E, which builds a strong reproductive system, improves endurance, and aids heart functioning. It is also beneficial to the liver and gallbladder. Poorly masticated wheat can cause indigestion, mucus, allergies, and poor health. Chew and salivate all grains very well, and watch your health improve and allergies vanish like magic. Wheat is used in bread, cereals, sprouting, noodles, pancakes, bulgur, and couscous.

The gluten in wheat will not cause allergies if the liver, kidneys, and eliminative channels are kept clean and free of toxic wastes. Many times allergies are caused not by wheat alone but by a system filled with milk, cheese, fats, and sugars. The gluten may react allergically in a body that is weakened by high-fat and high-sugar foods. Wheat has been used by all great civilizations and cultures throughout history. Allergies are unknown in wheat-eating cultures where there is no milk, sugar, and fatty food. Experiment on yourself; discontinue all fatty, oily, and sugared products, including dried fruit and tropical fruit, for several weeks. Then eat whole wheat for a few days, and observe the reaction in your body.

Legumes

Legumes take in the whole bean family, including peanuts, peas, split peas, and lentils. Legumes consist of both protein and starch. They are considered complex carbohydrates and are rich in vitamins and minerals, especially the B complex vitamins. All legumes should be eaten moderately more in winter than in summer. When cooking all beans, use about 3 cups of water to 1 cup of beans.

Adzuki Beans

Adzuki beans are good for general use and are used successfully in kidney disorders.

Black Beans

Black beans aid kidney functioning and sexual disorders, such as menstrual difficulties, frigidity, barrenness, low sex drive. Black bean juice (the liquid left over after cooking the beans; use 1 or 2 extra cups of water when you wish to make any bean juice) can be used for throat disorders such as laryngitis and hoarseness. Black turtle beans are excellent in soups and combined with rice or buckwheat.

String Beans

These beans are more like vegetables, but they contain more protein. They should be eaten in warm summer months, in season when available. They are good for constipation, rheumatism, acidosis, bladder, and kidney disorders. They are low in protein and rich in vitamins A, B_1, C, and B_2.

Soybeans

Soybeans and their products are high in protein. However, we generally recommend against eating soybeans regularly, as they contain substances that are difficult to assimilate, which have an adverse effect on the thyroid gland. Tofu, a soybean cheese, can be used occasionally. Miso and tamari sauce are made from soybeans and can be used more often during winter months for body warmth. These products are high in vitamin B_{12} and iron. They also help the body fight off the harmful effects of environmental radiation and fallout. They are beneficial to the thyroid gland.

Green Peas

Green (split) peas are good for the stomach and lungs. They contain many valuable vitamins and minerals. Green peas are highly nourishing and strengthening. They aid conditions of anemia, emaciation, and low blood pressure. They contain vitamins A, B_1, B_2, B_6, and nicotinic acid. They are good with most grain dishes and salads. Yellow split peas are excellent for all digestive disorders and are very easy to assimilate. They can be used at all times of the year for warmth and energy. Lentils have similar properties as split peas and cook the same way. They are all good sources of protein. Dried peas can be cooked without soaking overnight, in sixty to ninety minutes on the stove; in thirty minutes if pressure-cooked.

White Beans

White beans aid in discharging excess toxicity from the heart. They are a good all-around bean to eat with grains and vegetables.

Garbanzo Beans

These beans, also called chickpeas, are a good source of protein. They are used in many cultures around the world, including Greece, the Near East, and in most American restaurant salad bars. Chickpeas can be eaten in soups, salads, loafs, sauces, and dressings. They have a rich flavorful taste and are highly nourishing.

Pinto Beans

Pinto beans contain the highest RNA and DNA factors of almost all foods, except sardines. They have been used in the south and Mexico for many years, and they are usually combined with corn bread and other corn recipes. Pinto beans are also high in protein, vitamins, and minerals.

Kidney Beans

Shaped like the human kidney, these beans are said to strengthen the kidneys. They are rich in protein and are very warming and nourishing to the body. They can be used in salads, casseroles, and other grain dishes.

Lima and Butter Beans

These beans are very strengthening and building and can help to overcome emaciation and malnutrition. They are good sources of protein and iron and are easily digested and assimilated. They are good for anemia and weak digestive systems. They contain vitamins B_6, B_1, and B_2. Lima beans aid the discharge of toxins from the liver and build strength in that organ. They are good in casseroles, grain, and cooked vegetable dishes.

Germinated Seed and Nuts

Germinated seeds and nuts are alive with life; they have the power to grow and to create new life. And they can create a rebirth in your own body if used regularly. Three-thousand-year-old seeds found in Tutankhamen's tomb have been put in the soil and have grown. When two-hundred-year-old sunflower seeds found in old missions have been planted, they have grown. The seed is the element that contains the birth of a tree or a plant: the birth of fruits and vegetables. In the seed of the tree we have the pattern for the bark, the sap, the flowers, the fruit, and the full unfolding of the tree.

Seeds contain nearly every single food element that has been discovered and doubtless all the additional factors not yet identified. No other one food is so rich in nutrients, as the seed contains all the life forces needed to build a new generation. Seeds also have highly potent therapeutic values. They are one of the most potent sources of unsaturated fatty acids needed to maintain youthful and elastic arterial conditions.

Seeds and nuts are high in calcium, vitamin E, phosphorus, niacin, lecithin, fatty acids, iron, natural oils, and high-quality protein. The king of all nuts is the almond. Sunflower and sesame seeds are the queens of all seeds. Pumpkin seeds contain zinc, a hard-to-get mineral necessary for proper prostate functioning. Seeds are rich in vitamin A, B complex, and magnesium. Germinated seed and nut milks are an excellent substitute for regular milk and contain complete proteins of a superior biological value, capable of sustaining life in perfect health indefinitely.

Although seeds and nuts are full of essential nutrients for the body, mentioning them can generate the following kinds of reactions: "They make me constipated. They cause skin problems. They are indigestible." Yes, when seeds and nuts are eaten in the conventional way they can cause these problems. If they are eaten after a heavy meal, snacked on between meals, poorly chewed, ungerminated, salted, oiled, and preserved with chemicals, they can cause much harm to the liver and intestines. Seeds and nuts are very concentrated, so they must be eaten in small quantities.

Seeds and nuts are quite difficult to digest for most people, which means they pass through the body unassimilated. That is why we recommend soaking the seeds or nuts overnight in water or juice to maintain the protein elements that are needed for the daily acid/alkaline balance. The longer you sprout a seed or nut, the more alkaline it becomes and the less acid-reacting qualities it will have. Three- to seven-day-old sprouts are excellent alkaline foods, but they should be balanced with one-day-old soaked seeds or nuts.

Soaking and sprouting seeds and nuts makes them very easy to digest and assimilate. This method also converts them into complete protein, allowing the body to utilize up to 100 percent nutrition as a result. Unsoaked or ungerminated seeds and nuts contain only 20 to 30 percent nutrition: the rest being waste products, causing indigestion and cravings for junk food. Humans cannot derive complete nutrition from dried seeds and nuts. Undigested protein from these foods creates toxemia, which can cause the following conditions in time: falling hair, poor eyesight, anemia, diabetes, and weakness. They can become as disease-producing as devitalized foods, due to their indigestibility and poor assimilation.

If we could pick nuts and seeds right from the tree and eat them on the spot, there would be no need to soak them because the necessary moisture and life force would still be intact. In the dried state the life force is lying dormant; these foods require soaking to wake up the life force within them. The life force within the seed or nut is tremendously increased. Since we are living in an unnatural society and environment, we have to resort to these methods, which are in no way contrary to natural law. Also, as these foods were already tampered with through the process of early picking and storing, we are merely replacing the natural moisture that was taken out. We are simply bringing out their finer qualities and not detracting one iota from the health value.

Dr. Edward Howell, research biochemist in the field of nutrition and enzymes, states that any ungerminated raw seeds or nuts contain enzyme inhibitors. These inhibitors are necessary for the protection of the seed, to keep it from germinating prematurely and dying. As a result, raw seeds and nuts actually neutralize some of the enzymes our body produces. In fact, Howell states, eating foods with enzyme inhibitors causes a swelling of the pancreas. Raw peanuts and egg whites contain the most enzyme inhibitors. Most fruits and vegetables do not contain enzyme inhibitors; they are rich sources of living enzymes. Sprouting and germinating seeds and nuts destroys the enzyme inhibitors and also increases the enzyme content from a factor of three to six.

Germinating Seeds and Nuts

You can sprout anything that will grow from a seed. Try sunflower, pumpkin, and sesame seeds, almonds, filberts, pine nuts, walnuts, and pecans.

1. Make sure that you hull these seeds and nuts before soaking them. The seeds need only be soaked overnight. The heavier nuts can be soaked up to 24 hours for better assimilation and nutrition.

2. If you are planning to sprout seeds and nuts for a longer time, use a sprouting dish or a jar with a screen on the lid. Wash them with water 2 or 3 times a day; let the water drain over the sink, and in 3 to 6 days you will have some nutritious and delicious sprouts. The last day of sprouting, place the sprouts on the window ledge and the sprouts will turn green.

 ## Germinated and Blended Seed/Nut Milk

Seeds and nuts that have been soaked overnight become much easier to digest and assimilate when they are combined with sub-acid fruits. No more than 2 or 3 ounces should be eaten.

1. Soak seeds or nuts overnight in fruit juice or water, and the next morning or afternoon make a blended nut milk.
2. Add berries and juice along with 1 teaspoon of vegetarian protein powder; blend together and you will have a meal of total and complete nutrition.

After a few weeks on these super-nutritious foods, your complexion will glow and your blood count will rise. As health culturists, let us look the part, so that we may be an inspiration to everyone we meet. Remember, the proof is in the doing.

 ## Sprouts: Wonder Food

Sprouts are truly a miracle food. They are an excellent source of vitamins A, B complex, C, D, E, G, K, and U. Dr. Pauline Berry Mack, at the University of Pennsylvania, found that soybean sprouts grown for seventy-two hours contain more vitamin C than six glasses of orange juice. Sprouts also contain all eight amino acids that make up protein. To sprout legumes and grains (wheatgrass, lentils, mung beans, and alfalfa seeds), use the same technique as sprouting nuts and seeds.

1. The simplest container is a mason jar, with a wire mesh or cheese-cloth substituted for the lid. Place this in a large bowl since the jar should be at a forty-five degree angle to assure proper drainage.

2. Soak the seeds overnight in a warm dark place in about three times as much water as you have seeds. The water should be warm (70–80°F) and free of chlorine and fluorine, which can sterilize the tender embryo.

3. Pour the water off and rinse well to prevent mold. This water is excellent for juices and stock. Place the seeds in a warm, moist, dark container. Flush every 4 to 6 hours with water to clean them and assure adequate growth. Be certain the seeds drain well because they will sour and rot if you do not.

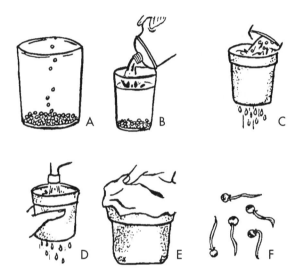

Fig. 10.3. Sprouting seeds for an individual portion

A. Put a ¼-inch layer of seeds in a water glass.

B. Fill glass about ¾ full of distilled water (do not use tap water). Let this soaking take at least 6 hours, or if done just before going to bed, let stand overnight in a warm place.

C. Pour contents of glass into a small flower pot that has small holes in the bottom. If it is a pot with one large hole, put cheesecloth or wire mesh over the hole.

D. Rinse seeds in flower pot thoroughly under running water.

E. Cover seeds with wet cheesecloth, or Turkish toweling. Repeat rinsing of seeds three times a day (step 4), replacing moist cloth over seeds.

F. Sprouts should look like this on the third day and be ready to eat.

4. In 3 to 6 days, depending on the temperature (80–90° is best) and seed variety, your seeds will have doubled or tripled and be ready for consumption. Sprouts reach their highest vitamin peak 60 to 80 hours after germinating.

5. If you expose your sprouts to indirect sunlight during the final several hours of growth, they will develop chlorophyll. The chlorophyll molecule is very similar to that of hemoglobin, and it consequently acts as a blood booster; the only difference between the two is that chlorophyll has magnesium at the center, while hemoglobin has iron.

Fruits for Beauty, Health, and Longevity

In a mysterious way the bioelectric forces of Earth, combined with the biomagnetic forces of the sun and atmosphere, produce fresh, ripe, blood-building fruit. Fresh wholesome fruit, taken in season and in moderation, provides the body with vital alkaline vitamins and minerals, the living building blocks so necessary for healthful robust living.

Living fruit, kissed by the basking rays of the energizing sun, absorbing drafts of magnetized air, attracting to itself all the vital elements necessary for its perfection, is a cosmic miracle, an electrochemical laboratory of nature (the Tao). Scientists can put all the chemicals of an apple into a chemist's dish, but they cannot construct an apple. They may probe and analyze all the elements of a cherry, but they are dumbfounded to know what makes them red. They may take apart and attempt to reconstruct a plum, and they will find that the plum will help support life, but the broken down chemicals do not. Fruit contains essential bioelectric principles, yin and alkaline elements, which, when eaten in addition to a well-rounded, balanced diet, will give the electric spark of life and vital health force.

Chlorophyll is not only found in the green element of vegetables but also in all fruits kissed by the sun. Fruits are also very abundant in organic vitamins, mineral salts, and purified distilled water, and they are refreshing and healthful. They are high in natural sugars and fruit acids. Most fresh fruits contain about 90 percent water, 10 percent carbohydrates, and less than 1½ percent protein. Fruit is more likely to be free from strontium 90 radiation fallout than other food grown close to the ground. A large fruit orchard will produce more than 100 times more pounds of fruit than meat in the same acreage.

Whose mouth does not water on seeing a luscious peach, cherry, or melon when hungry? The sight, aroma, and taste of fruit bring on an abundant secretion of digestive juices, making fruit very digestible on an empty stomach. Fruits are cooling and refreshing to the body because of their high water and organic acid content. A total fruit or eliminative diet can be used for a short period of time as a remedy to balance yang kidneys, liver, colon, and intestines.

Otherwise, use fruit in season and grown locally. Eat more fresh raw fruits in hot summer months when they are abundant; less in cold weather when they are not in season and less abundant. Apples or pears can be baked or steamed in the winter for warmth and variety. Fresh berries head the list as being the best of all blood-builders, containing a rich source of iron and vitamin B_{12}. Melons are a rich source of minerals and vitamins, but they should be eaten only in small quantities, especially in the case of expanded (yin) kidneys.

Fruits contain citric acid, malic acid, and tartaric acid. Citric acid is found in all citrus fruits and in other fruits such as cherries, currants, berries, pomegranates, and tomatoes. Malic acid is found mostly in pears, plums, apples, pineapples, and cherries. Grapes contain tartaric acid. Oxalic acid is found in small amounts in most fruits, but cranberries, spinach, and most greens are high in it.

Types of Fruit

BERRIES	MELONS	SEASONAL FRUITS	TROPICAL FRUITS
Blueberries	Watermelon	Cherries	Oranges
Blackberries	Cantaloupe	Grapes	Grapefruit
Strawberries	Honeydew	Apples, Figs	Tangerine
Raspberries	Casaba	Pears, Raisins	Pineapple
Huckleberries	Persian	Peaches	Mango
Gooseberries	Crenshaw	Apricots	Papaya
Elderberries		Plums	Lemons
Loganberries		Nectarines	Limes, Avocado
Boysenberries		Persimmons	Bananas, Dates

Sweet fruits are especially valuable for their delightful sugars, so easily digested (sometimes almost predigested), which sustain the body with so little energy expenditure for digestion. Fruits are easy to assimilate; if

Fig. 10.4. Seasonal fruits at Tao Garden

eaten moderately they do not overwork the pancreas, as do pastries, fats, and sugar products. Ripe fruit, in moderation, does not cause acid or toxic conditions in the body, nor does it cause diabetes or other diseases when used judiciously. In healthy people, fruits are alkaline in reaction in urine tests. All ripe fruits are alkaline-reacting within the system. These alkalines neutralize the acid poisons, uric acid, and acidosis, which usually come from a high-protein meat diet.

However, be advised that an excess of fruit will overalkalize the body and blood, and cause yin diseases such as hypoglycemia and diarrhea. Overeating of fruit, especially the citrus variety, will saturate the body with citric acid, which can cause serious calcium loss, mineral depletion, and an unbalanced blood chemistry resulting in yin arthritis, stiff joints, tooth decay, nervousness, nerve diseases, and toxic acidity. Sub-acid or acid fruits may aggravate a system that is already highly toxic or acidic; they will stir up the internal acids and cause pain or discomfort. Acid and yang conditions can benefit from the use of nonacid fruit, such as all melons, and neutral vegetables and their juices.

Fruits, especially cherries, grapes, prunes, figs, berries, and lemons, can help you overcome yang constipation. The acids of fruits increase the secretions of the intestines, move the bowels, and increase their peristaltic action. Fruit meets the bodily need for natural bulk and intestinal health. Since fruits are yin, overeating them can easily cause yin constipation (expanded colon and intestines). In this condition, eat less fruit, and increase consumption of cooked grains, vegetables, miso, and tamari, for a natural balance and healthy colon.

Most fruits contain phosphates and alkalines, together with acids,

Fig. 10.5. Seasonal melons

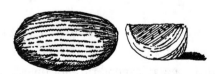

which increase the solubility of the blood, causing it to flow through the system more readily. A balanced diet, including fruit, so purifies the blood that even the craving for alcoholic drinks has been known to disappear. When the blood is purified and its pure nutrient stream bathes the cells and tissues, it will remove wastes, impurities, and dead cells, and leave behind strong healthy tissues. In time, an alcoholic can be completely purified and cleansed, and back in his or her right mind. Alcohol will then be repugnant after the cleansing period.

Eat Fruit Alone

Fruits should be eaten on an empty stomach and not as a dessert, after the appetite is satisfied and the digestion is already sufficiently taxed. Fruit taken in the morning, before the fast of the night has been broken, is very refreshing. In addition to its nutritive qualities, it serves as a stimulus to the digestive organs. Berries, cherries, melons, tropical fruits, apples, or pears are all excellent at this time. Fruit is best eaten half an hour before protein or starch meals.

To be most valuable, fruit should be ripe, sound, fresh, and of superb quality in every way, and it should be eaten raw or baked. If you live in the sub-tropics, you can pick and enjoy fruit directly from the trees almost all year long. Northerners will find apples, pears, peaches, and plums most enjoyable during the summer and winter months.

Many people believe that fruit does not agree with them. In such cases, the trouble may be traced to the abuse and misuse of the fruit or because of digestive weakness due to previous poor eating habits. Combined properly, fruits will not cause problems. Fruits eaten with starch or other junk foods will cause fermentation. Fruits eaten moderately and by themselves are easily digested.

Vegetables: Rich in Chlorophyll

Chlorophyll, as found in fruits and greens, is necessary for the health and well-being of all living creatures on this planet. The human system requires green chlorophyll for proper blood formation, which builds healthy cells and tissues. Vegetables, especially the nonstarchy greens, contain the greatest amount of blood-building chlorophyll and rank high as health builders and superior bowel regulators. Chlorophyll is composed of a combination of tiny molecules of a substance called pyrrole. These pyrroles are the building blocks of the animal blood pigment, hematin or hemoglobin. The pyrroles in plant chlorophyll are tied together by an atom of magnesium, whereas in human blood the mineral bond of these pyrroles is iron.

The color green, according to the ancient art of color therapy, is a healing agent and bone mender. Green vegetables are excellent sources of vitamins A, B_1, B_2, C, K, and E, as well as an abundance of organic mineral salts, alkaline elements, trace minerals, and enzymes. About 20 to 30 percent of the daily diet should consist of raw and cooked vegetables.

All raw vegetable greens can be easily utilized and assimilated by the system when they are juiced and consumed immediately. The rich green chlorophyll in vegetable juices is easily absorbed into the system within a matter of minutes. However, use juices moderately at all times. Eat small raw salads in warm weather and cooked vegetables in cold weather. A word of caution: consuming large salads daily will overwork the liver and stomach, causing digestive disorders. Too many raw vegetables will cause expansion (yin) conditions within the body. The best raw vegetables for salad-making are the tender juicy varieties such as alfalfa and mung sprouts, cucumbers, green and red sweet peppers, onions, radishes, celery, Romaine, Bibb, and Boston lettuces. Coarse, tough vegetables should not be used.

Root vegetables, cabbage, beans, peas, and squash should all be cooked for proper assimilation. Hardly a person exists that can properly digest and assimilate these foods without the aid of fire to soften the cellulose and tough fibers, substances that are indigestible for humans, and which are not acted upon by the digestive fluids, unless softened by heat. You can make delicious vegetable broth soups, steam a variety of starchy and mildly starchy vegetables such as potatoes, pumpkin, beets, carrots, broccoli, celery, and cabbage, or cook with grains such as brown rice, buckwheat, millet, or oats. Steam and cook your vegetables and grains in a stainless steel pressure cooker, steamer, or waterless cooker over a very low flame. This will ensure that the goodness and freshness of the cooked food remains intact when you serve it at the table.

Cultured Dairy Products

The long-lived Russians, Europeans, and Bulgarians believe strongly in the use of cultured dairy foods. Scientists have found that cultured dairy products help to increase the beneficial and friendly bacterial flora in the intestines, maintaining their cleanliness and health. Soured acidophilus milk rejuvenates the intestinal tract, improves digestive problems, and relieves constipation.

Those who want to use dairy food without the harmful effects of high-fat milk and cheese can consume the following low-fat dairy products in moderation: buttermilk, low-fat yogurt, cottage cheese, and skim milk. These products (except for low-fat cottage cheese, which is more yang) are not extreme yin or yang but are more neutral. Yogurt, which began its rise to fame many years ago in European countries, suddenly has become a super food of the world. It contains high-quality and easily digestible proteins, vitamins (including D and B_{12}), minerals, and enzymes. Because it flourishes with friendly bacteria it is almost a predigested food, quickly absorbed and assimilated into the bloodstream.

The sparing use of low-fat dairy products can add variety and nourishment to your natural food diet. However, that milk was originally intended for infants only. Use wise judgment in the dietary use of this food. Cultured dairy food should be used very sparingly in cold weather and moderately in warm weather.

FIVE ELEMENTS AND FOOD

As we have seen (in chapter 6), in five-element nutrition different flavors have different energetic effects and are used to balance each element.

> *Sweet:* this is actually the central flavor of the diet, which is full of sweet foods such as whole grains, beans, and root vegetables. The empty sweet flavor of sugars, honey, and fruit should be used more cautiously.
>
> *Pungent:* this flavor helps expel fluids and pathogens from the body. Thus, it is good to use this flavor when getting a cold or flu, and also to clear mucus and heat. Warming pungents are ginger, cayenne, and pepper. Cooling pungents include peppermint and radish.

Salty: this flavor is grounding. It can be used when we feel high or scattered, such as overexcited or having difficulty concentrating. Salty foods include sea salt, miso, and seaweed.

Sour: this flavor draws energy inward and so can be used wherever there is abnormal fluid leakage or prolapsed organs. Sour food includes lemons, limes, and pickles.

Bitter: this is the most cooling flavor and is excellent when there is body heat or fever. Many herbs used for fevers are extremely bitter indeed. Bitter foods include endive, alfalfa, bitter melon, and rye.

These principles of five-element nutrition have been incorporated into Tao Garden's kitchen. We grow as much food as possible on site in our organic gardens. In this way, we can preserve the chi of the food. Much chi is lost through storage and transportation of foods over long distances. In addition, many fruits are picked before they have been ripened by the sun, so that they do not rot before they reach the supermarket shelves. At Tao Garden we allow the fruit to ripen naturally in the sun and it is harvested only when it is ready for eating. Some of the food served at Tao Garden will have been picked only hours previously. This is called "living food," as its life-force energy is flourishing.

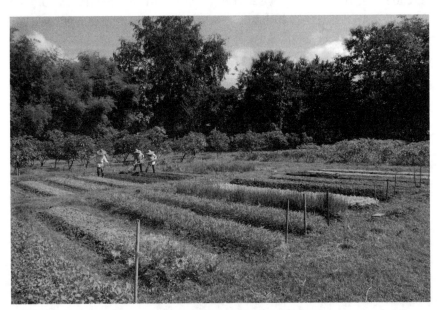

Fig. 10.6. Tao Garden's organic gardens

Balancing the five elements can become extremely complex. However, there is a lot you can do with careful choice of food to rebalance your own organs and health. First, look at the different internal and external climates and the foods that are beneficial:

Condition: Too windy
Season: Spring
Symptoms: Moving pains, wind, spasms, dizziness
Foods to Aid: Oats and pine nuts; chamomile tea, ginger, and fennel; fresh greens and salads bring a spring cleanse

Condition: Too hot
Season: Summer
Symptoms: Feeling hot, flushed skin
Foods to Aid: Raw foods, fruit, cooling herbs (mint); light eating

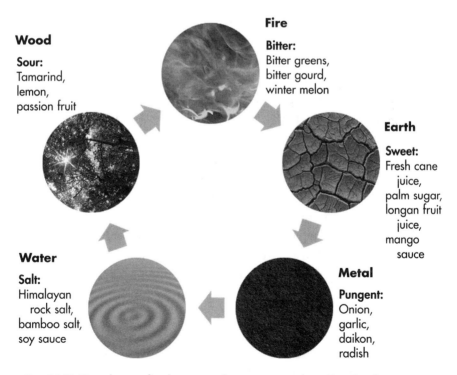

Wood

Sour:
Tamarind,
lemon,
passion fruit

Fire

Bitter:
Bitter greens,
bitter gourd,
winter melon

Earth

Sweet:
Fresh cane
   juice,
palm sugar,
longan fruit
   juice,
mango
   sauce

Water

Salt:
Himalayan
   rock salt,
bamboo salt,
soy sauce

Metal

Pungent:
Onion,
garlic,
daikon,
radish

Fig. 10.7. Five-element food tastes in the creation cycle at Tao Garden

Condition: Too dry
Season: Autumn
Symptoms: Dry skin, thirst, constipation
Foods to Aid: Soy products, nuts, seeds, dairy, psyllium, malva nuts, flaxseed tea

Condition: Too cold
Season: Winter
Symptoms: Feeling colder than people around you
Foods to Aid: Soups, casseroles, warming spices, ginger; warmth-building foods

Condition: Too damp
Season: Rainy season/ seasonal changes
Symptoms: Having too much mucus or phlegm
Foods to Aid: Avoid dairy and cold foods; mung beans, adzuki beans, garlic, pumpkin, to reduce damp

HEALTHY MENU PLANNING

It is very difficult to set down a specific dietary eating program for all persons under varying conditions on a daily basis. Menu plans need to be flexible and adaptable to meet individual needs and requirements. Each of us must use supreme judgment in choosing foods, recipes, and menus to fit our own personal and environmental needs. We have to devise our own pattern of how to eat, when to eat, where to eat, and what to eat. For example, people working physically hard outdoors all day long may require a more substantial breakfast to meet their energy demands. People not working as hard will require less food and calories.

The main thing to remember is to eat only when hungry in the morning and throughout the day. Keep in mind, however, that soon after waking the body is not fully awake and ready to absorb and assimilate a heavy meal. The ancient Taoists recommended that we eat more food at breakfast in cold winter weather and less food in the evening during warm summer months.

The suggested menus shared here should not be understood as a strict cut-and-dried calculation. Use them as approximations of what to eat, which should be adjusted according to climate, locality, and daily body requirements. Study the diets of various countries around the world. Many nations with a history of longevity and good health have a national staple based on legume and grain combinations, which are easily included in a vegetarian or transition diet.

Adjustments can also be made for people on special diets or with severe digestive disorders, such as blending salads or pureeing fruits and nut and seed milks. Weak digestive systems need much help, and they can greatly benefit from the use of blenders, juicers, and mixers. These life-saving dietary measures can be used whenever necessary.

Breakfast

At Tao Garden we strive to make breakfast the best start to the day. From 7 a.m. to 9 a.m. the stomach is active, and from 9 a.m. to 11 a.m. the spleen and pancreas. These are the main organs involved in digestion and in balancing blood sugar. If the wrong food is taken at this time, digestion becomes sluggish and blood-sugar levels may begin to rise and fall too fast, leading to crashing energy levels.

If your digestion is weak, choose warm foods for breakfast. If you are cleansing, choose fruit. Make or buy breads with whole grain flours.

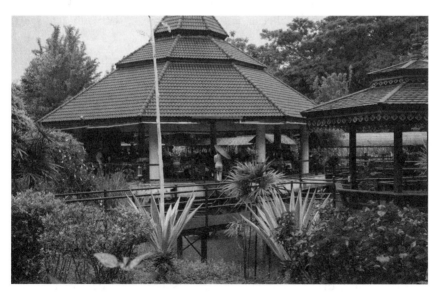

Fig. 10.8. Tao Garden's Kwan Yin Dining Hall

Goat's dairy is easier to digest than cow's dairy. If you choose cow dairy, opt for organic varieties. Minimize hidden sugars: check your cereal, bread, and spread ingredient lists. Use only sugar-free jams and spreads. If your blood-sugar levels tend to crash, be careful not to eat too much fruit and fruit juice for breakfast. Minimize heavy oils: cooked foods can be cooked in broth or grilled rather than fried in a lot of oil.

Before Breakfast

Upon arising, drink 2 ounces of any one of the following juices: apple, grape, cherry, fig, prune—mixed with 4 ounces of pure water. Or you may drink your favorite herb tea. Follow this with a light internal exercise program, deep breathing, and a short morning meditation.

Suggested Choices for Breakfast or Brunch

If not truly hungry for a protein or grain breakfast, eat a piece of fruit, such as apples, pears, peaches, berries, grapes. Eat melons alone. Or choose from among the following:

1. Seed or nut milk (germinated/soaked overnight), with berries, apples, or peaches. Best in summer.
2. Whole grain cereal with slice of rye or whole wheat bread and 4 ounces of cereal grain beverage. Best in cool or moderate weather.
3. Low-fat cottage cheese, yogurt, buttermilk, with sub-acid fruit. Best in summer.
4. Oatmeal cooked with a few raisins (soaked overnight) and a slice of corn bread. Best in cool weather.
5. Whole grain granola cereal. Pour warm water over cereal, add ¼ teaspoon licorice powder, lecithin granules, fresh wheat germ flakes; mix contents; cover bowl and let stand 10 minutes. Eat and enjoy. Best in cool to moderate weather.

Lunch

(Note: Lunch and dinner menus can be interchanged; be flexible.)

A healthy lunch consists of a vegetable salad (raw, best in warm weather), natural complex carbohydrates (grains and legumes), and your favorite health drink. Remember, salads should not be eaten before protein or starch but always with or after these foods.

Salad Suggestions (Raw)

Salads can be composed of choices from the following:

Celery, cucumber, tomatoes (sparingly)
Onions, garlic, red or green sweet peppers
Romaine, Bibb, or Boston lettuce
Alfalfa, mung, or other sprouts
Steamed beets
Avocado (sparingly)
Wheat grass

Complex Carbohydrates

Complex carbohydrates can be chosen from the following:

Grains: rice, barley, buckwheat, rye, wheat, millet, oats, corn
Legumes: Lima, soy, adzuki, navy, pinto, or kidney beans, split peas,
   lentils, chickpeas
Whole grain breads: wheat, rye, corn, bran muffins, rye crisp
Sandwich spreads: tofu, sesame, tahini, hummus
Soups: vegetable broth, miso soup, bean soup, pea or lentil soup, bar-
   ley soup, mushroom soup

Health Beverages

Beverages should be salivated thoroughly before swallowing; 2 to 4
ounces after meals is sufficient. They can be chosen from the following:

Fresh raw vegetable juice
Grain beverages
Herbal teas

MID-AFTERNOON SNACK
(ONLY IF HUNGRY)

Any health beverage of your choice, such as fresh carrot or celery juice,
or any fruit in season.

DINNER (FOR NOON OR EVENING)

A healthy dinner consists of vegetable juice one-half hour before dinner, a raw vegetable salad (in warm weather), one or two steamed or baked vegetables, natural complex carbohydrates and complete protein (grains and legumes).

Steamed or Baked Vegetables

Vegetables for steaming or baking can be chosen from the following:

Asparagus, corn, string beans, summer squash, winter squash
Beets and greens, onions, carrots, turnips, potato (sparingly), yam
Cauliflower, broccoli, brussels sprouts, sauerkraut
Peas, artichokes, mushrooms (sparingly), celery, okra
Dandelion greens, endive, kale, Swiss chard

Complete Protein Meals

Choose from among the following legume and grain combinations that provide complete protein.

1. Split pea or lentil soup with whole grain bread
2. Beans and corn bread
3. Chickpea falafel with whole grain pita bread
4. Beans and rice
5. Whole grain spaghetti with chickpea balls
6. Pea soup with corn bread
7. Buckwheat and lima beans
8. Tempeh (soy) and millet
9. Tofu spread and rye bread

Make your grain choices guided by the following seasonal indications.

Hot weather grains: corn, red millet, long grain brown rice
Cold weather grains: buckwheat, oatmeal, short grain brown rice, barley
Temperate weather grains: wheat, rye, yellow millet

Additional protein guidelines:

If you are on a transition diet away from meat products, use only lean
meats, such as white fish, halibut, trout, and chicken, 2 or 3 times
per week. Avoid pork, beef, or any other high-fat meats. Limit
eggs to 2 to 3 times per week.

Make sparing use of high-fat dairy such as cheddar, muenster, edam,
and Swiss cheese. If you can maintain good health without these
foods, do so.

Lacto-vegetarians can add buttermilk, goat milk, skim milk, cheese
(made with vegetable rennet), yogurt, kefir, clabbered milk, or
cottage cheese.

Complete vegetarians/vegans can supply their protein needs by choosing from among legumes, tofu, miso, germinated seeds (sunflower,
sesame, or pumpkin) and nuts (almonds and others), wheatgrass,
sprouts, buckwheat, alfalfa, spirulina, and seaweed products.

Cold Weather Menu Suggestions

Morning

It is good in cold weather to start the day with:

Cooked cereals, such as cream of wheat, rye, millet, rice, oatmeal,
seven-grain cereal

Whole wheat or buckwheat pancakes, waffles, drop biscuits, or
muffins

Scrambled tofu or tempeh; tofu bread pudding; marinated fried tofu

Baked stuffed apple, baked potato with gomasio

Beans

Midday

A good midday meal in cold weather consists of choices from among the
following:

Soups, such as vegetarian barley, miso, beans, brown rice, leek, chowder

Sandwich spreads, such as hummus, tofu

Cooked grains with beans

Veggie burgers
Pita bread with spreads and sprouts
All leftovers for quick and easy lunch

Evening

In cold weather a welcome hearty evening meal will be chosen from:

Soups
Vegetables stir fried, sautéed, steamed, curried, baked, and stuffed
Casseroles, baked cheese spaghetti; chili; rice curry; pasta with sauce
Soy dishes such as tofu quiche, tofu lasagna or stroganoff, baked
    tempeh, tofu enchiladas
Grains and beans
Nut loaves
Whole wheat pizza

Warm Weather Menu Samples

Mornings

It is good in warm weather to start the day with:

Fruit or fresh fruit compote, or applesauce
Vegetable juice or fruit smoothie
Whole grain cold cereal or granola
Seed or nut milk (with fruit, cereal, or alone)
Rice or bread pudding

Midday

A good midday meal in warm weather consists of choices from among
the following:

Salads, such as carrot-raisin, cucumber onion, tabouli, raw vegetables
    with sprouts, three-bean, macaroni, or potato
Soups, especially cold soups such as gazpacho, vichyssoise, fruit soups
Burgers and falafel
Stuffed tomatoes
Fresh fruit compote

Evening

In warm weather the evening meal should emphasize salads and raw vegetables; it should be light, chosen from among:

Beans	Salads	Vegetables
Grains	Soups	

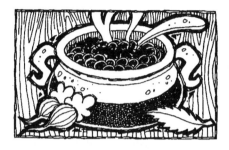

TAO GARDEN'S HEALING RECIPES

∞ THE PROFESSOR'S AMBROSIA: FOOD OF THE GODS MORNING CEREAL

(See color insert, plate 1)

Raisins, dried apricots, dates, or dried pineapple
Almonds, or pumpkin or sunflower seeds
Chopped apples or pears
Cinnamon
Rolled oats, millet, rye, or barley

1. Soak 2 or 3 dried fruits and seeds or nuts in a pot of water overnight.
2. In the morning boil the mixture with 2 or 3 pieces of diced fresh fruit and cinnamon.
3. After the mixture has boiled, remove from heat and let it sit.
4. Boil 3 cups of water to 1 cup of whole grain and add grain after the water boils. Then let it sit so the whole grain can absorb the hot water; for rolled oats, simply soak in the water.
5. After the water has been absorbed by the grain, add the fruit and seed/nut mixture, let it sit to marinate for an hour, and serve with honey if needed.

❧ TAO GARDEN CASHEW NUT BUTTER

Cashew nuts, 1 cup
Honey, 2 tsp

1. Dry-fry the cashew nuts in a wok, continuously moving them around to prevent sticking.
2. Cool slightly and then blend in a coffee grinder.
3. Add a little honey and blend in a normal blender.

❧ TAO GARDEN SESAME SEED BUTTER (TAHINI)

White sesame seeds, 1 cup
Sesame oil, 3 tsp

1. Dry-fry the seeds in a wok, moving around to prevent sticking. Watch as they change color and take on a golden hue. Remove from the heat before they burn.
2. After they have cooled down a little, blend the seeds in a coffee grinder.
3. Add a little sesame oil and blend in a normal blender.

❧ TAO GARDEN FRUIT COMPOTE (BUILDS DIGESTIVE FIRE)

(See color insert, plate 2)

Apple,* 1	Prunes (chopped), ½ cup
Orange,* 1	Chinese red date, ½ cup
Banana,* 1	Cinnamon, 1 tbsp
Raisins, ½ cup	Water to cover

1. Put everything in a saucepan over medium flame.
2. Stew together for 20 minutes until it all becomes very soft.
3. Serve warm as an accompaniment to another dish.

---

*You may substitute local seasonal fruit to make your compote.

℀ TAO GARDEN VEGETABLE BROTH (MINERALIZING AND ALKALIZING)

(See color insert, plate 3)

Celery/coriander roots, ¼ cup
White/red radish, 1½ cups
Pumpkin, 1½ cups
Gingerroot, ½ cup
Green papaya, 2½ cups
Onion, 1

Pandanus leaf, ¼ cup
Radish pickle, 2 tbsp
Water, 5 quarts
Black pepper (ground), 2 tbsp
Soybeans (rinsed), ¼ cup

1. Rinse everything well and cut vegetables into big pieces (you can leave seeds in and peels on). Bring water to a boil on maximum heat. Add all the vegetables, ground black pepper, soybeans, and coriander root to the water.

2. After the water returns to a boil, reduce heat and simmer for 3 to 4 hours with a lid on the pot. Skim the froth off the surface of the liquid from time to time using a strainer. When done, strain off the liquid to use as broth.

℀ TAO GARDEN BROWN RICE SOUP (KAO TOM TAN YA PEUT)

(See color insert, plate 4)

Vegetable stock, 1 quart
Cooked brown rice, 1½ cups
Sunflower seeds, 1 tbsp
Pumpkin seeds, 1 tbsp
Roasted white sesame seeds, 1 tbsp
Boiled sweet corn kernels, ½ cup

Soy sauce/tamari, 4 tbsp
Celery (chopped fine), 1 tbsp
Minced spring onion, 1 tbsp
Minced coriander, 1 tbsp
Fried garlic, 1 tbsp

1. Heat the vegetable stock until it comes to a boil. Add the cooked brown rice, reduce the heat, and cook for about 20 minutes.

2. Add the sunflower seeds, pumpkin seeds, white sesame seeds, and sweet corn kernels, and stir in well. Season according to taste with the soy sauce. Add the celery, spring onion, coriander, and garlic to the soup and turn off the heat.

✍ TAO GARDEN GOAT'S MILK YOGURT (COOLING AND PROBIOTIC)

(See color insert, plate 5)

Goat's milk
Vita-Ferment (or similar) yogurt starter

1. Bring goat's milk close to boiling point, about 180°F.
2. Let the milk cool down to 110°F. Mix in 1 pouch of yogurt bacteria until the ferment is dissolved. Pour into a sterilized container.
3. Close lid and place cultured milk into a warm place (about 110°F) for 6–8 hours.
4. During this time don't move or shake the fermented goat milk.
5. After fermentation period place yogurt in refrigerator for 12 hours.

✍ TAO GARDEN BROCCOLI SOUP (CALMING AND MOVES STAGNANT CHI)

(See color insert, plate 6)

Onion, 1, chopped	Vegetable broth, 2½ cups
Butter, 1 tbsp	Himalayan rock salt, 1 tsp
Broccoli, 3 cups	Ground pepper, ½ tsp

1. Sauté the chopped onion in the butter.
2. Add the broccoli cut into small pieces.
3. Add the vegetable broth, salt, and pepper.
4. Cook until the broccoli is soft.
5. Blend to a smooth consistency.

✍ TAO GARDEN TOM YAM SOUP (STIMULATES STAGNANT CHI)

(See color insert, plate 7)

Vegetable broth, 6 cups	Lemongrass, 2 sticks
Soy sauce, 2 tbsp	Kaffir lime leaf, 2 leaves
Lime juice, 2 tbsp	Small red chilies, 4
Coriander root, 6 pieces	Mushrooms (3 kinds), 2 cups
Shallots, 8 bulbs	Coriander leaf, 1 sprig

1. Warm the vegetable broth over medium heat until it begins to boil.
2. Add the soy sauce and lime juice to taste.
3. Add the coriander root, shallots, lemongrass, kaffir lime, and chili.
4. Add the three types of mushrooms.
5. Cook together and serve with a sprig of coriander placed on top.

⌘ TAO GARDEN PUMPKIN SOUP (BUILDS DIGESTIVE FIRE)

(See color insert, plate 8)

Pumpkin, 2½ cups	Vegetable stock, 1½ quarts
Onion, ½ cup	Light soy sauce, to taste
Butter, 2 tbsp	

1. Clean the pumpkin and chop into pieces.
2. Stir-fry the onion in the butter (those on a fat-free diet can soften the onion by cooking it in a little water).
3. Add the vegetable stock and pumpkin.
4. Boil until the pumpkin is soft. Add soy sauce to taste.
5. Allow to cool slightly and then process in a blender until smooth. Heat until hot and serve.

⌘ TAO GARDEN GREEN PAPAYA SALAD (ANTIPARASITE REMEDY)

(See color insert, plate 9)

Green papaya, 1 cup	Peanuts (optional), 50g
Carrot, 2 tbsp	Soy sauce, 2 tbsp
Tomato, ¼ cup	Tamarind paste, 1 tbsp
Chilies, 2	Palm sugar, ½ tbsp
Garlic, 2 cloves	Lime juice, 2 tbsp
String beans, 3	

1. Peel and shred fresh green (unripe) papaya and carrots. Slice tomato thinly.
2. In a clay mortar, pound the fresh chilies (whole) and peeled garlic. Add string beans, sliced tomato, and roasted peanuts, and pound lightly (do not overcrush).

3. Add soy sauce, tamarind paste, palm sugar, and lime juice. Add these items spoon-by-spoon, and taste as you go. Lightly pound (optional).

4. Add shredded papaya and carrot and pound together until mixed well. Serve with fresh cabbage on the side.

TAO GARDEN STIR-FRIED MIXED VEGETABLES (EASILY DIGESTIBLE)

Mixed vegetables, 3 cups

Coconut/sesame oil, 2 tbsp

Vegetable stock, 2 tbsp

Soy sauce, to taste

Fresh cane juice, to taste

Garlic (optional), ½ tsp

Cashew nuts, ½ cup

1. Wash and prepare your vegetables. Cutting vegetables energizes them (because you add some of your chi as you cut them). There are many different ways to cut vegetables, each giving different energetic properties. Smaller pieces have more energy, making grated vegetables highly energizing. Whole vegetables retain their wholeness and complete energy and will take longer to cook.

2. Pour a little oil and vegetable broth into a wok over a high heat.

3. When the mixture is hot, add the vegetables and condiments, and stir with a wooden spatula. Keep the vegetables moving so that they do not stick. Cook for a few minutes and serve while the vegetables are still warm.

TAO GARDEN RICE (BALANCING)

(See color insert, plate 10)

Rice (rinsed), 1 cup

Cold water, 2 cups

Himalayan rock salt, ¼ tsp

Mixed seeds (optional), ½ cup

1. It is preferable to soak the rice (or any grain) in water for 8–12 hours before cooking. This breaks down the enzyme-inhibitors and makes the grain more alkalizing. Place the rice, water, and salt into a pan. Cover with a tight-fitting lid and bring to a boil over full heat.

2. Turn heat to low and simmer until the water has been absorbed (roughly 12 minutes for white rice; 20 minutes for brown).

3. Stir in the mixed seeds if desired and serve hot.

⮑ TAO GARDEN BAKED FISH
(WITH TURMERIC, ANTI-INFLAMMATORY)

(See color insert, plate 11)

Turmeric, 1 tsp	Red (sweet) chilies, 2
Galangal, 1 tsp	Soy sauce, 1 tbsp
Garlic, 1 clove	Fresh filleted fish, 1 medium
Lemongrass, 1 tsp	

1. Preheat oven to 220°F.
2. Blend the turmeric, galangal, garlic, lemongrass, and one of the chilies in the soy sauce. Cut three long diagonal lines along the length of the fish, on both sides.
3. Pour all of the sauce over the fish and put into a preheated oven in a baking tray (lined with aluminum foil). Bake for 1 hour.
4. Slice the remaining chili and add over the top of the fish and serve.

⮑ TAO GARDEN CURRIED CHICKEN WITH
STRING BEANS (WARMING)

(See color insert, plate 12)

Vegetable oil (optional), 2 tbsp	Skinless chicken breast, 1½ cups
Chicken stock, ½ cup	String beans, 1 cup
Curry paste, 1½ tbsp	Kaffir leaves, 3
Cane sugar, ½ tbsp	Red pepper (sliced), 1
Soy sauce, ½ tbsp	

1. Heat the oil or a small amount of the chicken stock (for an oil-free version). Add curry paste, cane sugar, and soy sauce.
2. Heat at low temperature.
3. Add chicken and (the rest of) the stock.
4. Increase to medium temperature and cook until the water has evaporated.
5. Add string beans, kaffir leaf, and red pepper.
6. Continue to cook until beans are just tender. Serve with rice.

TAO GARDEN FRIED EGGPLANT WITH TOFU (MOVES STAGNANT BLOOD)

Green eggplant, 2 large
Sea salt
Firm tofu, 9 oz.
Miso paste, 2 tbsp
Cooking oil, 1 tbsp
Unrefined brown sugar, ½ tbsp

Soy sauce, to taste
Freshly ground pepper, ½ tsp
Vegetable stock, 3 tbsp
Chilies (cut diagonally), 5 pieces
Fresh sweet basil leaves, 10

1. Cut the eggplants into long strips and sprinkle with sea salt. Leave for 20 minutes and then rinse the salt off.
2. Grill the eggplant (both sides) until it is soft. Set to one side.
3. Cut the tofu into 1-inch cubes and steam until cooked.
4. Stir-fry the miso paste in hot oil until fragrant. Add sugar, soy sauce, pepper, vegetable stock, steamed tofu, and eggplant.
5. Add chilies and basil, stir and serve.

TAO GARDEN FRIED NOODLES (PAD THAI) (CELL BUILDER)

(See color insert, plate 13)

Rice noodles, 2 oz.
Tofu or shrimp, ½ cup
Chinese green chives, 1 tbsp
Bean sprouts, ¼ cup
Shallot (minced), 1 tbsp
Garlic (minced), 1 tsp

Sesame oil, 3 tbsp
Chicken/vegetable broth, 2 tbsp
Tamarind juice, 3 tbsp
Ground chili pepper, ½ tbsp
Egg, 1
Crushed peanuts, 1 tbsp

1. Soak dry noodles (15 minutes). Chop tofu, chives. Rinse the bean sprouts; mince shallots and garlic together.
2. Stir-fry the shallots, garlic, and tofu in the sesame oil until they start to brown. Add broth, tamarind juice, and chili pepper. Stir.
3. Crack the egg into the wok and scramble. Fold egg into the noodles.
4. Stir a few more times while adding bean sprouts and chives.
5. Pour onto a serving plate and sprinkle with crushed peanuts.

⤳ TAO GARDEN SALAD DRESSINGS (MOISTEN AND ENHANCE FLAVOR)

(See color insert, plate 14)

Where quantities are not noted, use proportions according to your personal taste. To make each sauce, blend ingredients in food processor and chill.

Tamarind Sauce

Tamarind paste

Miso paste

Coconut milk

Ginger Sauce

Minced ginger

Soy sauce

Sesame oil

Soy bean paste

Onion

Mango Sauce

Mango (ripe)

Himalayan rock salt

Chili sauce

Lemon juice

Raw cane juice/maple syrup

Passion Fruit Sauce

Passion fruit juice (juice
only; not the seeds)

Raw cane juice/maple syrup

Himalayan rock salt

Chili sauce

Lemon juice

Sesame Sauce

Sesame spread (tahini)

Himalayan rock salt

Water

Lemon juice

The Professor's Confection Sauce

Green onions, 1 bunch,
   chopped in food processor

Safflower oil, 1 cup

Tahini, 3 tbsp

Water, 1 cup

Juice of 1 lemon

Tamari, 1 cup

Cayenne, few dashes

Honey, 2 tbsp

TAO GARDEN SALAD TOPPINGS

Mix and add to suit your own taste. You can also experiment with adding local nuts, seeds, herbs, and roots to your salads.

Pumpkin seeds (soaked for 4 hours and drained): Rich in zinc and thus helpful for impotence, prostate swelling, bladder problems, parasites. (See color insert, plate 15)

Sunflower seeds (soaked for 4 hours and drained): Chi energy tonic, lubricates intestines and clears constipation. (See color insert, plate 16)

Garlic: Expels worms and parasites, reduces candida, clears colds and other infections, detoxifies the body. Use cautiously; can cause overheating. (See color insert, plate 17)

Ginger: Aids digestion by boosting the digestive fire (Kidney yang) and for any cold condition. Use cautiously; can cause overheating. (See color insert, plate 18)

Turmeric root: Anti-inflammatory and anti-oxidant qualities, protects liver from toxins, helps break down tumors. Good for gallbladder cleanse. (See color insert, plate 19)

Dried seaweed and sesame seeds: Provide a very mineral-rich alternative to salt. Sesame seeds are extremely rich in calcium. Increase alkalinity of body, assist in elimination of toxins. (See color insert, plate 20)

Limes/lemons: Highly alkaline-forming once digested; good for balancing body pH and removing toxins. Good for liver and gallbladder cleansing and to move stagnant liver chi. (See color insert, plate 21)

THE PROFESSOR'S PENETRATING SPLIT PEA SOUP

Green/yellow split peas, 2 cups	Celery, 2 stalks
Onion, 1 medium, sliced	Other vegetables, as desired
Water, 5 cups	Parsley, few sprigs
Carrots, 2 medium, diced	

1. Cook peas and onion in 4 cups of water until soft (about 35 minutes).

2. Separately, cook together carrots, celery, and other vegetables in 1 cup of water (20 minutes).

3. Puree peas and combine with cooked vegetables. Serve garnished with chopped parsley.

❧ THE PROFESSOR'S ENERGIZING GAZPACHO

Carrot, 1	Vinegar (apple cider), 2 tbsp
Celery, 2 stalks	Red pepper, to taste
Garlic, 2 cloves, minced	Whole cumin, ½ tbsp
Fresh tomato, 2 cups	Tamari, 1 tbsp
Parsley, 2 sprigs	Zucchini, sliced
Lemon juice, 3 tbsp	Tofu (cubed), 1½ cup
Safflower or olive oil, ½ cup	Green onions, finely sliced

1. At high speed, blend the carrot, celery, garlic, 1 cup tomato, and parsley. Pour into bowl.

2. Blend lemon juice, oil, vinegar, pepper, cumin, tamari, and 1 cup tomato; add to first mixture.

3. Add some sliced zucchini and red pepper, along with the tofu cubes. Refrigerate. Garnish with finely sliced green onions.

❧ THE PROFESSOR'S VITALIZING HUMMUS SPREAD

Dried chickpeas, 1½ cup	Chives or basil, 2 tbsp
Tahini, 2 tbsp	Tamari, ½ tbsp
Garlic, 3 cloves, minced	Cayenne, ¼ tsp
Parsley flakes, 3 tbsp (½ cup fresh)	Lemons, 2
Salt, 1½ tbsp	Scallions, minced, ¼ cup

1. Soak chickpeas overnight; boil until soft (45 minutes).

2. Cool the chickpeas, then mash to a thick paste.

3. Combine everything and chill.

THE PROFESSOR'S CONFECTION
WHOLE WHEAT PIZZA

Warm water, ⅓ cup
Dry yeast, 1 pkg
Safflower or olive oil, 2 tbsp
Unbleached flour, 1¼ cup
Whole wheat flour, ¾ cup

Sesame seeds, ¼ cup
Soy flour, ¼ cup
Prepared spaghetti sauce
Tomato paste
Toppings

1. Combine water and yeast. Let stand until yeast bubbles up to surface. Add oil.
2. Sift flours together, then add to yeast liquid a cup at a time along with the seeds. Knead and let rise, covered, in a warm place, for about an hour.
3. Punch down, knead, and roll out dough for pizza crust. Put on pizza pan or cookie sheet.
4. Add your favorite spaghetti sauce with extra tomato paste to thicken.
5. Garnish with desired toppings, such as sautéed mushrooms, garlic, onions, peppers, tofu, and sun cheese.
6. Bake at 400° for 20 minutes.

THE PROFESSOR'S CLARIFICATION
LEMONADE

Lemon, 1
Organic maple syrup, 1 tbsp

Cayenne, ⅛ tsp
Pure water, 1 glass

Squeeze lemon into glass of pure water with syrup and cayenne.

THE PROFESSOR'S LIBERATION
LIMA BEAN SOUP

Dried lima beans, 1 cup
Garlic, 3 cloves, minced

Scallions, minced, 1 cup
Pure water, 3 cups

1. Soak lima beans overnight.
2. Boil in 3 cups water with chopped garlic and scallions. Let simmer until beans are tender (but not mushy). Then cool slightly and serve.

∾ THE PROFESSOR'S PERFECTION THAI COCONUT ICE CREAM

Fresh coconut milk, 1 cup   Salt, ¼ tsp
Fresh coconut meat, ⅓ cup   Cane sugar, ½ cup
Pure water, ¼ cup

Mix all ingredients together and freeze.

∾ THE PROFESSOR'S TITILLATION DIP AND HORS D'OEUVRE

Dip
Organic almond butter, 1 bowl
Dr. Bragg's Amino Acids, ¼ cup
Lemon (squeezed), 1

Hors d'oeuvre
Dried smoked salmon, ½ cup   Radishes, ½ cup
Pickled cucumbers, ½ cup   Boiled shrimp, ½ cup
Daikon (chopped), ½ cup   Celery, 6 stalks
Green onions, ½ cup   Carrots, 6 sticks

1. Mix all ingredients for dip.
2. Prepare vegetables and fish and enjoy dipping.

∾ TAO GARDEN MUNG BEANS (THUA KHIAW TOM NAM TAAN)

(See color insert, plate 22)

Mung beans, 1 cup   Unrefined brown sugar, ¼ cup
Water, 2 cups   Gingerroot, 2 tbsp

1. Soak the mung beans overnight.
2. Add the beans to water, bring to a boil, and cook until the beans are soft.
3. Add the sugar and chopped gingerroot and continue to stir.
4. Serve warm.

TAO GARDEN RICE BALLS IN COCONUT MILK (BUALOI)

(See color insert, plate 23)

Glutinous rice flour, 1½ cups
Flour, 2 tbsp
Water, ½ cup
Pumpkin (steamed/pureed), 1 cup
Taro (steamed/pureed), 1 cup

Coconut milk, 3 cups
Coconut cream, 1½ cups
Palm sugar, 1½ cups
Himalayan rock salt, ¼ tsp

1. Mix the flours with enough water to make a firm paste.
2. Mix half the paste with the pureed pumpkin, then mix the rest of the paste with the pureed taro. Knead well and then form pea-sized balls.
3. Bring a large pot of water to a boil, toss in the balls, and remove when they float to the surface. Drain.
4. Bring the coconut milk and cream to a boil; add palm sugar and salt.
5. Stir constantly to prevent it from separating.
6. Add the flour balls.
7. When the mixture returns to a boil, remove from heat.
8. Serve as a dessert in small bowls.

Tao Garden's Condiments

At Tao Garden we make and serve the following healthful condiments.

Rice Vinegar with Fresh Ground Green/Red Chili: Dissolves mucus, warms stomach, and increases blood flow to the face and brain.

Red Chili Sauce: Helps digestion, restores alkaline condition to blood, prevents and cures cancer, boosts immune system.

Dried Papaya Seeds: Papaya seeds are ground with seaweed, sesame seed, and a little sea salt. Good for the brain. Contains iodine (thyroid/metabolism).

White Sesame Seeds: High in calcium and fatty acids. Contain very similar amounts of essential amino acids as red meat.

Black Sesame Seeds: Strengthen kidneys and liver and provide food for the brain.

Wheat Germ: High protein, high fiber, and contains vitamin E.

Dried Banana Powder: Nice energy booster and natural sweetener.

Dried Papaya Powder: Aids body to remove undigested proteins and putrefactive materials.

Stevia Leaf: Sweetener that helps the body regulate blood sugar, correcting both high and low blood sugar. It appears to lower blood pressure, without affecting normal blood pressure. It inhibits growth and reproduction of harmful bacteria and infectious organisms, and those causing gum disease and tooth decay. It can also be used in concentrated form to help heal skin problems including acne, seborrhea, dermatitis, psoriasis, burns, cuts, and eczema without scarring.

Pandanus Leaf: Helps to expel urine; nourishes the heart with a cooling effect. Good remedy for diabetes when used for cooking and tea.

Olive Oil: Best used raw or lightly heated. Assists in gallbladder cleansing (with lime juice). Essential fatty acids help remedy heart disease.

Coconut Oil: Enables rapid breakdown in digestion. Helpful in thyroid disorders, candida, and digestive disorders. Because of its stable nature it can be used at high temperatures.

Sesame Oil: Stable oil can be cooked at higher temperatures without risk of becoming rancid.

Nut Butters: Freshly and powerfully ground each day.

Tao Garden's Organic Fresh Sprouts

The sprouts we grow and serve are loaded with protein and other life-supporting factors.

Adzuki: 25% protein, high in calcium, niacin, iron, and amino acids.

Alfalfa: 35% protein, chlorophyll, vitamins A, B, C, D, E, F, K, U.

Buckwheat: 12% protein, high in lecithin, rutin, and minerals.

Fenugreek: Blood, liver, and kidney cleanser; mucus remover.

Garbanzo: 20% protein, high in iron, calcium, vitamins A and B.

Lentil: 25% protein, vitamins E, C, and B, iron, and phosphorus.

Peas: 22% protein, magnesium, chlorophyll, and amino acids.

Pumpkin: 30% protein, high in B vitamins, phosphorus, iron, and zinc.

Radish: Vitamin C, calcium, and potassium.

Sesame: 18% protein (1125 mg), vitamins E, B_1, niacin.

Sunflower: Vitamin B complex, D, E, and all minerals and zinc.

Tao Garden's Organic Herbal/Flower Teas and Juices

A wide variety of healthful drinks can be made from various leaves, seeds, roots, and fruits.

Safflower (with Stevia Leaf): Cleans the blood, dilutes it, and lowers cholesterol and high blood pressure. Makes a dark orange tea.

Lemongrass (with Stevia/Pandanus Leaf): Activates the thymus (improving the immune system) and helps ward off mosquitoes and insects. Mildly green tea.

Ginger (with Stevia/Pandanus Leaf): Warms the stomach (aiding digestion) and helps blood flow.

Lingzhi (with Stevia Leaf): Lingzhi is a kind of mushroom, said to strengthen the heart.

Chrysanthemum (with Buddha Fruit): Helps the throat, clears mucus, and cools the system.

Bael Fruit: Common Thai herb, which the locals say improves your sex appeal when consumed after dark.

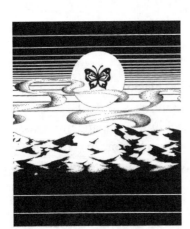

Fig. 10.9. Happiness is like a butterfly. The more you chase it, the more it eludes you. But if you turn your attention to other things, it comes and softly sits on your shoulder. This is the Way of the Tao.

Green Jasmine: Has some caffeine and will wake you up a bit. It is best not to drink this tea in the evening.

Mint Leaf: Served with lime.

Ginkgo Biloba: Improves circulation to the brain.

Mulberry (with Stevia/Pandanus Leaf): Harmonizes construction, assisting the middle burner.

Roselle: When made into a tea, this is a cooling blood purifier.

Ginger/Ginseng: Freshly prepared daily. Stimulates, warms, and energizes; helpful for fighting off colds and influenza viruses.

Senna (with Tea): One part Senna mixed with three parts of your favorite fresh tea makes a mild laxative and cleansing drink, which aids bowel contractions.

Japliang: This ancient blend of Chinese herbs assists in cooling the body.

Soymilk (with Pandanus Leaf): A digestive delight and refreshing wholesome drink.

Yogurt: Made from Thai goat's milk, it is effective in increasing the levels of beneficial bacteria within the large intestine.

Green Vegetable Juice: This juice, made from Chinese cabbage, scallion, pandanus leaf, pennywort, parsley, lettuce, sprouts, lime, and cane sugar juice, has natural enzymes, chlorophyll, and vitamins that alkalinize blood and cleanse the system of putrefactive debris.

Rice Milk: Contains the building blocks for DNA production. At Tao Garden four to seven grains are used to produce this milk fresh every evening.

Dragon-eye (Longan): This fruit is the traditional Thai way to sweeten food. Contains fruit sugar and so blood sugar is balanced.

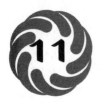

Harmonizing Your Life with the Tao

BALANCING YIN AND YANG

Just as physical objects, food, and climate are classified into yin and yang, there are also psychological aspects, mental characteristics, societal conditions, and individual tendencies of yin and yang. Yin and yang is the law of polarity or the law of opposites: nothing can exist except in relation to its opposite. Without mountains there can be no valleys. Without shadows there can be no perception of light. If only masculinity existed we would have no perception of feminine beauty. There would be no such thing as evil unless we were able to compare it with good. Without wisdom, there can be no ignorance. Without age there can be no such thing as youth.

Persons who are extreme, either with deficient yin or excessive yang, are not in conscious control of their physical and psychological forces. They are tossed about by outer circumstances because they have unbalanced their physical and mental yin and yang polarities. Yin and yang balanced individuals consciously flow harmoniously with the natural forces of life as daily situations arise. They are poised in every undertaking, whether it is working in a factory or selling insurance. Nothing disturbs their center of balance or their energy. They do not use the forces of nature or their own power to gain advantages over other persons. They know that any coercion or force will bring dire consequences for themselves and misery for others.

Yin and Yang Manipulate Each Other

Taoist wisdom teaches that the wise man seeks everything in himself; the ignorant man tries to get everything from somebody else. The essential difference between the controlled/balanced yin and yang person and those who are extreme yin or extreme yang is in the degree of conscious awareness. In the former the inner mind and soul are consciously balanced with the outer physical body, while the latter are unbalanced and totally controlled by desires, habits, and physical environment.

Essentially we live on a material plane, or in a yin-type world. Right from birth we are trained to be yin, to be materialists enough to support ourselves, to keep alive by adapting to the needs of existence. That is why there is no such thing as a totally yang person. We are trained by society to react yin to outward circumstances. And since yin is decay and death, we are more schooled in the art of dependence and confusion (yin) than in the art of healthful living and clear thinking (yin/yang balance). Yin needs. Yin is also dominated. That is the whole mystery of it in a nutshell.

Excessive and uncontrolled desires are the cause of much pain and heartbreak. Need someone or something excessively and you will become extreme yin. Let it affect you mentally, physically, emotionally, and spiritually, and you will become useless to everyone, including yourself. Crave something uncontrollably, and you are its slave. Psychologists say that you are on your way toward becoming an alcoholic as soon as you tell yourself, "I need a drink." Alcohol itself is an extremely yin substance and it tends to expand or make the body and brain more yin. Respond to something and you are in sympathy with it; you are a part of it. Respond to worry (yin) and you will have more worries.

A true relationship is based on mutual love and respect, where both people have totally balanced natures. If we enter into a relationship with a controlled attitude, without attachment or possession, we are considered balanced. An unbalanced relationship is generally emotional and possessive, which develops into jealousy, self-pity, and loss of self-confidence. In most modern-day relationships there is the lover (yin) and the beloved (yang). The lover pursues and attempts to possess the beloved, who in many cases is indifferent or unattached to the lover. A person is considered extreme yin in a relationship if he or she possesses, holds, or becomes emotionally crippled with uncontrolled attachment and desire. Extreme yang people consciously use yin passive people for their own ends and thus create a hell on Earth for themselves and others. By doing this, they set the wheels of cause and effect in motion and eventually reap what they sow: pain, grief, and suffering.

Allow financial worries to take you over and you cannot possibly lick them. Put yourself in the position of craving, lusting, and excessively worrying about money, and you will never get enough of it, because you are not ruling money, you are letting money rule you. If you are ruled by money, you are yin. Excessive miserly greed is extreme yang. Neither condition is healthy. Creditors are yang. They have control over your money if you allow it. You are yin and have created a need for something beyond your immediate capacity to buy. If you want peace of mind, owe no debts. Money in itself is neither yang nor yin; it is just a manifestation. The right attitude about money is to agree to its worth but not to crave it excessively; let the world see that you do not lust after it and you will get all you need. It works 100 percent if you give it a try.

Success comes from creating a need in others. For instance, advertising is the biggest business in the world. Its success comes from making others need (yin) things (a lot of which they do not really need). In a business sense advertising is yang. People who believe the propaganda are yin. A salesman can sell things to people that they do not really need. In that case, he is extreme yang and they are extreme yin. A person in yin and yang balance always uses good judgment in all purchases and is never duped by false advertising.

When you ask for sympathy, you are becoming more yin; you are putting yourself into the power of another. Like attracts like. Feel sorry for yourself (yin reaction to circumstances) and the only person who will sympathize with you is somebody else who is feeling sorry for himself (yin). Do not expect a disappointed lover to sympathize with your money troubles, unless she has lost sums of money in her pursuit of love. Those who have suffered much understand others who are still suffering. The less someone has, the more (in proportion) he is likely to give you. The millionaire who has never known suffering or poverty will not understand your need for money. The Way of the Tao is to take from those who have more than enough and give to those who do not have enough. But the typical way is to take from those who do not have enough and give to those who already have too much.

There is no such thing as absolute security in this finite, ever-changing material world. Nothing ever remains the same. Everything in life constantly changes; it is dynamic, not static, and the wise person flows smoothly with these changes. The only true security in this world is to live in harmony with the Tao or the natural laws of life. Balancing your yin and yang nature in all of its aspects will automatically lead you to peace of mind.

Mastering the Yin and Yang World

It seems a general rule that we always get a thing when we no longer want it, when our attitude is indifferent toward it. If you are a writer, you will have difficulty getting an agent until such time as you no longer need one. An agent will not start handling you for free until you have proved your ability (on your own) to sell manuscripts. Then he will agree to handle you for a commission, or what he can get out of you, because then he needs (yin) you. Set a price on yourself (whether for your services or your integrity) and nobody will want you. Refuse to set a price on yourself and people will swarm to you because they will know you can be trusted.

Show a manufacturer that you need her product and she will raise its price. Walk away from her product, be indifferent to it, and she will come running after you. If we continue to allow the oil companies to sell us gas at exorbitant prices, the price will continue to rise. If everyone in the world stopped using their cars and machines for a week or two, the oil barons would come running after us to buy their oil, dirt cheap.

Strikes succeed because they are controlled by extreme yang forces (the ability to walk away from something) and the manufacturers have to give in (yin) to the demands (yang) of labor because they need (yin) the workers to produce their products. As long as your employer needs you, your job is safe. Demand and complain (extreme yin) that you need a raise, and he will pretend that he did not hear you. Demonstrate to him that you are wanted by another company for a higher salary, and he will probably give in to your demands.

You may ask why millionaires continue to make money, if they are not dominated by money and therefore extreme yin. That question answers itself. Most millionaires are not motivated to manage investments and big business deals because of lack. They made their money to assert their egos, to prove their ideas to themselves first, and to others secondly. They do not worry about making big deals or losing a few thousand dollars here and there. It is all a discussion of theory and inventive reasoning, of outsmarting the competitor or getting him to react. The money is merely incidental. It's the excitement and adventure of pulling a fast one that motivates them, not security.

Overcoming Temptations and Becoming Free

Have you ever found yourself at a table with others who loved to eat rich foods and lived to eat? They will tell you to forget your silly health diet and eat up, assuring you that you can start back on your diet tomorrow. They are slaves (yin) to food and want to make sure that you are as enslaved as they are. Slaves do not want other people to be free. When in Rome, do as the Romans do: if you are surrounded by yin food gluttons, they will ostracize and deride you if you do not eat and act like them. Yin people dislike others who think for themselves in a controlled yin and yang manner. Since they are not free of their rebellious habits, they despise others who are free.

Since the majority of the human race has been trained to be yin, and is yin wholeheartedly, there are very few people who can bring themselves to believe that there are, indeed, enlightened and self-realized sages, saints, and holy men and women now living on this planet. The world has its vices (yin enslavements, yin needs, yin habits) and is convinced that the holy person must have his or her own vices also. Maybe he conceals them, they think, but he still has them. So what do they do? They try to tempt him.

He does not like rich food. "Just give me the simple things of life," he informs them. They will tempt him with goodies and try to force him into a craving (yin) for them. As long as he can honestly reject them, he is safe. If you are yin and yang balanced and demonstrate that you can do without anything, you will have it thrust upon you. When you demonstrate that you disdain something that the masses lustfully crave, you will be totally overwhelmed by it, because you will be a challenge to the whole materialistic (yin) world.

A vain nature invites diverting pleasures and must suffer accordingly. A person who is unstable within indulges indiscriminately in the pleasures of the world, thus giving them a powerful influence. As such a person is swept along, it is no longer a question of danger, of good fortune, or misfortune. Once a person has given up direction of her own life what becomes of her depends on chance. No one is forcing the slave to remain the slave. If a person insists on retaining his vices, if he insists on being dominated by his desires and those of society, there is no hope of helping him unless he is willing to be helped.

We all have a tendency to let ourselves become slaves—the herd instinct. We all want to follow some sort of leader or authority without question, allowing somebody else to do our thinking for us and take over our personal responsibilities. We want a certain thing because we've acquired the habit (yin) of it and we lack discipline and courage to break the habit. A long life is only the blink of an eye. If you seek only material things and earthly pleasures, the mirror will reflect your own pale face and the degeneration of your body. Material things may fill the valley, but possessions cannot last. The idea is to never need anything so badly that you cannot do without it.

Buddha knew the secrets of life when he said desire is the source of all pain. A philosopher once said that contentment consists not in great wealth, but in few wants. The best method of all is to stop needing so much. Stop letting yourself be dominated by outward circumstances. If you develop a little guts and gumption by being more independent, you can easily master this life in due time. The person who knows that enough is enough will always have enough.

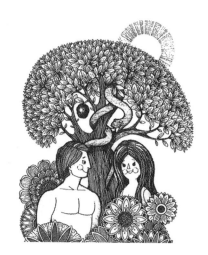

Fig. 11.1. Conserve your powers. Cravings deplete your inner peace; through them, vital waters are wasted in the barren soil of material things. Wrong desire is the greatest enemy of happiness. Be like the expansive ocean, which quietly absorbs the rivers of the senses.

Take a look at all the slaves of fashion (who try to get you to have your hair clipped off in the latest style) and the slaves of decoration (who try to persuade and seduce you into stocking your house with all sorts of dust-catching objects). It is those who are independent of fashion who become its leaders. All the latest fashion designers achieved success and reputation by being innovative, creative, and unique, not by following the trend. We revere Lincoln, Washington, Einstein, Edison, and Shakespeare because they dared to be different, to be individualists and first in their field.

The universal laws of life are exact in their operation. As you sow, so shall you reap. For every action, there is an equal and opposite reaction. It is the law of cause and effect on the physical plane. Like begets like. Plant a rose and you will not get rice. Sow yin, harvest yin. Sow hate, harvest hate. Sow friendship, harvest friendship. Sow love, harvest love. Sow war, harvest war. Sow politics, and all you get is more politics. A good person contributes toward a good family; a good family contributes toward a good nation; good nations contribute toward a good world.

An extreme yang attitude is likely to bring an overwhelming extreme yin reaction in others, perhaps even hatred or destruction. Extremes are to be avoided at all times. The key is to balance your yin and yang polarities through proper diet, sufficient exercise, attention to the needs of others, kindness, and spiritual development. Extremes in any endeavor only create pain, suffering, disease, and trouble.

What the world calls repose, the sage does not. The repose of the sage derives from a mental attitude that becomes the mirror of the universe. Nothing disturbs her tranquility; hence her repose. The sage cares not for herself but responds to the needs of others. Be good to people who are good. To those who are not good also be good. Thus goodness is achieved. Be sincere to those who are sincere. To people who are not sincere also be sincere. This is the Way of the Tao.

Balancing Individual Qualities

To balance the elements in one individual, it is well to understand that there is no mental characteristic found in men that is wholly absent from women. There is no mental quality found in women that is not possessed in some measure by men. This is on the human plane. On the spiritual plane there is no gender distinction. The spiritual person possesses masculine and feminine qualities in balance.

In music, certain notes, when struck separately, make discord. The same notes, when struck together, can make harmony. The same law applied to the characteristics given in the table below will produce like results. In electrophysics negative and positive currents produce a circuit. The feminine elements and the masculine elements, balancing each other, create harmony and complete the circuit of life on the human plane. To bring about this balance or harmony, the two elements under the heading of feminine and masculine need to converge into each other until the fusion is complete in consciousness and demonstrated in life and power.

YIN FEMININE QUALITIES		YANG MASCULINE QUALITIES
Feeling	is balanced by	Intellect
Love	is balanced by	Wisdom
Meekness	is balanced by	Self-value
Caution	is balanced by	Courage
Freedom	is balanced by	Responsibility
Patience	is balanced by	Aggressiveness
Tenderness	is balanced by	Stability
Joy	is balanced by	Moderation
Faith	is balanced by	Understanding
Gentleness	is balanced by	Strength
Intuition	is balanced by	Logical reasoning
Generosity	is balanced by	Economy
Repose	is balanced by	Energy
Zeal	is balanced by	Reflection
Ambition	is balanced by	Unselfishness
Charity	is balanced by	Justice
Candor	is balanced by	Tactfulness
Aspiration	is balanced by	Judgment
Benevolence	is balanced by	Discrimination
Liberty	is balanced by	Obedience to law

Success, health, and peace are the perfectly natural culmination of harmonious development, which brings the fulfillment of our desires, whether in the material or the spiritual world. If we have completed our

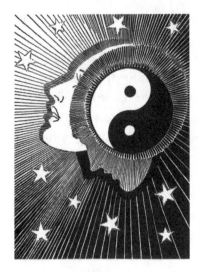

Fig. 11.2. The yin and yang within

development, no earthly force can stop us. We are certain of achievement, for no one with complete harmony of being can fail. It is as impossible to visualize failure as it is to imagine the failure of the sun to appear in the heavens. Let us be thankful and joyful that we have the opportunity to achieve all that we have yearned for during a lifetime. A high purpose is magnetic and attracts rich resources.

Marriage of Truth and Love (Yin and Yang)

In the Divine Mind, truth and love are indissolubly wedded. All human undertakings that count for anything exemplify this union. The forces of evil try to divorce truth and love in human consciousness and to make us believe that truth can be advanced through war and strife, carried on with motives of anger, hatred, revenge, self-interest, or self-justification.

To counter this, problems of importance must be discussed and settled in our families, in our business relations, and in the larger negotiations of politics, law, diplomacy, government, and religion. In these discussions, let us defeat evil through understanding and by bearing in mind that, by no amount of argument, however valid, and by no amount of force of any kind, can we successfully promulgate truth, unless, during our efforts, we purposely and habitually exercise the spirit of good will, right feeling, and right purpose.

In dealing with others, reasoning and goodwill are like the wings of a bird. If a bird tries to fly with only one wing, he whirls round and round, to his own confusion, making no headway; but, using both wings, he will make much progress in his flight. Only when the male principle, truth, and the female principle, love, are wedded in our consciousness can we obey the spiritual command: be fruitful (of righteous thoughts and deeds), and multiply (them), and replenish the earth (with them), and subdue it. Truth will go no further and no faster than love leads as a companion.

CULTIVATE A POSITIVE MENTAL ATTITUDE

We build our future, thought by thought,
for good or ill, and know it not.
Yet so the universe is another name for fate,
choose then thy destiny and wait,
for love brings love, and hate brings hate.

Discouragement is a disease. It leads to failure, narcotics, prostitution, gambling, and anger; it destroys confidence and faith in oneself. To feel inferior, and to think that you are nobody, is to be your own worst enemy. Negative thoughts must be overcome if you are seeking a positive mental attitude and inward calm.

Stop grumbling. Stop feeling sorry for yourself! Let go of that gloomy attitude. No one likes to be around such a person. Self-pity destroys health and happiness. Instead of complaining about your life and environment, be thankful for what you already possess in life. There are people in far worse circumstances than you! Seek beauty in everyone and everything wherever you may be. The loving, cheerful person beams with vibrant health and happiness. Life will never smile upon those who whine, murmur, criticize, and constantly find fault with life. They are repulsive people who drive all the wonderful and beautiful things of life away. Conversely, the happy, cheerful individual attracts all the grand and lovely things of life.

Keep in mind that you are a child of the Tao. You are the light of the world, a great being. Why not act like one? Perhaps up until now you have failed, or experienced many reverses in your life, and you think that you cannot succeed. But you can turn things around right now! Failure is no reason to give up. Use failure as a stepping-stone to a higher and better achievement. Start again. Never give up. You cannot be defeated unless you allow failure to defeat you. No matter how dark the clouds in your life may be, or how many obstacles may stand in your way, do not give up. Keep on with persistence and determination, and you will succeed beyond your fondest dreams.

Stop making excuses. Quit feeling sorry for yourself! Instead, believe that you can and will be a success. Feel deep down in your heart that you are already a complete success! Believe, know, and have faith that your dreams will come true. Cultivate a taste for beautiful classical music. Visit places of culture and refinement and beauty. Make your life beautiful. Spread hope, kindness, and sunshine everywhere.

All that we are is founded on our thoughts; it is made up of our thoughts. If a man speaks or acts with an evil thought, pain follows him,

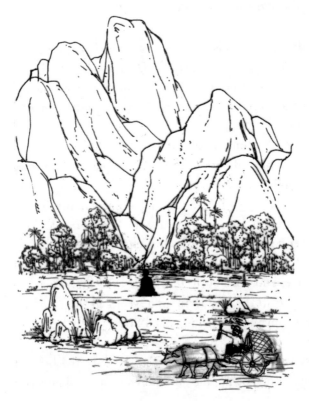

Fig. 11.3. As a wheel follows the foot of the ox that draws the carriage

as a wheel follows the foot of the ox that draws the carriage. If you are discouraged and depressed, give yourself thoughts of confidence, courage, and love. Believe in your heart that these wonderful attributes are yours. Make a list of positive inspiring words or phrases, then read them out loud to yourself, especially when feeling discouraged, distressed, or blue. Repeat these words with as much feeling and power as you possibly can. The habit of reading them aloud to yourself will give you courage, confidence, and faith; it will help you to overcome shyness and timidity.

Positive, inspiring affirmations seed your subconscious mind with the qualities you require for a successful, harmonious life. Here is a list of affirmations. Repeat them with deep sincerity from your heart and mentally visualize yourself as you wish to be.

1. I am master of my surroundings; nothing disturbs me adversely; I am master of my situations.
2. I am well poised, calm, and self-controlled always.
3. I surround myself with an atmosphere of shining success, happiness, and love.
4. I have perfect mastery over my temper, emotions, and passions.
5. I am pure in thought and deed and no evil shall befall me, as the Divine is in my body and watches over me.
6. I ask for strength and guidance, and to be surrounded by the white light of Divine protection.
7. With the Creator's help, I am master of my destiny.

As you repeat these inspiring affirmations, the subconscious mind will pick them up and you will begin to feel more positive and happy. Then and only then should you discontinue the affirmations for the time being. At first you may need to repeat them up to an hour before you feel relaxed and at peace. Afterward repeat the affirmations only when the inner need arises.

This follows the natural rhythm cycle; there is no need to affirm confidence or peace when you are already in those states of consciousness. When you are already in a positive frame of mind, and you continue to affirm more positive thoughts, it causes mental and physical exhaustion. When reading these positive affirmations, do not become over-emotional or overjoyous to the point of losing self-control. If you affirm positive (yang) thoughts and actions in the extreme, you will revert to the other extreme (yin): tiredness, depression, and unhappiness.

The true positive attitude is to be content and balanced, with calm self-controlled emotions, neither extremely happy nor sad. Positive thoughts have ten times the power when we have a controlled mental and emotional poise. Be still for a few minutes each day and feel the presence of the Tao; this will help you to be in control, physically, mentally, emotionally, and spiritually, with very little effort.

Repeating the following positive words and character-building qualities makes it easier for the body to eliminate its toxins, as they relax the system, mentally and physically.

Words and Qualities That Stimulate Positive Thought

Affection	Forgiveness	Poise
Alert	Freedom	Politeness
Beauty	Gentleness	Power
Bravery	Gladness	Relax
Charm	Happiness	Relaxation
Cheer	Harmony	Self-control
Compassion	Health	Sincerity
Confidence	Honesty	Strength
Consideration	Hope	Success
Courage	Humility	Sympathy
Decisiveness	Humor	Tact
Dependable	Joy	Thankful
Determination	Kindness	Tolerance
Dignity	Love	Trust
Dynamic	Loyalty	Understanding
Ease	Magnetism	Unselfishness
Encouragement	Mercy	Virility
Energy	Optimistic	Vitality
Enthusiasm	Patience	
Faith	Peace	

Discontinue These Negative Faults and Thoughts

Anger	Gloominess	Needless talking
Bully	Greed	Pessimism

Complaining	Grief	Selfishness
Discouragement	Grumbling	Self-pity
Dominating	Hate	Shouting
Doubt	Inferiority	Sorry
Fault-finding	Jealousy	Superiority
Fear	Nagging	Vengeance

Be courageous. See no evil in another. See only the good and beautiful. Do not even hint at the bad. Charge the atmosphere with sunshine, cheerfulness, and loving-kindness. You will be rewarded well. Positive traits build the magnetic personality.

Majesty of Inward Calmness

Do you constantly worry? Do the smallest problems get you down? Does life seem hopeless? Are you full of fear and doubt? Do you make mountains out of molehills? Do you get angry over nothing? Are you nervous and irritable? Are you constantly grumbling, criticizing, and complaining? Are you envious of the success of others? Are you plagued by the green-eyed monster, jealousy? Do you carry grudges, trying to get even with other people? If you are a slave to any of the above habits, you can never have mental peace. Confusion in the mental kingdom disorganizes the body and poisons the blood. Worry, fear, hate, and all negative thoughts lead to enervation and finally to disease.

We all know that worry is a great destroyer of health and happiness. But how many of us can stop worrying about our problems and the problems of the world? Perhaps you cannot sleep nights because of your problems, so you worry not only about the problem but because you cannot sleep. If you are a victim of fears and worries, say this to yourself: "So what?" Your troubles will dwindle in size. Stop tormenting yourself with useless questioning and imaginary doubts. You cannot carry the whole world on your back. Do the best you can with what you have as working tools. Get in harmony with the laws of life. Love your neighbor and forget about the troubles of the world today. Say, "So what?" and fall off to sleep. When morning arrives you will be refreshed and filled with zest for living. Then your real problems can be easily solved, and the imaginary ones will fade out of existence.

Worriers are not realists; their perceptions are very narrow; they do not have a universal view of life. They are dwelling on their own small individual problems, without seeing the whole picture of existence. Those who think broadly are philosophers; they relinquish their small ego to the larger spiritual force (the Tao), which creates and sustains the limitless universe.

Very few individuals in this world possess that great treasure: peace of mind. Would you like to be at peace with yourself and the world, overflowing with joy and happiness? Of course you would. To be poised in both mind and body is the quality of a great person. You will be looked up to as a leader and teacher. The person who cultivates inward calm will always possess self-control and be moderate in all phases of living. This is a sign of a magnetic personality.

Law of Personal Magnetism and Attraction

Magnetism is attraction, repulsion is the opposite. Each type of person has his or her own power of attraction and each individual has a per-

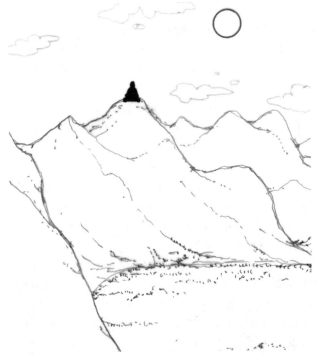

Fig. 11.4. Personal magnetism in the Tao

sonal magnetism or influence, either pleasing or displeasing, uplifting or depressing. Magnetism used for evil purposes is hypnotic. A rattlesnake or a blood-thirsty tiger is hypnotic. A soulless, heartless, evil, and power-hungry person is hypnotic, whereas a saint is magnetic. If you feel humble, insignificant, stupid, strange, inferior, mean, nervous, or angry in the presence of a man or woman, he or she is not the one for you. If you become lustful and familiar in the presence of your chosen one, it is not magnetic love, nor affinity magnetism. That which you then mistake for love is nothing but stormy, amatory infatuation, which is very dangerous to your future happiness. That special kind of magnetism in a woman or in a man that enlarges your mind and soul is the right kind of affinity magnetism for you. Affinity magnetism and magnetic love exalt and broaden all your powers.

Taoist Secrets of Personal Magnetism and Peace in Life

1. Seek beauty in everyone and everything.
2. Love unselfishly.
3. Speak in a positive manner or be silent.
4. Maintain calmness and poise at all times.
5. Do unto others as you would have them do unto you.
6. Cultivate a charming, pleasing disposition.
7. Develop a personality that wins, holds, and attracts others.
8. Improve your life by learning something new each day.
9. Get interested in people, life, or a hobby.
10. Cultivate a pleasing, magnetic voice, cultured and flexible.
11. Always lend a helping hand to those in need.
12. Be clean and neat in your dress and appearance.
13. Always be polite and courteous to everyone.
14. Avoid affectation and veneer; be your natural self.
15. Be thoughtful and considerate of others.
16. Never gossip, criticize, nag, or scold others.
17. Past forgotten, do not worry about the future; live in the now.
18. Praise and flatter others with sincerity and with good taste.
19. Avoid arguments, physical violence, and hostility.
20. Assert yourself positively but graciously.
21. Eliminate self-pity, fear, anxiety, nervousness, and doubt.

22. Be dignified and poised, without stiffness.
23. Acquire a flexible, healthy, attractive body.
24. Develop a wholesome, positive, active mind.
25. Be a gentleman or lady at all times.
26. Cultivate mastery over your mind and emotions.
27. Think clearly before you act and speak.
28. Have a daily objective and a goal for life.
29. Improve yourself in small ways while waiting for big opportunity.
30. Never let a day go by without doing something constructive.
31. Take prompt right action when the opportunity presents itself.
32. Express yourself in a poised, confident manner.
33. Eat foods that agree with your body and nerves.
34. Maintain order in your home and belongings.
35. Develop self-confidence. Affirm aloud to yourself daily that you are now healthy, happy, and successful.
36. Enjoy every task you perform and complete each one before going on to the next one.
37. Practice moderation in all activities. Stop before your limit. All things are accomplished by following the middle path.
38. Forgive everyone who has done wrong to you. Never hold a grudge. If you forgive, you will be forgiven. Release all those who have wronged you, and peace will flow into your life. Love all.
39. Allow others to live their own lives; expect nothing from others and you will never be disappointed. Do not try to change people against their will, as you would not like to be changed against your will. Enjoy people for their company and friendship. Avoid fault-finding or criticizing, and you will always have dedicated and true friends.
40. Meditate daily until you feel the peace and presence of the creative force of the universe flowing through the Tao.

GAINING INFINITE VISION

There are many billions of suns in the sky, circled by billions of worlds known as planets. Such worlds could also contain millions or billions of people. Our sun is a small star. Earth is a small planet. As compared with the trillions of other worlds in the sky, Earth is like a grain of sand on an endless shore. How much more tiny are we in comparison! We worry over small trifles, yet the great universe operates in perfect order.

Seen with that greater vision, Earth has passed from a state of rock to a state of fertile soil as in the twinkling of an eye, yet it has revolved on its axis billions of times and circled the sun a hundred million years. Still this vast lapse of time seemed as nothing. A century is reeled off so quickly that it is too small a trifle to arrest the attention; yet a woman giving birth to a child looks upon the hours of suffering as an age of duration. But millions are born year in and year out; new beings are opening their eyes to the wonders of earth; they grow, they build, they accomplish gigantic tasks, and they pass on.

The remotest event of history is not six thousand years old, while the earth is more than a hundred million years of age. Cities that contain massive structures will some day be rolled under the crust of this earth,

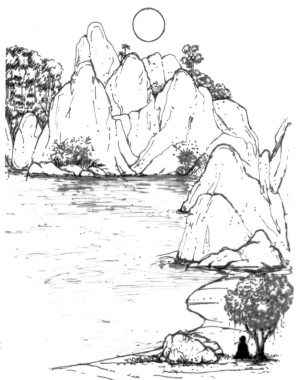

Fig. 11.5. Winds of
freedom in the Tao

and not one trace of them will be found by the peoples who shall come here six thousand years hence. To the greater eye this world is rushing on with whirling speed; weeks, months, and years are too slight to be counted; nothing but eons are worthy of attention; and yet an eon witnesses the rise of peoples, the writing of a few thousand years of history, then the wiping of the slate to erase everything.

One hundred years from now you will be wholly forgotten. Every year many millions like you pass to their sleep in earth. They have been going and coming for eons. They will keep coming and going for eons yet. If your greatest achievements were to surmount the tasks of the past, they and you would disappear and be wholly lost in the melting changes of time and nature. What is the use of worrying when there is nothing at stake for you? You think and fear that a given trifle is fearfully and terribly wrong. The spot on your clothing, the loss of a dollar, the breaking of the glass, the ill remark of an acquaintance, this, that, or something else, racks your mind and depresses your buoyancy.

The rich man who loses all his wealth is to be pitied. The calamity that has overtaken you may be worse. But what does it matter? We humans are but insects, ants that swarm to and fro on the surface of the world. The span of the longest life is but a second of time on the clock of the universe. In a century it will not matter what you win or lose, what you accomplish or suffer. Look upward and outward, now downward and inward. Then you will worry no more. Toothaches, earthquakes, disasters, holocausts are seemingly great evils, but what difference will it make when the surface of the earth is rolled up as a scroll and a new eon is under way?

The view of ancient Taoist philosopher Chuang Tzu is that the source of worry and confusion is the apparently real world, with all its pressures and entanglements. The truly wise person, realizing that these may well be an illusion, does not take them too seriously. Thus she is free to achieve harmony with nature. She does not need to worry about obtaining true knowledge about the state of the world.

The universe never hurries. Nature plans her activities slowly and patiently, without hurry. Hurry always shows a lack of proper planning and method, as well as confusion and anxiety in the mental realm. Hurried and arrogant ambition can ruin the best of projects. The intelligent person never hurries, but is always thoughtful and calm before undertaking the task at hand. Failures usually run full steam into projects and soon give up in despair; they lack thought and planning. Hurry creates distress, disease, tension, and a multitude of physical and mental ills. A hurried, worried, and anxious attitude will never bring good health, long life, and peace of mind.

People hurry for wealth, not caring about their health. They seek to attain some ambition to satisfy their ego at the expense of truth and spiritual attainment. A hurried, diseased person relies on pills and drugs to get well, but this method never results in good health. Health improvement and maintenance requires patience, deep thought, study, and proper application over a period of time. Those who are ill demand quick release from suffering, and it never comes, because nature works ever so slowly and surely in returning us to health. The hurried person does not care about health, does not live according to the laws of health, and therefore does not achieve it.

Hurry takes us away from the flow of Tao in our lives; it is the opposite of a calm, dignified, and poised attitude. All great projects in life are the result of slow growth, patient and careful planning, correct and proper action at the right time. The oak takes years to reach maturity, but it lives for decades; weeds sprout and die quickly. We cannot cause the sun to set or rise ahead of its time; it moves in exact cycles. If we desire success we must accept slow growth and realize that we will reach our goal in due time, after we have paid our dues in proper study and work and patience. We should do the best we can at the moment and let the future take care of itself.

SELF-RELIANCE: KEY TO SUCCESS

A person can be very self-confident, yet lack self-reliance. Self-confidence sees possibilities and opportunities; self-reliance actualizes them. We must all work out our own salvation, financially, emotionally, morally, mentally, socially, physically, and spiritually. We can be our own best friend or our own worst enemy. We must learn to save ourselves from our arrogance and ignorance. All books, all words, all religious teachings, all health teachings are but guides, tools, and theories. The self-reliant individual functions beyond the letter of the word by relying on the still, small voice within. Such a person is friendly, compassionate, and kind to

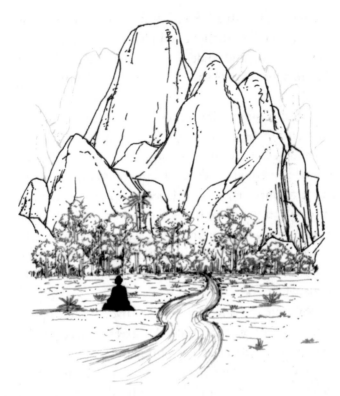

Fig. 11.6. Self-reliance in the Tao

all. With no ax to grind, the self-reliant one is beyond argument, anger, and self-righteousness. Such a person seeks to follow no one and does not seek a following.

If we do not rely on ourselves, we drift through life without direction, waiting for someone else to give us a push. The weak, dependent individual blames others for his failures. He thinks society is against him and that no one will listen to, appreciate, or recognize him. He thinks no one has suffered failure and poverty as much as he. The self-reliant person seeks only to discover and conquer her own shortcomings, failures, and weaknesses that keep her from success and happiness. She goes to the power source within to find reliance to overcome the influences around her.

Opportunities are there for the asking; we must be ready and prepared for them at the right time, and we must then take the proper action. We must develop our own talents and rise to meet the challenges or opportunities that present themselves. No one can give us good health but ourselves; no one can eat for us, exercise for us, breathe for us, or study for us. Attaining good health requires knowledge, time, and personal application; no institution or professional can do it for us. No external advantages can supply the place of self-reliance. The force of our being, if it has any force, must come from within. We can never safely imitate another, nor by following in the footsteps of another can we ever gain distinction or enjoy prosperity.

The spirit of self-help is the root of all genuine growth in the individual. We are all in life alone, and we must make decisions to reach our goals alone, from within the temple of the inner soul. Help from without is often enfeebling in its effects, but help from within invariably invigorates. Our freedom and independence are in proportion to our self-reliance and our power to sustain ourselves from within. In order to be successful in all areas of life we must be self-reliant. We do not have to know all things, but we must be self-reliant in our own profession. When we draw from our inner strength to overcome the trials and tribulations of life, we don't need anyone to hold us up. Create your own life and circumstances. Think for yourself, act for yourself, and depend on yourself. Be a strength to others by living the example of self-reliance. As you become stronger, you will be able to help others in their crisis of weakness.

The self-reliant realize that there is light at the end of the tunnel, that sunshine always comes out of darkness, that storms are only temporary, that cold winter blasts give way to warm summer sunshine. When storms are brewing, they are calm and peaceful and sail unharmed to the quiet waters beyond the storm. Such people are not conceited or aloof; they dare to stand apart from the crowd and think and speak their mind. They are oaks, not weeds, offering others support and inspiration, but not craving or desiring it. They are independent, not dependent.

Humanity does not care whether you fail or succeed; it pays little heed to the individual. However, it acknowledges and recognizes the self-reliant and successful. If you desire success, strength, and the ability to perform, do not envy others, or wish you had their ability. Emulate the process of success in others, train for it, rely on yourself, and you may develop equal power. Look upon yourself as a deep well of infinite possibilities and opportunities; dig deep and bring up from within your depths your hidden talents and powers, then develop and cultivate them to their fullest. Grow from within, outward. Progressing in an upward spiral brings harmonious growth to mind, body, and soul.

Happiness Comes from Within

Happiness grows from within. It does not come from possessions, people, or money. It consists not of getting something, but of being, enjoying the moment, finding total contentment and peace within the heart, regardless of outward conditions. We create our own happiness and misery. Excessive cravings and desires are the root of all unhappiness and discontent. We are satisfied and content when we are thankful and grateful for the things we have. False appetites and illusory desires destroy our poise and inner peace. If we attempt to find happiness in material things, disappointment will follow. Happiness is soul-satisfaction, not the stimulation and satisfaction of the mind and body. Happiness is an intangible, spiritual possession.

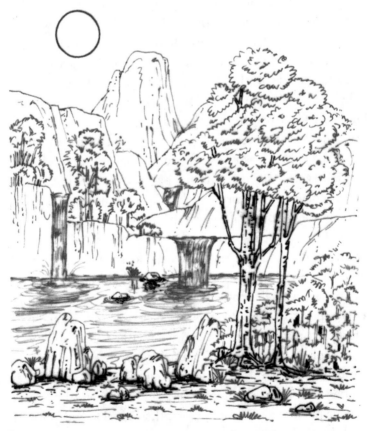

Fig. 11.7. Happiness comes from within.

No one who criticizes, complains, or hates can ever attain inner happiness. True happiness of the soul allows us to overcome obstacles and trials with a calm joyous heart. A happy person does not struggle or worry but seeks to place the happiness of others above his own. True happiness is egoless; it is optimistic, faithful, loving, honest, and simple.

Golden Stairs in the Tao

A clean life, an open mind, a pure heart, an eager intellect, an unveiled spiritual perception, a brotherliness for all, a readiness to give and receive advice and instruction, a courageous endurance of personal injustice, a brave declaration of principles, a valiant defense of those who are unjustly attacked, and a constant eye to the ideal of human progression and perfection depicted by the sacred science: these are the golden stairs up which the learner may climb to the temple of divine wisdom.

RIGHT ACTION LEADS TO HARMONY

A decisive positive attitude leads to health and happiness. A negative confused attitude creates disease and unhappiness. You must choose your own lifestyle. You have been given free choice to chart a destiny during this life. No one else can alter or chart a course for you. No one can live your life for you. There are no magic pills, no potions, no masters, no gurus, no books that can take action for you. Only you can make your decisions and take the necessary action that will eventually bring forth the blessings of health, happiness, and success to your life. By cleansing your blood and body of impurities, eating wholesome natural foods, purifying your mind, and thinking positive optimistic thoughts, you will lose the basic fears that plague humanity.

Unselfish Service: Key to Happiness

Unselfishness, service to others, or a high ideal is the key to happiness. Forget yourself and help those around you. This is the key to the gates of Heaven. Accomplish good because it is the correct thing to do. You do not have to tell anyone of your good deeds; we are judged for our

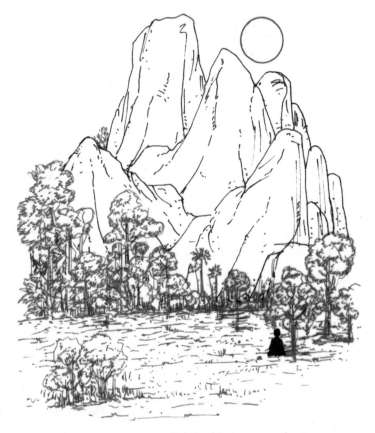

Fig. 11.8. Right action leads to harmony in the Tao.

good or bad deeds whether others see us or not. The Tao sees to it that we get back exactly what we give out. If we are discontent, unhappy, or dissatisfied, we can blame no one but ourselves. We cannot put happiness into someone else; our mate, parents, or children cannot confer it upon us. We can cultivate happiness by patience, self-reliance, honesty, good deeds, and unselfishness. When we follow these higher ideals, we do not have to search for happiness at the end of the rainbow; it will be with us forever.

Honesty Is the Best Policy

Can you always be depended upon to do what you say you shall do? Honesty and dependability are two of the greatest character traits you can possibly possess. To give your word and not keep it is to lose self-respect and your influence over others. You will never be truly respected. The person who keeps his word is always admired and respected. When a person is honest and dependable, her voice is always full of love and sincerity. She is sympathetic to all people. Oh, what a tangled web we weave, when at first we practice to deceive. The dishonest person might seem successful at first, but in the long run the honest person will acquire peace, happiness, and success. He will then display a clear conscience for all the world to see. Make it your policy to be honest.

Cleansing Power of Forgiveness

Do not go to bed any night feeling that you have an enemy in the world. Spend a few minutes each night forgiving everyone who might have committed a transgression against you. Let go of your hates, anxieties, and problems, then ask for divine guidance for your life. You will find a change in your life for the better. Real calmness will set in. Just as it is necessary to cleanse the physical body through fasting to attain a state of good health, so is it necessary to cleanse the heart and mind. Forgiveness is the best means of cleansing. You will never have perfect health or peace of mind while holding a grudge or seeking revenge. Thoughts are things, and they will come back to you just as sure as the sun rises in the east. When you forgive, you release a tremendous amount of tension.

No matter how badly anyone has treated you, you must forgive. If you do not, you are the one who suffers. This is why the ancient sages and saints all have taught us to love one another. As you mentally bless and forgive others, and include yourself, a heavy weight will be released from your mental shoulders. As you cleanse your mind of hate, vengeance, envy, and jealousy, peace and love will flow right in. You will experience a peaceful bliss and feel uplifted. Send out thoughts of love to everyone. Forgiveness is the great mental nerve tonic and is unparalleled in bringing about a state of inward calm.

Peace through Individual Freedom

The easiest thing in the world is to give advice; the most difficult is to know thyself. Advice is like salt; it should be given only when asked, and only in small doses. When we attempt to change others against their own will, we stifle the Tao within them. We stop their personal growth and experiences. Realize that the same Tao that is guiding your life is guiding others' lives. Many people have lost touch with their inner voice, or the Tao within, and they consequently live against the grain of their own being, experiencing much suffering as a result.

The enslaved and tyrannical individual, not free himself, attempts to dominate others or force them into his way of living and thinking in order to justify his own enslaving habits. He does not allow others the freedom to live out the experiences they really need in life. Parents attempt to mold their children into their own image; marriage partners try to make each other perfect; friends tend to criticize each other's faults; congressmen attempt to legislate morality. This cannot be done. These enslaving efforts only stifle and suppress the freedom and divine power in others.

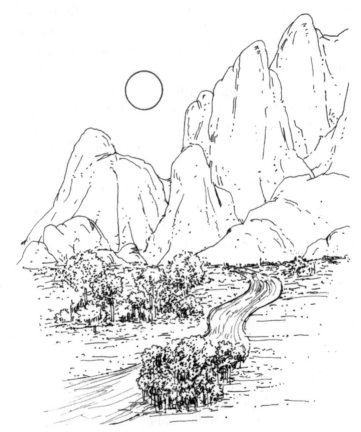

Fig. 11.9. Peace and harmony of the Tao

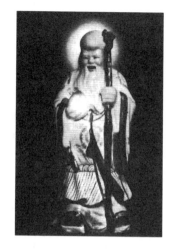

Fig. 11.10. Lao-tzu, Taoist sage, author of the *Tao te Ching*

The ancient sage Lao Tzu said that there is nothing worse than the desire to change others against their will. When Confucius came to Lao Tzu and announced that the leaders of the world would not listen to him on how to make the world peaceful, even though he gave them the greatest wisdom and advice, Lao Tzu answered, "That is good, because your advice would have stirred up more suffering and trouble for the nation." He added, "The more laws you make, the further you take the nation's people away from the Tao within. You remove the last speck of individual creativity from their soul. Leave them alone and do not interfere with their life force. If you stir muddy water, it becomes muddier. When the water is still, the mud will fall to the bottom; the water will clear by itself."

Each and every day, we must extend total freedom to every person in the universe, including our family members and close friends. Let them live their own lives. Stop trying to change the world and other people's habits against their will. Let every person make his or her own decisions, good or bad. No one wants to be fenced in; we all want to be free. The Tao forces no one, for love cannot compel, therefore it is a thing of perfect freedom. The natural way of spreading ideas calls for more than ridding ourselves of name-calling, propagandizing, telling others what to think or how to act, and other such actions. It suggests that the soul be cleansed of any such notion, for it is clear that we can no more improve another person than we can alter the heavens above.

Give up self-assertion and relax. Let go! Give up all efforts to be important or superior to your fellow humans. Quit trying to make carbon copies of others; instead, give them something to copy. Realize that you cannot improve another; all you can do is inspire. This is where the old saying that an example is worth more than a thousand sermons holds true. When you give up the bad habit of dictating another's life, you open up the channel of love between individuals. Peace will then be yours. You will attract more friends, and your acquaintances and family will find boundless joy and happiness in your presence.

Sympathy and Compassion Unlock Hearts

We are all alike in that we all want to be loved, appreciated, caressed, and understood. Sympathy is the key that unlocks the door to every heart. To develop sympathy and compassion for others, practice listening to them sympathetically and with attention. Speak softly; this helps the other person to relax and listen. Try to understand the ideas and

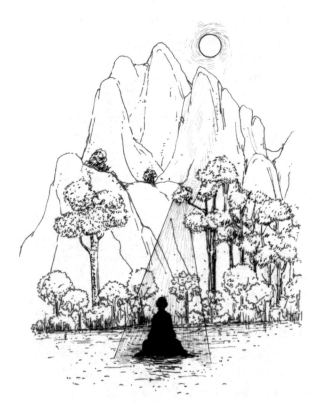

Fig. 11.11. Sympathy and compassion unlock hearts.

thoughts of others. Never argue, but agree on common ideas. Look with understanding eyes; people can see your sympathy in your eyes. Without compassion you cannot be happy; give it to others and you will receive it in return. The person of humility does not attempt to reform others or to make them good, but he or she always loves and makes others happy, for in so doing, they become good. With this spiritual attitude, self-righteousness cannot be present, because you will be at one or in harmony with those around you.

It Is More Blessed to Give

The average person always thinks in terms of getting. Too many people believe that getting is what brings happiness, but giving is the true answer that leads to joy, happiness, and life without strain. Try living opposite the way of the world; instead of clinging and holding on to what is yours, learn to give. This will enable you to relax and let go of tensions, thereby letting the universal divine supply flow into your life.

If you hold and cling on to what you have, you will find yourself in difficult situations. You may at times feel that the world is against you; this is the time to stop wanting your own way and reverse your objective. Go out of your way to help someone in need. Be of service to humanity. Give of yourself for a change. Give your best to the world and the world will give its best back to you. Do a good deed without seeking a reward. Give of yourself unselfishly and you will attain physical, emotional, mental, and spiritual happiness.

THREE TREASURES OF TAO

Kind Gentle Nature

The universe is a great whispering gallery; it whispers back to us the echoes of our thoughts and deeds. It is like a mirror; when we frown, it frowns back; when we smile, it smiles back. When we hold negative, cruel, or hateful thoughts and wish them upon others, they come back to us like a boomerang and deprive us of happiness and a joyful life. This is the universal law of cause and effect: whatever we sow, so shall we reap. Forceful, critical, and aggressive people, by their very attitude, create for themselves much trouble, suffering, and unhappiness. Being kind, we can be brave; being moderate, we gain ability; not venturing to go ahead, we become great. Whatever troubles come to you in life, if you react to them with a kind gentle nature, they will be much easier to master.

Calmness is the key to success, happiness, and love in life. If we are calm and gentle, we likewise attract to us other people of the same spiritual quality. If our nature is harsh, irritable, or unfriendly, we not only repel those around us, but we also cause suffering to ourselves and others. If we use our clever intellect to outwit or cheat someone, in like proportion we attract to ourselves people of the same cleverness who will try to outwit or cheat us. It is that simple. What we give out, good or bad, comes back to us tenfold. If we use physical or mental force to dominate others and get our way, we will meet with a similar force in return. Even if we always get our way, we still lose, because people are generally repelled by and dislike forceful and dominant characters. On the other hand, if we are fair, considerate, and well mannered, others will likewise be fair, kind, and honest with us.

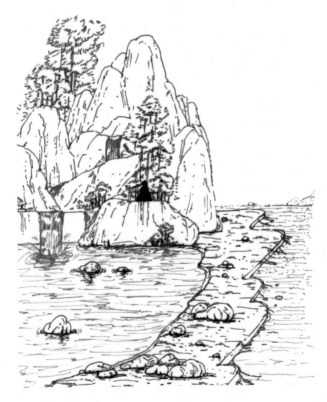

Fig. 11.12.
Developing a
kind, gentle nature
in the Tao

The ancients teach that we are one with the Tao. The gentle, kind person allows life to flow with the Tao and always radiates peace and love. But we cannot be kind or gentle when we are tensed or stressed. The key to relaxation is to totally let go of mental and physical problems. Dwelling on the past or worrying about the future takes us away from doing our best in the present. Allow yourself a few minutes a day for meditation. Feel your muscles relax; relax your forehead, neck, abdomen, pelvis, legs, and feet. Throw your cares to the wind and let the universal force, the Tao, guide your life.

Be Still and Listen

The human body and mind are finite, yet they are a manifestation of the Tao (Infinity). The limited conscious mind often attempts to solve the difficult problems of life. If we learn to let go and relax, the Tao will show us the answers that we seek. Cultivate quiet moments throughout the day; still your thoughts and body movements; feel the presence of the Tao within your consciousness and in the universe. The Tao is everywhere—as close as our breath and to the end of the galaxies.

When we let go of our problems, then the mind becomes open to the inner voice, or the Tao within, which guides us in the right direction. "Be still, and know that I am" applies to stilling the mind and listening for inner guidance. A heavy mind bogged down with worries, problems, uncontrolled desires, and emotions slams the door in the face of the Tao and shuts us off from true answers to our problems. A mind that is light, relaxed, and at peace is always open for divine guidance. Such a mind overcomes worries and problems by not thinking about them or struggling with the lower mind to solve them.

Struggling, overworking, and becoming heavy in mind and body does not create high-level health mentally, physically, or spiritually. When we learn to relax and be gentle, we create a Heaven right here on Earth. Trust in the universal force and it will never fail you. Ask, and you shall receive; seek, and you will find; knock, and the doors (of wisdom) shall be opened unto you. When the lower mind and fleeting passions and desires are transcended, the Tao operates through us for the good of all.

Love versus Power

A wise, loving person in a leadership position commands without exercising any authority or egotistic force. He has mastered himself and has harmonized his consciousness with the creative force. The Tao is love; this is the ultimate reality in the universe; therefore, the wise person is kind, gentle, and tender. He gives love without seeking it in return, because he knows that everyone needs to be understood and loved. The power of love overcomes all harshness, fear, and weakness. If you would be perfect in knowledge, wisdom, and principles, be perfect in love, compassionate in heart, and calm in mind. Only then will you banish sorrow, suffering, and grief.

People engage in heated controversies and foolishly imagine they are defending "truth," when in reality they are merely defending their own petty interests and perishable opinions. The follower of self takes up arms against others. The follower of "truth" takes up arms against himself. Truth, being unchangeable and eternal, is independent of your opinion and of mine. We may enter into it, or we may stay outside, but both our defense and our attack are superfluous and are hurled back upon ourselves.

Men and women, enslaved by self, passionate, proud, and condemnatory, believe their particular creed or religion to be *the* truth and all other religions to be error, and they proselytize with passionate ardor. There is but one religion, the religion of truth. There is but one error, the error of self. Truth is not a formal belief; it is an unselfish, holy, and aspiring heart, and one who has truth is at peace with all and cherishes all with thoughts of love.

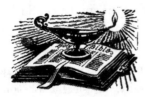

Fig. 11.13. Seek the truth and the truth shall make you free—free from suffering, sickness, limitation, and distress.

MODERATION, BALANCE, AND SIMPLICITY

Our goal in life is to develop all of our forces: mental, physical, emotional, and spiritual. By blending these forces into one, we perfect, harmonize, and realize the completion of our being. This will lead us to a true understanding of creation, peace of mind, the sense of beauty, and the appreciation of our real inner self. One quality is almost useless without another. Intelligence can be of no real value unless there is physical strength to carry out its ideas. Inversely, health alone is valueless unless it is accompanied by mental and spiritual development. A criminal may be intelligent, but he is not well balanced. He lacks the moral and aesthetic sense, and he very often is poor in health. Complete wholeness and harmony are necessary for the perfect life.

The code to this unifying principle is very simple: moderation and balance. Following the middle path of life activity and diet and avoiding extremes will automatically create a yin and yang balance, leading to harmony in body, happiness in mind and soul, and success in life. The more the fundamental laws are followed, the more we will be guided in life by the supreme force or Creator.

Moderation and simplicity have been taught by all of the great sages, saints, mystics, and religions throughout history. A moderate simple life is one of balance and equanimity. An immoderate person lives life in extremes: overworking, too much talking and useless chatter, excess or lack of exercise, reading and studying to the point of mental and physical exhaustion, and dietary extremes.

The little mind clamors after selfish desires and ego aggrandizement. It seeks excitement in sophisticated immoderate pleasures, such as drinking, smoking, mind-expanding drugs, and laziness. The greater mind seeks only to maintain balance and simplicity. Many modern diseases have developed due to our unnatural and immoderate habits of living, thinking, and eating. Extremes in living lead to nerve exhaustion; fatigue and exhaustion cause mental depression, in which we selfishly and constantly dwell upon our problems, making them larger and more complicated than they really are, resulting in failure, suffering, and unhappiness.

Life and being are simple. The universe is simple. The laws of life are simple. We complicate the original simplicity with our secret vices, lusts, desires, passions, and opinions about this or that; we remain ignorant in the university of wisdom, though we attain many college degrees. The simple and moderate life is where true joy resides. Only when we learn to listen to our inner voice—and are guided by it in all of our life's activities of eating, sleeping, playing, meditating, exercising, singing, and working—can we master this life. By cultivating moderation and simplicity, we will be at one with the Tao and enjoy a peaceful and happy life without strain.

THANKFUL, HUMBLE ATTITUDE

Be thankful and humble, and your mind will be clear and sharp. You will then know the joy of creativity, happiness, success, and harmony in life. You will attract to you all that is necessary for your health and well-being. Western religion says, "He who exalts himself shall be humbled; he who humbles himself shall be exalted." Eastern and Taoist religions more than five thousand years ago said, "He who is first is last. He who is last is first." The philosophy is identical.

When we strive to be self-assertive and act important, we become exalted and our ego puffs up. An overblown ego can be easily deflated or humbled. A humble person does not over- or underestimate herself. She does not brag, show-off, complain, criticize, or suffer a deflated ego. Her attitude is humble and thankful. She is free from envy, jealousy, greed, self-pity, and self-conceit. She does not seek ego gratification, nor desire to be the first in the eyes of others, or to exalt her talents to prove herself. If a person is wise and talented, people will find out through that person's every deed, action, and word.

If we continually strive after wealth, scheming, toiling, and saving, we create a self-made prison. Greed, selfishness, ingratitude, and pride all lead to a life of loneliness and misery. If we are unhappy because others possess the wealth we do not have, we are stricken with the problem of envy. If we are to be happy and dispel envy, we should feel joy and goodness about the success of others. A thankful humble attitude places us in harmony with life and the Tao. By this attitude, we flow with the grain of life and not against it; the good that we send out will come back to us.

Dwelling on our past actions and feeling sorry for ourselves because we are not yet successful, happy, or healthy causes us more suffering and trouble. Gratitude and thankfulness can lead us out of this self-pitying attitude. If we are thankful 2 percent of the time, we will be happy only 2 percent of the time. If we are thankful 100 percent of the time, we will always be happy. The universe pays us back exactly what we give out. In fact, the more we grumble and complain, the tougher and more difficult our life will become. The selfless, humble person who lives a life of giving and sharing, and is kind and encouraging to all, will have peace of mind and a life of happiness.

Thankfulness and humbleness is true prayer. Be thankful for the home you live in, the friends you have, the food you eat, and all the good things of life. Realize that no matter how much we own, how highly degreed we are, or how much discipline we have applied in our religious beliefs, we are not better or higher in the eyes of the Tao. To think otherwise is to miss the mark. When pride comes, a fall comes. No matter how much intellectual understanding of the Tao we may have, how beautiful a temple we pray in, or what religion we profess, we are all on equal grounds with the person who prays and meditates with sincerity and thankfulness in a humble ghetto shack or a barren desert.

The kingdom of Heaven is within us. We need not go anywhere to pray. We can simply bow our heads and ask the creative force for guidance and with that attitude we can live a heavenly joyous life, even during difficult and troubled times. Your good is here. Accept it. Your joy is near. Embrace it. Your power is within. Harness it. Your victory is now. Claim it. Your freedom is real. Declare it. Your abundance is overflowing. Share it. Your prosperity is good. Receive it. Your problem is purposeful. Bless it. Your spirit is divine. Free it. Your love is great. Give it. Your faith is mighty. Use it. Your song is beautiful. Sing it.

LIFE IS A STAGE

Life is a stage and we are all acting out a part. The stage is set. You have been given a role to play. It is now your time to go into action and to utilize the props and scenes that the Creator has so generously given you to perform with: natural foods, air, water, and sunshine. These are the fundamental Taoist secrets that no man or woman can ever do without. They are part and parcel of life itself. Our function is to learn how to play our role in life superbly well and become the star attraction we were all designed to be.

Through the understanding and application of natural law—physical, mental, emotional, and spiritual—we become an acting part of the creative force that has brought us to this earth stage. We urge you to seek this path to health, beauty, and spiritual evolvement; sincerely believe in it, and inspire others to follow your message and example.

We trust that we have shed some light on the subjects of health, happiness, fitness, and longevity. May this book wing its way across the earth to those in need of help, inspiration, and hope. Our sincere intention is to help others, so that they may help themselves.

May you live in love and peace, and may the Tao be with you always. Life is just a manifestation of energy. If you have complete energy, you have a fuller life. If your energy is incomplete, you only enjoy part of life. It does not matter whether you are rich or poor. What matters is the good virtue found inside of you, such as honesty, sincerity, patience, and courage. It is particularly important to cultivate these basic virtues with a positive attitude. The virtue of life is by no means external or artificially contrived. It is deeply rooted within your being.

The way you will look and feel tomorrow depends on what you do today. For things to get better you have to get better. For things to change you have to change. We are all the controller of our own destiny because we are all divine with our understanding of the Tao. We come from nothingness, we belong to nothingness, and we are destined for nothingness (the Tao).

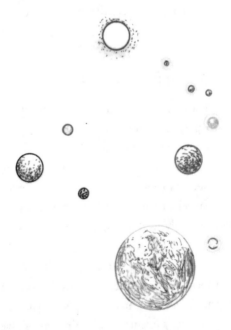

Fig. 11.14. We are destined for nothingness (the Tao).

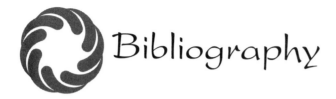 # Bibliography

Abehsera, Michel. *Zen Macrobiotic Cooking.* New York: Avon Books, 1971.

Airola, Pavvo. *Are You Confused?* Phoenix: Health Plus Publishers, 1973.

———. *Health Secrets from Europe.* New York: Arco Books, 1972.

———. *How to Get Well.* Phoenix: Health Plus Publishers, 1974.

Allen, James. *The Way of Love.* Lakemont, Ga.: CSA Press, 1971.

Austin, Mary. *Acupuncture Therapy.* New York: ASI Publishers, 1972.

Bethel, May. *The Healing Power of Herbs.* Los Angeles: Wilshire Book Co., 1968.

Bogert, Jean L. *Diet and Personality.* New York: The Macmillan Company, 1934.

Bragg, Paul C. *The Miracle of Fasting.* Burbank, Calif.: Health Science, 1965.

———. *Super-Brain Breathing.* Santa Ana, Calif.: Health Science, 1963.

Brodsky, Greg. *From Eden to Aquarius.* New York: Bantam Books, 1974.

Carque, Otto. *Rational Diet.* Mokelumme Hill, Calif.: Health Research, 1971.

Carrington, Hereward. *Vitality, Fasting and Nutrition.* New York: Rebman Co., 1908.

Carroll, David. *The Complete Book of Natural Medicines.* New York: Summit Books, 1980.

Chang, Stephen. *The Book of Internal Exercises.* San Francisco: Strawberry Hill Press, 1978.

Chia, Mantak. *The Alchemy of Sexual Energy: Connecting to the Universe from Within.* Rochester, Vt.: Destiny Books, 2009.

———. *Chi Self-Massage: The Taoist Way of Rejuvenation.* Rochester, Vt.: Destiny Books, 2006.

———. *Healing Light of the Tao: Foundational Practices to Awaken Chi Energy.* Rochester, Vt.: Destiny Books, 2008.

———. *The Inner Smile: Increasing Chi through the Cultivation of Joy.* Rochester, Vt.: Destiny Books, 2008.

———. *Living in the Tao: The Effortless Path of Self-Discovery.* Rochester, Vt.: Destiny Books, 2009.

———. *Simple Chi Kung: Exercises for Awakening the Life-Force Energy.* Rochester, Vt.: Destiny Books, 2011.

———. *The Six Healing Sounds: Taoist Techniques for Balancing Chi.* Rochester, Vt.: Destiny Books, 2009.

———. *Taoist Cosmic Healing: Chi Kung Color Healing Principles for Detoxification and Rejuvenation.* Rochester, Vt.: Destiny Books, 2003.

Clark, Linda. *How to Improve Your Health.* New Canaan, Conn.: Keats Publishing, 1979.

Clark, Percival Lemon. *How to Live and Eat for Health.* Chicago: The Health School, 1923.

Claunch, Stanford Kingsley. *Exploding the Germ Theory.* Pacific Grove, Calif.: Self-published, 1960.

Cott, Allan. *Fasting: The Ultimate Diet.* New York: Bantam Books, 1975.

Crampton, Ward C. *Physical Exercise for Daily Use.* New York: G. P. Putnam's Sons, 1924.

Davis, Adelle. *Let's Eat Right to Keep Fit.* New York: Harcourt, Brace, Jovanovich, 1970.

Deier, Gerhard, W. *Light to Healthy Living.* Winnipeg, Manitoba: Health Book Supply Co., 1976.

De Smedt, Evelyn. *Lifearts: A Practical Guide to Total Being, New Medicine and Ancient Wisdom.* New York: St. Martin's Press, 1977.

Donsback, Kurt W. *Preventive Organic Medicine.* New Canaan, Conn.: Keats, 1976.

Doyle, Rodger P., and James L. Redding. *The Complete Food Handbook.* New York: Grove Press, 1980.

Ehret, Arnold. *Mucusless Diet Healing System.* Beaumont, Calif.: Ehret Literature Publishing Co., 1970.

Empringham, James. *Intestinal Gardening for the Prolongation of Youth.* N.p.: Health Education Society, 1938.

Estes, St. Louis. *Raw Food and Health.* Chicago: Estes Health Club, 1923.

Fryer, Lee, and Annette Dickinson. *A Dictionary of Food Supplements.* New York: Mason/Charter, 1975.

Gach, Michael Reed, and Carolyn Marco. *Acu-Yoga.* Tokyo: Japan Publications, 1981.

Gaines, Thomas R. *Vitalic Breathing.* New York: Thomas Gaines, 1926.

Garten, M. O. *The Health Secrets of a Naturopathic Doctor.* New York: Parker Publishing Company, 1967.

Graves, W. H. *Banish Constipation and Colitis.* Columbia, Calif.: Self-published, 1953.

Hall, Manly P. *Questions Answered on the Problems of Life*. Los Angeles: Philosophical Research Society, 1965.

Hass, Elson M. *Staying Healthy with the Seasons*. Millbrae, Calif.: Celestial Arts, 1981.

Hills, Christopher. *Secrets of Spirulina*. Boulder Creek, Calif.: JNM Books, 1980.

Hyde, Emily M. *Physical and Mental Rejuvenation*. Milwaukee, Wis.: Super Science, 1926.

Iijima, Kanjitsu. *Buddhist Yoga*. Tokyo: Japan Publications, 1975.

Inches, Howard V. H. *Brother, Heal Thyself: A Textbook of Natural Healing*. Cleveland, Ohio: Phoenix Press, 1938.

Jackson, Robert G. *How to Be Always Well*. Toronto: Print Craft Limited Publishers, 1927.

Jensen, Bernard. *Nature Has a Remedy*. Provo, Utah: Bi-World Publishers, 1978.

———. *Unfoldment of the Great Within*. San Marcos, Calif.: Bernard Jensen International, 1992.

———. *Vital Foods for Total Health*. Los Angeles: Mason-Springs Corp., 1959.

Jordan, William George. *The Majesty of Calmness*. University of California Libraries, 1900.

Kellogg, John H. *The Health Question Box*. Battle Creek, Mich.: The Modern Medicine Publishing Co., 1930.

———. *How to Have Good Health through Biologic Living*. Battle Creek, Mich.: The Modern Medicine Publishing Co., 1932.

Kirschner, H. E. *Nature's Healing Grasses*. Riverside, Calif.: H. C. White Pub., 1970.

Kime, Zane. *Sunlight Can Save Your Life*. Penryn, Calif.: World Health Pub., 1979.

Kirschmann, John D., and Nutrition Search, Inc. *Nutrition Almanac*. 6th ed. New York: McGraw-Hill, 2007.

Kloss, Jethro. *Back to Eden*. Riverside, Calif.: Lifeline Books, 1973.

Kroeger, Hanna. *Old Time Remedies for Modern Ailments*. N.p.: Self-published, 1971.

Kulvinskas, Viktoras. *New Age Directory*. Woodstock Valley, Conn.: Omangod Press, 1981.

———. *Survival into the 21st Century*. Woodstock Valley, Conn.: Omangod Press, 1976.

Kushi, Michio. *How to See Your Health*. Tokyo: Japan Publications, 1980.

Lappe, Frances M. *Diet for a Small Planet*. New York: Ballantine Books, 1976.

Lindlahr, Henry. *Philosophy of Natural Therapeutics*. Chicago: The Lindlahr Publishing Co., 1921.

Liu, Da. *The Tao of Health and Longevity*. New York: Schocken Books, 1978.

Lucas, Richard. *Secrets of the Chinese Herbalists*. New York: Cornerstone Library, 1978.

Lust, John. *The Herb Book*. New York: Bantam Books, 1976.

Macfadden, Bernarr. *Home Health Library*. New York: Macfadden Book Company, 1940.

Malstrom, Stan. *Own Your Own Body*. New Canaan, Conn.: Keats Publishing, 1989.

Mann, Felix. *Acupuncture: The Ancient Chinese Art of Healing and How It Works Scientifically*. New York: Vintage Books, 1973.

Minick, Michael. *The Kung Fu Exercise Book*. New York: Bantam Books, 1974.

Muramoto, Naboru. *Helaing Ourselves*. New York: Avon Books, 1973.

Ni, Hua-Ching. *The Taoist Inner View of the Universe and the Immortal Realm*. Malibu, Calif.: The Shrine of the Eternal Breath of Tao, 1979.

Nichols, Joe D., and James Presley. *Please, Doctor, Do Something*. Atlanta, Tex.: Natural Food Associates, 1972.

Null, Gary, and Steve Null. *The Complete Handbook of Nutrition*. New York: Dell Books, 1972.

Nyoiti, Sakurazawa. *You Are All Sanpaku*. Translated by William Dufty. New York: Citadel, 2002.

Ohsawa, George. *Practical Guide to Far Eastern Macrobiotic Medicine*. Oroville, Calif.: George Ohsawa Macrobiotics Foundation, 1976.

Ott, John N. *Health and Light*. New York: Pocket Books, 1976.

Palos, Stephen. *The Chinese Art of Healing*. New York: Herder and Herder, 1963.

Price, Weston A. *Nutrition and Physical Degeneration*. Los Angeles: The American Academy of Applied Nutrition, 1942.

Reuben, David. *Everything You Always Wanted to Know About Nutrition*. New York: Avon Books, 1978.

Rodale, J. I. *Complete Book of Food and Nutrition*. Emmaus, Pa.: Rodale Press, 1961.

Scheimann, Eugene. *Doctor's Guide to Better Health through Palmistry*. New York: Parker, 1986.

Shaftesbury, Edmund. *Life Electricity*. Plymouth, Mich.: Universal Books, 1978.

Shelton, Herbert M. *Basic Principles of Natural Hygiene*. San Antonio, Tex.: Dr. Shelton's Health School, 1949.

———. *The Hygienic System, Orthotrophy Vol. II.* San Antonio, Tex.: Dr. Shelton's Health School, 1947.

Tilden, John H. *Toxemia Explained.* Mokelumni Hill, Calif.: Health Research, 1970.

Tilney, Frederick. *Young at 73 and Beyond.* New York: Information, 1968.

———. *Your Wishes Realized.* Hollywood, Fla.: 1938.

Van Lysebeth, Andre. *Yoga Self-Taught.* San Francisco: Weiser Books, 1999.

Veith, Ilza, trans. *The Yellow Emperor's Classic of Internal Medicine.* Berkeley: University of California Press, 2002.

Wade, Carlson. *Magic Minerals.* New York: Arc Books, 1971.

Watts, Alan W. *The Two Hands of God.* New York: Collier Books, 1963.

About the Authors

MANTAK CHIA

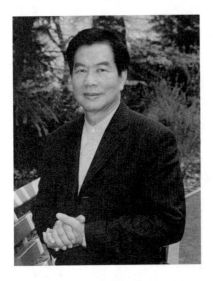

Mantak Chia has been studying the Taoist approach to life since childhood. His mastery of this ancient knowledge, enhanced by his study of other disciplines, has resulted in the development of the Universal Healing Tao system, which is now being taught throughout the world.

Mantak Chia was born in Thailand to Chinese parents in 1944. When he was six years old, he learned from Buddhist monks how to sit and "still the mind." While in grammar school he learned traditional Thai boxing, and he soon went on to acquire considerable skill in aikido, yoga, and Tai Chi. His studies of the Taoist way of life began in earnest when he was a student in Hong Kong, ultimately leading to his mastery of a wide variety of esoteric disciplines, with the guidance of several masters, including Master I Yun, Master Meugi, Master Cheng Yao Lun, and Master Pan Yu. To better understand the mechanisms behind healing energy, he also studied Western anatomy and medical sciences.

Master Chia has taught his system of healing and energizing practices to tens of thousands of students and trained more than two thousand instructors and practitioners throughout the world. He has established centers for Taoist study and training in many countries around the globe. In June of 1990, he was honored by the International Congress of Chinese Medicine and Qi Gong (Chi Kung), which named him the Qi Gong Master of the Year.

WILLIAM U. WEI

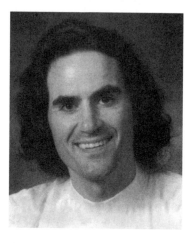

Born after World War II, growing up in the Midwest area of the United States, and trained in Catholicism, William Wei became a student of the Tao under Master Mantak Chia in the early 1980s. In the later 1980s he became a senior instructor of the Universal Healing Tao, specializing in one-on-one training. In the early 1990s William Wei moved to Tao Garden, Thailand, and assisted Master Mantak Chia in building Tao Garden Taoist Training Center. For six years William traveled to over thirty countries, teaching with Master Mantak Chia and serving as marketing and construction coordinator for the Tao Garden. Upon completion of Tao Garden in December 2000, he became project manager for all the Universal Tao Publications and products. With the purchase of a mountain with four waterfalls in southern Oregon, USA, in the late 1990s, William Wei is presently completing a Taoist Mountain Sanctuary for personal cultivation, higher-level practices, and ascension. William Wei is the coauthor with Master Chia of *Sexual Reflexology*, *Living in the Tao*, and the Taoist poetry book of 366 daily poems, *Emerald River*, which expresses the feeling, essence, and stillness of the Tao. He is also the cocreator with Master Mantak Chia of the Universal Healing Tao formula cards, Chi Cards (six sets of over 240 formulas), under the pen name "The Professor—Master of Nothingness, the Myth that takes the Mystery out of Mysticism." William U. Wei, also known as Wei Tzu, is a pen name for this instructor so the instructor can remain anonymous and can continue to become a blade of grass in a field of grass.

The Universal Healing Tao System and Training Center

THE UNIVERSAL HEALING TAO SYSTEM

The ultimate goal of Taoist practice is to transcend physical boundaries through the development of the soul and the spirit within the human. That is also the guiding principle behind the Universal Healing Tao, a practical system of self-development that enables individuals to complete the harmonious evolution of their physical, mental, and spiritual bodies. Through a series of ancient Chinese meditative and internal energy exercises, the practitioner learns to increase physical energy, release tension, improve health, practice self-defense, and gain the ability to heal him- or herself and others. In the process of creating a solid foundation of health and well-being in the physical body, the practitioner also creates the basis for developing his or her spiritual potential by learning to tap in to the natural energies of the sun, moon, earth, stars, and other environmental forces.

The Universal Healing Tao practices are derived from ancient techniques rooted in the processes of nature. They have been gathered and integrated into a coherent, accessible system for well-being that works directly with the life force, or chi, that flows through the meridian system of the body.

Master Chia has spent years developing and perfecting techniques for teaching these traditional practices to students around the world through ongoing classes, workshops, private instruction, and healing sessions, as well as books and video and audio products. Further information can be obtained at www.universal-tao.com.

THE UNIVERSAL HEALING TAO TRAINING CENTER

The Tao Garden Resort and Training Center in northern Thailand is the home of Master Chia and serves as the worldwide headquarters for Universal Healing Tao activities. This integrated wellness, holistic health, and training center is situated on eighty acres surrounded by the beautiful Himalayan foothills near the historic walled city of Chiang Mai. The serene setting includes flower and herb gardens ideal for meditation, open-air pavilions for practicing Chi Kung, and a health and fitness spa.

The center offers classes year round, as well as summer and winter retreats. It can accommodate two hundred students, and group leasing can be arranged. For information on courses, books, products, and other resources, see below.

RESOURCES

Universal Healing Tao Center
274 Moo 7, Luang Nua, Doi Saket, Chiang Mai, 50220 Thailand
Tel: (66)(53) 495-596 Fax: (66)(53) 495-852
E-mail: universaltao@universal-tao.com
Website: www.universal-tao.com

For information on retreats and the health spa, contact:
Tao Garden Health Spa & Resort
E-mail: info@tao-garden.com, taogarden@hotmail.com
Website: www.tao-garden.com

Good Chi • Good Heart • Good Intention

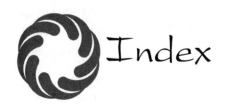

Index

BOOKS OF RELATED INTEREST

Simple Chi Kung

Exercises for Awakening the Life-Force Energy

by Mantak Chia and Lee Holden

Cosmic Detox

A Taoist Approach to Internal Cleansing

by Mantak Chia and William U. Wei

Healing Light of the Tao

Foundational Practices to Awaken Chi Energy

by Mantak Chia

Chi Self-Massage

The Taoist Way of Rejuvenation

by Mantak Chia

Healing Love through the Tao

Cultivating Female Sexual Energy

by Mantak Chia

The Six Healing Sounds

Taoist Techniques for Balancing Chi

by Mantak Chia

Iron Shirt Chi Kung

by Mantak Chia

Living in the Tao

The Effortless Path of Self-Discovery

by Mantak Chia and William U. Wei

INNER TRADITIONS • BEAR & COMPANY
P.O. Box 388
Rochester, VT 05767
1-800-246-8648
www.InnerTraditions.com

Or contact your local bookseller